The Handbook of Psychiatry

The Handbook of Psychiatry

Residents of the UCLA
Department of Psychiatry

Senior Editor:
Barry Guze, M.D.

Editors:
Steven Richeimer, M.D.
Daniel J. Siegel, M.D.

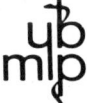

YEAR BOOK MEDICAL PUBLISHERS, INC.
CHICAGO · LONDON · BOCA RATON · LITTLETON, MASS.

Copyright ©1990 by The Regents of the University of California. All rights reserved. No part of this publication may be reproduced, stored in a retrieval system, or transmitted, in any form or by any means—electronic, mechanical, photocopying, recording, or otherwise—without prior written permission from The Regents of the University of California. Printed in the United States of America.

Permission to photocopy or reproduce solely for internal or personal use is permitted for libraries or other users registered with the Copyright Clearance Center, provided that the base fee of $4.00 per chapter plus $.10 per page is paid directly to the Copyright Clearance Center, 21 Congress Street, Salem, MA 01970. This consent does not extend to other kinds of copying, such as copying for general distribution, for advertising or promotional purposes, for creating new collected works, or for resale.

6 7 8 9 0 R P 98 97 96

Library of Congress Cataloging-in-Publication Data

The Handbook of psychiatry / [edited by] Barry Guze, Steven Richeimer, Daniel Siegel.
    p.   cm.
  Includes bibliographies and index.
  ISBN 0-8151-3644-7
  1. Psychiatry—Handbooks, manuals, etc. I. Guze, Barry.
II. Richeimer, Steven. III. Siegel, Daniel, 1957-
  [DNLM: 1. Mental Disorders. 2. Psychiatry. WM 100
  H233682]
RC456.H36 1989
616.89—dc19   89-5549
DNLM/DLC   CIP
for Library of Congress

Sponsoring Editor: Richard H. Lampert
Associate Managing Editor, Manuscript Services:
    Deborah Thorp
Production Project Coordinator: Karen Halm
Proofroom Supervisor: Barbara M. Kelly

Contributors

All contributors were residents of the UCLA Department of Psychiatry.

Miguel Arias, M.D.
George Bartzokis, M.D.
Anthony Bassanelli, M.D.
Alexander Beebee, M.D.
Nicolas Carosella, M.D.
Chris Chang, M.D.
Connie Corson, M.D.
Kathy Dong, M.D.
Alison Doupe, M.D.
Noel Gardner, M.D.
Barry Guze, M.D.
Alison Hall, M.D.
Gregory Hanna, M.D.
Elisa Hoffman, M.D.
Nancy Hornstein, M.D.
Rebeka Howland, M.D.
Maga Jackson, M.D.

Vivian Kleinman-Burt, M.D.
Brian King, M.D.
James Landen, M.D.
Stuart Levine, M.D.
Jay-Jo Portonov, M.D.
William Reichman, M.D.
Steven Richeimer, M.D.
Nicolas Rosenlicht, M.D.
Todd Sadow, M.D.
Daniel J. Siegel, M.D.
Martin Szuba, M.D.
Rick Trautner, M.D.
William Wirshing, M.D.
John Wynn, M.D.
Douglas Ziedonis, M.D.
Bonnie Zima, M.D.

Every effort has been made to ensure that diagnostic and therapeutic recommendations, including drug dosage schedules, contained herein are accurate and in accord with the standards accepted at the time of publication. However, as new research and experience broaden our knowledge, changes in diagnosis and treatment occur. Therefore, the reader is advised to check current authoritative reference sources, including product information sheets for each drug he or she plans to administer. With regard to drugs, the reader should be certain that changes have not been made in the recommended dose or in the contraindications. Opinions expressed herein are not necessarily those of the UCLA Neuropsychiatric Institute, the Department of Psychiatry or The Regents of the University of California.

Preface

Contemporary psychiatry presents its house officers and students with an ever-increasing amount of information about the assessment, diagnosis, and treatment of the wide array of disorders that fall within its boundaries. Those psychiatrists and primary physicians responsible for helping the perplexing patients who suffer the anguish of cognitive disturbances, emotional pain, behavioral disorders, addictions and dependencies, physiological imbalances, psychological turmoil, and troubled interpersonal relationships, are confronted by a confusing myriad of theories and therapies, and are obliged to search their way through a maze of sometimes contradictory points of view.

The residency program at the UCLA Neuropsychiatric Institute and West Los Angeles Veterans Administration Medical Center has always tried to foster an educational attitude of scholarly open-mindedness, to train residents to practice a comprehensive version of psychiatry that most highly values humane care to patients, and to encourage empirically sound and pragmatic problem-solving approaches to the specific sources of suffering that patients have incurred. House staff are strongly urged to critically evaluate the science and the dogmas on which various shibboleths of psychiatric practice have been based, and to craft their psychiatry from a thoughtful synthesis of the best ideas and models currently available, regardless of the specific ideologies or schools of thought from which they were derived. In our view, the best way to help patients and their families is to take the most effective perspectives and interventions available anywhere, and to weave them into individually designed plans for workup and intervention.

This handbook represents the efforts of psychiatric residents and fellows trained at UCLA to extract the essence of such a comprehensive and practical psychiatry, and to make it available to others who deal with psychiatric patients in emergency room, general hospital, psychiatric inpatient, and both psychiatric and primary care office and clinic settings. The editors are accomplished young psychiatrists who were chief residents and fellows at UCLA. The authors they have assembled have focused on the basic "need to know" information required by all who deliver competent psychiatric care: practical aspects of assessment, diagnosis, and differential diagnosis; sophisticated psychopharmacology; a clear delineation of the basic elements of the psychotherapies that outlines the central ingredients and components of each in clear language; and some special problems that present frequently in psychiatric and primary care settings. The authors present most of their information in outline form without excess verbiage. Technical terms are kept to a minimum but are defined precisely when used. This book should be of great help to house staff and practitioners in psychiatry and primary care fields, to medical students, and to allied health professionals who work in psychiatric settings. Many will want to keep it handy, and will find themselves reaching for it often in the daily course of their work.

Joel Yager, M.D.

Contents

Preface **vii**

PART 1: EVALUATION AND DIAGNOSIS 1

1 / Initial Psychiatric Assessment **2**
Anthony Bassanelli and Nicolas Carosella

2 / Medical Illness Presenting as Psychiatric Illness **20**
John Wynn

3 / Psychological Testing **37**
Alexander Beebee

4 / Psychiatric Rating Scales **55**
Kathy Dong

5 / The Use of EEG in Psychiatry **81**
Noel Gardner

PART 2: PSYCHIATRIC DISORDERS 93

6 / Affective Disorders — 93
Barry Guze, Daniel J. Siegel, Steven Richeimer, and Maga Jackson

7 / Schizophrenic Disorders and Other Nonaffective Psychoses — 105
Miguel Arias

8 / Psychiatric Aspects of Alcohol Abuse — 115
Bonnie Zima

9 / Organic Brain Syndromes — 139
William Reichman and Nicolas Carosella

10 / Eating Disorders — 171
Todd Sadow

11 / Factitious and Somatoform Disorders — 203
Brian King

12 / Dissociative Disorders (or Hysterical Neuroses, Dissociative Type) — 216
Nancy Hornstein

13 / Axis I Disorders in Children and Adolescents — 231
Daniel J. Siegel

14 / Axis II Disorders in Children and Adolescents — 272
Daniel J. Siegel and James Landen

15 / Personality Disorders — 281
Noel Gardner

Contents　xi

16 / Sleep: Its Order and Disorder　**304**
Elisa Hoffman and Nicolas Rosenlicht

17 / Pain　**317**
Stuart Levine

PART 3: PHARMACOTHERAPY　*329*

18 / Neuroleptic Antipsychotic Medications　**330**
Alexander Beebee and George Bartzokis

19 / Antidepressants　**369**
Alison Hall

20 / Lithium and Other Antimanic Agents　**379**
Alison Doupe and Martin Szuba

21 / Benzodiazepines　**396**
Barry Guze

22 / Stimulants　**405**
Alexander Beebee

23 / Extrapyramidal Symptoms, Neuroleptic Malignant Syndrome, and Their Treatment　**414**
Nicolas Rosenlicht

24 / Psychotropic Drug Use and Pregnancy　**426**
Barry Guze

25 / Drug Treatments in Child Psychiatry　**432**
Gregory Hanna

26 / Geriatric Psychopharmacology　**441**
Rick Trautner

Contents

27 / Electroconvulsive Therapy — 454
Martin Szuba and Alison Doupe

28 / Interactions Between Psychotropic and Other Drugs — 465

PART 4: PSYCHOTHERAPIES — 474

29 / Choosing the Appropriate Psychotherapy — 475
Daniel J. Siegel

30 / Psychodynamic Psychotherapies — 504
Connie Corson

31 / Behavioral and Cognitive Therapies — 514
Rebeka Howland

32 / Family Therapy — 538
Douglas Ziedonis

33 / Group Therapy — 552
Alexander Beebee

34 / Relaxation Training, Biofeedback, and Hypnosis — 561
Nicolas Rosenlicht

35 / Acute Crisis and Intervention — 571
Vivian Kleinman-Burt

36 / Short-term Individual Psychotherapies: An Overview — 584
Daniel J. Siegel

37 / Psychotherapy With Difficult Patients — 594
Kathy Dong

38 / Psychotherapy With Children and Adolescents *Daniel J. Siegel*	**607**
39 / Psychotherapy With the Elderly *William Wirshing*	**627**

PART 5: SPECIAL TOPICS 633

40 / Forensic Psychiatry *Stuart Levine*	**634**
41 / Seclusion and Restraint *Brian King*	**647**
42 / Abuse *Jay-Jo Portonov*	**653**
43 / Transcultural Psychiatry *Chris Chang*	**667**
Index	**681**

I
Evaluation and Diagnosis

1
Initial Psychiatric Assessment

I. **Introduction.** The evaluation of a psychiatric patient consists of two parts:

1. The subjective information that the patient relates.

2. The objective information obtained through the observation of the patient.

This is the basis for a psychiatric assessment. This is true for individual patients, children, adults, couples, and families. What follows is a guideline to be used in obtaining and organizing information about a patient.

II. **The psychiatric history.** The psychiatric history consists of the patient's chief complaint, history of present illness, past psychiatric history, family psychiatric history, past medical history, family medical history, history of alcohol and drug use, occupational history, and developmental and social history. These data can be obtained by listening to the patient, as well as by direct questioning. An attempt should be made to obtain this information during the first interview with the patient. The following outline is a customary format for writing a psychiatric evaluation.

A. **Chief complaint.** This is the patient's presenting problem for which he/she is seeking help. An attempt is made to record this accurately as a brief declarative statement in the patient's own words, e.g., "I can't seem to stop crying."

B. **History of present illness.** This is obtained by posing open-ended questions to the patient. The patient is encouraged to relate the history in his/her own words. The interviewer should attempt to listen to the patient while expressing concern and interest, and simultaneously observing the patient's behavior. It may be helpful to make brief notes of the patient's history. However, this should not inhibit the patient or interfere with establishing rapport.

C. **Past psychiatric history.** This includes the prior psychiatric symptoms and diagnoses that a patient may have had; the number, location, and length of psychiatric hospitalizations; history of suicide attempts; types of psychotropic medications prescribed and maximum dosages reached; duration of medications' use and effect achieved; and types of outpatient psychotherapy and their length.

D. **Family psychiatric history.** The same information listed above is determined for the patient's family members.

E. **Past medical history.** The patient's medical history must be well characterized. The effect of medical illness and medicines on a patient's mood, thinking, and behavior is discussed in Chapter 2. Any history of head trauma is determined.

F. **Family medical history.** The same information listed above is determined for the patient's family members. In particular, any history of atherosclerosis, strokes, dementia, and metabolic or genetic disorders is determined.

G. **History of alcohol and drug use.** Describe the patient's use of alcohol, cocaine, marijuana, phencyclidine hydrochloride (PCP), and any other substances in terms of quantity, duration of use, frequency, and desired effect. Look for temporal relationships between

4 *Evaluation and Diagnosis*

the presenting problem and use or withdrawal from substances.

H. **Occupational history.** Describe the patient's exposure to organic solvents, heavy metals (lead, antimony, or arsenic), and gaseous compounds (carbon monoxide); also note history of job injuries, and occupational responsibilities and function.

I. **Developmental and social history.** This is a brief biographical sketch of the patient from birth to the present, including the following details: difficulty during the patient's prenatal development or birth; timing of major developmental milestones; characterization of relationships with parents, siblings, and peers; types of schools attended and highest level of education achieved; work, legal, and military histories; history of interpersonal relationships; interests and hobbies; current marital status; number of children; living situation; and means of financial support.

III. **The mental status examination.** The assessment begins with the first interaction with the patient and includes the manner in which the patient presents and conducts himself/herself. The format of a mental status examination varies, but it should include the following information. Below is a customary format for writing and organizing the data.

A. **General appearance and behavior.**

1. **Physical appearance.** Note grooming, hygiene, dress, and overall physical health.

2. **Motor activity.** Assess the patient's activity:

a. **Psychomotor agitated**—Handwringing, pacing, generalized restlessness, and discomfort.

b. **Psychomotor retarded**—Expressionless face, decreased spontaneous hand or body movements, and slowed speech and thoughts.

c. **Abnormal motor and/or vocal activity**—Tremors of hands, mouth, arms, or legs; abnormal tongue or jaw movements; hip or truncal thrusting; vocal grunts or shrieks *(vocal tics)*; facial or other motor tics; abnormal postures *(dystonias)*; and other *dyskinesias*.

3. **Attitude toward interviewer.** The ability of the patient to establish eye contact, cooperate, and respond to questions. Example: "The patient maintained a fixed gaze on the interviewer and did not respond spontaneously to questions."

B. **Speech.**

1. **Rate.** Describe as slowed, rapid, or pressured; the latter refers to speech that is uninterruptible and usually rapid.

2. **Rhythm.** Common rhythms are as follows:

a. **Fluent**—Smooth patterns of speech.

b. **Halting**—Unusually placed breaks in speech.

3. Presence or absence of *dysarthria*.

C. **Sensorium.**

1. Level of consciousness and degree of alertness; note any fluctuations.

2. **Orientation.** Usually assessed by directly asking the patient for the day, date, month, year, location, and his/her understanding of the situation or problem. Orientation is commonly recorded as "oriented to person, place, time, and situation" or simply "oriented in all four spheres."

3. **Attention.** Assess ability of patients to focus and maintain concentration on the interviewer and the questions put to them. Additional helpful tests include:

a. **Digit span**—The patient repeats strings of digits forward and backward. The string of digits is gradually increased from 3 to 7. The normal range is at least seven forward and five backward.

b. **"A" test**—The interviewer reads a list of letters; the patient is instructed to raise his/her hand with every "A."

c. **Serial 7's**—(See calculations below.) This also tests attention and concentration.

D. **Intellect.**

1. **General fund of knowledge.** Assess the patient's knowledge of current news events, naming the President, reciting capital cities, or giving directions to cities.

2. **Memory.** Assess the patient's recall of both recent and remote events:

a. **Recent memory**—Patient is told three objects and asked to repeat them aloud (which tests *immediate recall*); then, patient is instructed that he/she will be asked to repeat them again in a few minutes. Results are recorded "three out of three objects at 5 minutes." (It may be necessary to cue the patient with categories or multiple choices; this should be recorded.)

b. **Remote memory**—Patient names the Presidents backward or relates past historical events.

3. **Calculations.** Simple addition and multiplication problems are given. Instruct the patient to subtract 7's serially from 100 or 3's serially from 30.

4. **Constructions.** Instruct the patient to write his/her name; write a sentence; copy objects, such as those shown in Fig 1–1; and draw a clock face with the numbers and give a specific time to draw with the hands of the clock.

5. **Abstraction.** This intellectual function is highly dependent on the patient's cultural and educational background. Therefore, it is important to know about the patient's background when assessing a patient.

a. **Proverbs**—Simple slang expressions, idioms, and proverbs of increasing complexity are given, and the patient is asked to interpret, e.g., what is meant by a "warm heart," "a cold shoulder," "don't cry over spilt milk," "the squeaky wheel gets the grease," and "people who live in glass houses shouldn't throw stones." Some verbatim responses are recorded.

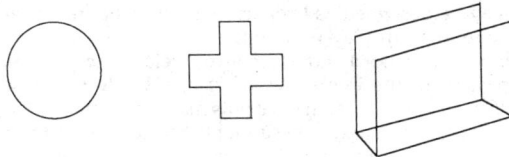

FIG 1–1.
Objects for patient to copy as part of test of intellect.

b. **Similarities**—Patient is instructed to tell how pairs of objects are similar, e.g., knife/fork, table/chair, apple/orange, bicycle/airplane, rough/smooth, and night/day.

Responses are usually assessed as good or concrete.

6. **Judgment.** This is best assessed by an evaluation of the patient's recent behavior. It can also be assessed by problems posed to the patient and the patient's ability to demonstrate appropriate goal-oriented solutions, e.g., "What would you do if you found a sealed, addressed, stamped envelope on the street?" or "What would you do if you were on a trip and lost your luggage?"

7. **Insight.** Evaluate the patient's understanding of his/her problem.

E. **Mood and affect.**

1. **Mood.** This describes the overall pervasive emotional tone of the patient, e.g., anxious, depressed, sad, belligerent, silly, euthymic, or expansive.

2. **Affect.** This describes the range of emotional tones displayed by the patient. Affect is considered to be more objective, i.e., the observed demonstration of emotion, whereas mood is often the patient's subjective report of his/her emotional state. Depressed patients usually display sad or depressed feelings with very few displays of laughter or smiles. Since the range of emotion displayed is limited to depressed feelings, affect

may be described as "constricted." Schizophrenic patients may display a vacant, expressionless face and mood with no demonstration of feelings despite the content of the interview; affect may be described as *"flat"* or *"absent."* Manic patients may demonstrate silly, giddy laughter and then suddenly become irritated and angry. Patients with frontal lobe syndromes may demonstrate exaggerated laughter and quickly shift to exaggerated tearfulness. These are examples of *"labile"* affect.

Note whether the mood and affect are congruous with the content of the patient's history or appropriate to the situation, e.g., a patient who is talking about the recent death of a spouse with a smile and occasional laughter demonstrates affect that is *inappropriate* to the content.

F. **Thought.**

1. **Form.** Describe the patterns in which the patient's thoughts are constructed:

a. **Circumstantiality**—Overinclusion of irrelevant information; the patient eventually completes the initial thought.

b. **Tangentiality**—Patient begins a thought and then talks about a related topic and does not complete the initial thought.

c. **Loosened associations**—Thoughts expressed by the patient are poorly connected and often difficult for the interviewer to follow.

d. **Blocking**—The patient's expression of thoughts suddenly stops and then begins moments later.

e. **Perseveration**—Repetition of the same thoughts regardless of questions posed to the patient.

f. **Flight of ideas**—The patient rapidly relates many thoughts that have little connection; thoughts are generally more related than in loosened associations.

2. **Content.**

   a. **Poverty of content**—Markedly diminished thought output or descriptions.

   b. **Delusions**—Ideas tenaciously embraced or believed by the patient that do not have any factual basis. Types of common delusions:

   (i) **Grandiose**—The patient believes that he/she possesses unusual powers, intelligence, or strength.

   (ii) **Religious**—Unusual ideas of religion and spirituality that are not common to the patient's cultural and family background.

   (iii) **Somatic**—Unusual ideas about their health or body.

   (iv) **Paranoid**—Ideas that individuals or agencies are organized in some way to harm the patient.

   c. **Ideas of reference**—The actions of others and even inanimate objects have special meaning only for the patient.

   d. **Obsessional thoughts**—Intrusive thoughts whose content is particularly upsetting to the patient and seem to enter the patient's mind "out of the blue." Obsessional thoughts are commonly associated with the presence of compulsive, repetitive, ritualistic behaviors, and when obsessional thoughts are present, the patient should be questioned for the presence of these behaviors.

   e. **Ruminative thoughts**—Excessive, repetitive worrying or thinking about past conversations, experiences, and problems. These are especially associated with syndromes of depression and anxiety.

   f. **Homicidal ideation**—The patient expresses feelings of harming or killing particular individual(s). When present, the intent and any plan of action must be determined.

   g. **Suicidal ideation**—This is usually characterized as follows:

(i) **Active**—The patient is actively considering killing himself/herself. When present, one must always ask about a plan or method of suicide and determine the patient's intent, level of perturbation, and lethality of the act.

(ii) **Passive**—The patient "wishes" that he/she were dead but has no plan or intent to actively kill himself/herself.

G. **Perception** This refers to disturbances in sensory experiences of the environment, usually described as follows:

1. **Auditory hallucinations.** These are characterized as to frequency, types of sounds, and when they occur; if they are voices, then how many and whose; and word-for-word accounts of something the voices say should be obtained. In particular, it is important to ask the patient if the voices *command* the patient to hurt himself/herself or others.

2. **Visual hallucinations.** These should be described as completely as possible; they are most commonly associated with organically based disorders.

3. **Olfactory hallucinations.** Note specific instances and types of odors perceived. These, too, are commonly associated with neurologic disease.

This basic format of a mental status assessment is by no means all-inclusive or complete. It is meant to be used as a guideline to approaching patients and formulating a tentative psychiatric diagnosis. Findings can be investigated in more detail in later meetings with the patient. For a further explanation of the terminology and phenomena discussed above, see the references at the end of this chapter.

IV. **Neurologic assessment.** It is important to evaluate all areas of neurologic function (cranial nerves, motor and sensory reflexes, coordination, and gait) because of the possible association between mental status or behavior aberrations and distinctive neurologic abnormalities.

Cranial Nerves:

I: Olfactory examination can be done with peppermint or coffee. Test one nostril while pinching the other nostril.

II: **Acuity**—Use a "near-card" or standard distance well chart.

Fundi—To evaluate for signs of papilledema, atherosclerosis, or embolic plaques.

Fields—Usually done by confrontation. Can be more accurately done by perimetry.

III, IV, and VI: **Extraocular movements**—Look for dysconjugate gaze, loss of horizontal/vertical gaze, or nystagmus.

Pupils—Carefully look for pupillary response to light directly and consensually and to accommodation.

V: Testing the sensation of the face in the three subdivisions of the trigeminal nerve (ophthalmic, maxillary, and mandibular branches) and the strength of the masseter muscle.

VII: **Acuity**—The ticking of a watch, the rubbing of fingers, or a quiet whisper.

Weber test—Done with tuning fork of 512-Hz frequency placed at the center of the forehead. It should be heard equally in both ears.

Rinne test—Done with tuning fork of 512-Hz frequency placed on mastoid process behind ear. Ask the patient to signal when bone vibration sensation ends. The patient should be able to still hear the active air vibration sound. Air conduction is better than bone.

IX and X: Examine gag reflex, upper palate movement. Note if hoarseness is present.

XI: Note the strength of the trapezius muscle with shoulder shrug and the sternocleidomastoid muscle with the head turning against resistance.

XII: Note the range of motion of the tongue and any deviation on protrusion.

Motor system:

Strength: Note the strength in all proximal and distal muscle groups.

Tone: Note any increased tone, including spasticity, or cogwheeling.

Limb drift: Used to find lateralized weakness; helpful when weakness is subtle.

Movement abnormalities: Including chorea, ballismus, tremor, tic movements, athetosis, and myoclonus.

Sensory system:

Pain: Utilizing a safety pin, broken Q-Tip, or "pin"-wheel.

Temperature: A tuning fork usually retains a cool sensation and is very effective.

Vibration: Done with a tuning fork of 512-Hz frequency or lower.

Position: With patient's eyes closed, test position sense of toes and fingers.

Double simultaneous stimulation: With patient's eyes closed, touch one extremity, the other, and then both. Often, there is a lack of simultaneous sensation in parietal disease.

Two-point discrimination: With calipers/two pins. Normal caliper of 208 mm on fingertips, greater on the forearm (approximately 4.0 cm).

Reflexes:

Jaw jerk: With jaw partly open, it is often considered the "normal" reflex of a patient and is useful for comparing the other reflexes as follows:

Biceps

Brachioradialis
Triceps
Abdominal
Patellar
Ankle

Plantar responses: Leg must be fully extended to consider it a satisfactory test. Look for plantar extension. Techniques include the Babinski sign (stroke sole of foot upward along lateral edge), the Chaddock sign (stroke along lateral aspect of dorsum of foot in upward direction), and the Oppenheim sign (noxious stimulation by pressure along tibia toward foot).

Abnormal reflexes:

Grasp: Stroke palm of hand. Patient's grasp will be difficult to release.

Root: Stroking of cheek elicits turn of face toward stimulus.

Snout: Light tapping of philtrum, eliciting outward movement of lips in snout shape.

Palmomental: Stroking of palm of hand, eliciting ipsilateral contractions of muscles of the chin.

Coordination: Tests of coordination are affected by cortical, subcortical, and cerebellar disease.

Finger-to-nose: Look for past-pointing, intention tremor, and/or asymmetry.

Heel-to-shin: Abnormal "rocking" movement most notable over first 12 in. of leg.

Rapid alternating movements: Test with rapid finger movements, hand movements, and/or foot tapping.

Gait/station: Test ability to walk in routine fashion, with tandem gait, standing, heel walking, and toe walking. Note if spasticity, limp, or other abnormal movements are present.

Evaluation and Diagnosis

Body awareness:

Right/left orientation: Does patient know his/her left from right side?

Body part identification: Stroke victims are often unable to recognize their paretic side (neglect). Other possible areas of disturbance include finger identification (finger agnosia).

Praxis: Defined as the ability to perform actions. Test both right and left sides of body if possible.

Limb command: Ask the patient to show how he/she might light a cigarette, comb hair, and/or put on shoes.

Limb imitation: Have the patient imitate your movements.

Limb object: Have the patient use an object in the environment (such as the telephone).

Oral/lingual: Have the patient pretend to eat an apple and/or blow out a candle or match.

Whole-body movement: Have the patient perform a task that involves whole-body coordination, such as serving in tennis and/or swinging a golf club or baseball bat.

"Frontal systems" tasks: Abnormal findings would include an impaired ability to perform complicated voluntary activities in the appropriate manner or sequence.

Hand sequences: Have patient perform three-step movements ("slap-fist-cut").

Rhythm tapping: Have the patient tap his/her fingers in a specific pattern shown by examiner.

Reciprocal tapping: Have the patient perform a certain rhythmic pattern when another pattern is performed by the examiner (e.g., three taps for two taps and two taps for three taps).

Language: A multifaceted area of evaluation. Testing will involve cognition, memory, and receptive and expressive language function.

Spontaneous speech: Includes fluidity, quantity, quality, construction, neologisms, paraphasias, grammatic structure, and emotional content.

Comprehension: Includes ability to follow directions and to understand a "story" that might be read to the patient.

Repetition: Ability to repeat statements, such as "tongue twisters."

Naming: Ability to identify common objects in the environment (e.g., tie, watch, or pen).

Word list: Have the patient name as many animals/mammals as possible in a given time frame (such as 30 seconds).

Automatic speech: Have patient name the days of the week and months of the year. Look for differences in quality/quantity between this type of language (involving memorization) and spontaneous language output (controversial speech).

Singing: Preserved in some types of dysfunction when spontaneous speech is abnormal.

Figure 1–2 shows two types of patterns that are useful as tests for perseveration (often seen in patients with frontal lobe pathology). Have the patient attempt to

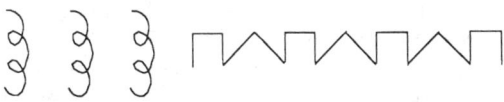

FIG 1–2.
Two types of patterns for patient to copy as part of test for perseveration.

copy the objects. Look for distortion or alteration in the patterns.

V. **Child assessment.** Psychiatric assessment of the child is approached in the same general format as the adult. Adolescents can be expected to give a good account of their presenting problems and their past psychiatric, medical, and developmental histories, and they can be directly questioned for mental status testing. However, younger children or children with autism, mutism, or severe degrees of mental retardation are limited in their capacity to give a narrative account of this information. Furthermore, an assessment of their mental status will often rely more heavily on the observational skills of the interviewer.

For these patients, it is necessary to obtain historical information from parents and other family members, guardians, schoolteachers, school records, pediatricians, and medical and psychiatric charts, if they exist. As noted in the past history of adults, it is especially important to note any significant medical history, medicines prescribed for the patient now or in the past, problems during the child's prenatal history and delivery, birth weight, and substances used by the mother during pregnancy. The child's developmental history should be characterized as fully as possible as follows: who cared for the patient since birth; whether the patient was breast-fed or bottle-fed; and ages when the patient smiled, sat up, walked, spoke first words, used words together, achieved toilet training, and any particular personality attributes (temperament) generally ascribed to the patient. Furthermore, the child's ability to play with peers and siblings is determined.

The mental status examination obviously needs to be tailored to the age and cognitive level of the child. It may often be difficult to establish rapport with the child. Therefore, a very useful technique is the use of toys and age-appropriate games. In so doing, this allows the interviewer to engage the patient and observe his/her behavior, range of affect, and spontaneous use of language and expressions. Gradually, the interviewer may then be more able to begin to discuss the presenting problem with the child.

VI. **Family assessment.** Families are usually referred for therapy because of a family member with a particular psychiatric disorder. A family may be defined as the "identified patient" and the one or more persons most intimately involved with the patient. Although there is an "identified patient," it is important to keep in mind that the patient's disorder may be a symptom of the family transactional style. Therefore, the organizational structure and transactional style of the family are assessed in an initial interview. Listed below are some of the important observations to be noted:

1. Seating arrangement assumed by the family.

2. Which family member(s) begins conversation or assumes role of spokesperson.

3. Which member(s) remains silent or appears to be withdrawn.

4. Overall emotional tone of the family and level of emotion that is openly expressed within the family.

The family therapist should attempt to engage each member of the family. The most illustrative manner in which the therapist can observe the style of interaction of the family is for them to create a scenario for the family to play out in their natural style while the therapist observes. For a further discussion of working with families, see Chapter 32; also, see references at the end of this section.

VII. **Transcultural issues.** It is essential to keep in mind the cultural background of patients. The way in which patients experience their environment, other people, and themselves are strongly biased by numerous cultural factors. As the United States continues to evolve into a "melting pot," increasing numbers of culturally diverse people have begun to seek medical care. However, many cultures, including our own, may attach a stigma to psychiatry, which strongly influences the feeling that these patients have when they seek mental health services.

Cultural factors also influence the manner in which patients talk about their problems. For example, some cultures may speak about their psychic pain only in terms of physical pain, while others may place great emphasis on remaining silent or stoic and expressing neither psychic nor physical discomfort. This can lead to much difficulty in determining a diagnosis, such as depression vs. somatization disorder. Furthermore, there may exist important differences in the manner in which different sexes within a culture express themselves.

One area of particular difficulty is that of delusions. Since delusions are beliefs that have no factual basis, one must have a grasp for the cultural realities to determine whether or not the beliefs are truly delusional. For example, voodoo beliefs may sound delusional in the United States, but they are culturally consonant in Haiti. Therefore, the psychiatrist must approach each patient with an inquisitive attitude about the patient's cultural heritage and background to establish rapport and empathy and to formulate an accurate psychiatric assessment. For a fuller discussion, see the Chapter on Transcultural Psychiatry.

REFERENCES

1. Cummings JL: *Clinical Neuropsychiatry*. Orlando, Fla, Grune & Stratton, 1985, pp 5–15, chap 1.
2. DeGowin EL, DeGowin RL: *Beside Diagnostic Evaluation*. New York, Macmillan Publishing Co, Inc, 1976, pp 759–822.
3. Gregory I: in Smeltzer DJ (ed): *Psychiatry Essentials of Clinical Practice*, ed 2. Boston, Little Brown & Co, 1983, pp 4–12.

4. Kaplan I: in Sadock BJ (ed): *Comprehensive Textbook of Psychiatry/IV*, ed 4. Baltimore, Williams & Wilkins, 1985, pp 482–549. Examination of the Psychiatric Patient.
5. MacKinnon RA, Michels R: *The Psychiatric Interview in Clinical Practice*. Philadelphia, WB Saunders Co, 1971.
6. Minuchin S: *Families and Family Therapy*. Cambridge, Mass, Harvard University Press, 1974.
7. Strub RL: in Black FW (ed): *The Mental Status Examination in Neurology*. Philadelphia, Davis Co Publishers, 1977.

2 | Medical Illness Presenting as Psychiatric Illness

I. **Introduction.** The primary medical expertise of the psychiatrist lies in the examination and characterization of the mental state. Discrimination of organic from psychiatric mental dysfunction is usually straightforward, but occasionally difficult.

Confusing organic mental states will frequently be due to (1) intoxication/withdrawal from abused or prescribed substances; (2) endocrinopathy; (3) systemic and/or central nervous system (CNS) infection. Agitation, confusion, disorientation, and diminished sensorium should always suggest the possibility of an organic mental disorder (OMD); bizarre thoughts, auditory hallucinations, affectively laden (grandiose, euphoric, persecutory, and/or depressive) hallucinations, and well-performed yet irrational behavior may be seen in either psychiatric disease or OMD.

The possibility of OMD must always be kept in mind. The mental status and findings from physical examinations may raise suspicion or provide confirmatory evidence, but the diagnosis of organic illness usually proceeds from the history.

A. **History.** Given a chance, most patients (with the help of their friends or family) will tell the astute clinician what is wrong. Establish the premorbid state, the onset, and the context of the disturbance in mental function; consider the course of the illness and its temporal relation and similarity to previous episodes.

1. **Onset.**

a. Acute or gradual.

b. Sudden acceleration of a gradual deterioration with or without psychosocial precipitant.

2. **Context.**

a. Premorbid functioning.

b. Temporal relation to physical complaints.

c. History of medical illness.

d. Habitual intoxication.

e. Recent trauma.

f. **Recent exposure**—new pet, travel, and/or hobby.

g. **Medication**—new or recently changed withdrawal or noncompliance.

h. **Family history**—endocrine, neurologic, and psychiatric.

3. **Review of systems**—Special attention to

a. Change in appetite or weight,

b. Sleep disturbance, including nightmares, and

c. Change in level of daytime activity, i.e., work or

d. Recreational.

B. **Examination of the patient: signs of OMD.** Every psychiatric patient must have a *thorough* screening, i.e., *general physical* and *neurologic examinations*. Medical illness is more common in the psychiatric population, and the stigma of psychiatric illness often leaves these patients with inferior medical attention. In addition to the important routine examination, special note should be taken of the following, with a ready inclination toward medical/neurologic consultation. Consider especially:

1. **General appearance.**

   a. Habitus.

   b. Attention to hygiene.

   c. Clothing.

   (i) Cleanliness.

   (ii) Appropriateness to season.

   d. Undue fatigue or anxiety.

   e. Tremulousness and incoordination.

   f. Speech and thought process.

   (i) Depressed, manic, or schizophrenic patients should not be disoriented, lethargic, tremulous, or aphasic.

   (ii) Memory and higher cortical functions should be intact.

   (iii) Any change in mental status in the hospital (especially new irritability, belligerence, confusion, or disorientation) should suggest occult substance abuse and/or withdrawal.

   (iv) There should be little variation in the patient's ability to cooperate from moment to moment.

Advanced mania, psychotic agitation, or severe depression may preclude the concentration necessary to perform tests of cortical function. The cognitive dysfunction of depression (see Chapter 9) brings the frequent response, "I don't know," or long pauses followed by, "What was the question?." Demented patients are more likely to try and cover their deficits.

Every attempt should be made to clarify why the patient cannot answer a question: disorientation, sympathomimetic intoxication, anomia, and lethargy may be confused with ambivalence, pressured thought, thought blocking, and psychomotor retardation. It may be quite difficult to distinguish a thought disorder from a focal deficit, i.e., a "functional" from an "organic" disorder.

"Functional" or "Organic"?

The loci, mechanisms, and physiologic sequelae of subtle brain function remain unknown. The increasing sophistication of our theories belies the persistence of our essential ignorance, despite great progress in neuropsychopharmacology.

We remain committed to the thesis that schizophrenia, affective disorders, and personality disorders are essentially like stroke, neurosyphilis, and hyperosmolar coma: the change in behavior represents a change in brain parenchyma.

So, there is no meaningful etiologic significance to the distinction between "organic" and "functional" mental illness. The patient is first a human being, troubled by an alteration in homeostasis.

The distinction we make in this chapter is between the etiologically defined and the yet-to-be-understood disorders of brain function, i.e., between organic and psychiatric illness.

II. **Thyroid disease.**

A. **Hyperthyroidism.** May present as mild agitation to severe psychosis.

B. **Hypothyroidism.** Most commonly presents with depression.

1. **History.** Patient may report changes in appetite, energy, weight, heat/cold tolerance, diarrhea/constipation, perspiration, and/or texture of skin and hair. Elderly patients especially may present with "apathetic hyperthyroidism," i.e., depression and psychomotor retardation in the hyperthyroid state.

2. **Examination.** Consistent with above. Note especially:

a. **Blood pressure and pulse**—Increased pulse pressure or atrial fibrillation may be the only physical sign of thyroid illness.

b. **Size and texture of thyroid gland.** Mental

24 *Evaluation and Diagnosis*

status examination may be consistent with agitation/mania/psychosis/coma in hyperthyroidism; depression (with attendant cognitive deficits, see Chapter 9) in hypothyroidism.

III. Adrenal disease.

A. Hyperadrenocorticism (Cushing syndrome). This may present with depression, affective lability, decreased libido, irritability, suicidality, cognitive impairment, and sleep disturbance. Exogenous corticosteroid excess may more commonly result in excitement, euphoria, and mania, with an increased appetite and libido.

B. Hypoadrenocorticism (Addison disease). This often is associated with an insidious onset of alterations in personality and behavior suggestive of endogenous depression. Acute hypocortisolism may present as frank psychosis, with delusions and/or hallucinations.

   1. **History.** Any exogenous steroid preparation is suspect, but patients with chronic illness (systemic lupus erythematosus [SLE], renal transplant, rheumatoid arthritis, or temporal arteritis) who are receiving long-term steroid therapy are at greatest risk for steroid excess or acute addisonian crisis. Possible presentations include insidious onset of apathy, fatigue, psychomotor retardation, dementia, affective lability, weakness, anorexia, and/or weight loss.

   2. **Examination.** Hypotension with any psychiatric disturbance should suggest hypocortisolism*; weakness and easy fatigability, especially in proximal musculature; moon facies, buffalo hump, acne, and truncal obesity in Cushing syndrome; and/or diffuse hyperpigmentation in Addison disease.

   3. **Laboratory findings.**

   a. **Cushing syndrome**—Hypokalemic metabolic alkalosis.

---

*Postural hypotension is a common side effect of many psychotropic drugs, especially antipsychotic and antidepressant therapy.

b. **Addison disease**—Hyponatremia with a high urine sodium level or low specific gravity despite hypotension.

4. **Diagnosis.** Check A.M. and P.M. cortisol levels and dexamethasone suppression test results.

IV. **Alcoholism.** Acute confusional states and/or sleep disturbance in the first two weeks of hospitalization may be due to alcohol withdrawal. Many investigators suspect that prolonged alcohol abuse may result in a state clinically indistinguishable from chronic schizophrenia. Otherwise, there are four well-defined syndromes:

A. **Wernicke-Korsakoff syndrome.** Chronic thiamine deficiency may present acutely with Wernicke encephalopathy, classically including confusion, ataxia, and extraocular muscle dysfunction. These three are all present in only 20% of cases; apathy, confusion, or coma may be the sole presenting complaint. This may progress insidiously through a stage of confabulation and on to include a variety of cognitive deficits; these may or may not be related to the classic losses of memory and learning.

B. **Hepatic encephalopathy.** This is seen exclusively in the setting of severe liver disease, not uncommonly with choreoathetosis, dysarthria, cerebellar ataxia, and tremor; level of consciousness waxes and wanes, with intermittently intact orientation (delirium).

C. **Pellagra.** Remember the three D's.

1. Dementia.
2. Diarrhea.
3. Dermatitis.

Chronic niacin deficiency may result in depression, fatigue, anorexia, irritability, paranoia, and frank hallucinations; dermatitis is only present in patients exposed to sunlight.

D. **Marchiafava-Bignami syndrome.** Gait ataxia, spasticity, rigidity, and frontal release signs, associated with irritability and confusion, are seen in 45- to 60-year-old malnourished male alcoholics with cirrhosis who favor Italian red wines. Diagnosis: Computed tomographic (CT) scan shows callosal atrophy. (Please see the discussion of alcohol withdrawal in Chapter 8.)

V. **Perceptual deficits.** These are often overlooked in elderly patients who may hide their problems, e.g., progressive loss of visual and/or auditory acuity may lead to isolation, depression, and psychosis. Correction of perceptual deficits after appropriate testing may reverse severe confusion, depression, and psychosis.

VI. **Water, electrolytes, and gases.** Diagnosis is made by clinical setting (i.e., history) and the appropriate laboratory studies. Note that *in general the elderly are much less tolerant of metabolic disturbances.* Suspicion should rise with a history of anorexia, diarrhea, and emesis; abuse of cathartics, diuretics, or enemas; dialysis; diabetic ketoacidosis and its repair; and known disease of the parathyroid and adrenal glands, kidney, or intestines.

A. **Dehydration and water intoxication.** This is rarely chronic but may develop insidiously in the elderly diabetic or as a sign of psychiatric illness (psychogenic polydipsia).

B. **Serum electrolytes.** Electrolytes definitely involved in mental status abnormalities include sodium, potassium, calcium, magnesium, bicarbonate, and phosphorus.

C. **Blood gases.**

1. Acid/base. The brain is much more tolerant of acidemia than alkalemia: pH greater than 7.50 may lead to confusion, delirium, seizures, and/or coma.

2. Hypoxemia. Acutely, this is a frequent cause of confusion in emergency rooms; chronic nocturnal hypoxemia (chronic obstructive pulmonary disease and upper airway obstruction) may go unrecognized and lead to significant dementia.

D. Hypercarbia. This is more acute; note that confusion is uncommon in psychiatric illness.

VII. Hypovitaminosis/hypervitaminosis.

A. Thiamine and niacin. See IV. in this chapter and Chapter 8.

B. Folate. Dietary folate deficiency is seen in vegetarians and bizarre diets, as well as in the setting of chronic alcoholism; it may be seen without hematologic abnormalities but present with delirium or more subtle affective or cognitive dysfunction. Diagnosis by serum level must be made before patient departs from his/her usual diet.

C. B_{12}. Intermittent or relapsing depression, confusion, withdrawal, and disorientation may be seen in patients with no hematologic or obvious neurologic disorder.

VIII. Brain tumors: frontal and temporal lobe syndromes. Insidiously progressive alterations in personality may include the development of depression, emotional incontinence, rage, and/or disinhibition of social and sexual behavior. Personality disturbances are less commonly seen (20%) in temporal lobe disease. Patients with a frontal lobe tumor may demonstrate a facile, jocular attitude with euphoria or irritability. Always speak with someone who has known the patient over several years. Insight and judgment may be impaired well before obvious cortical deficits develop; these cortical deficits may include perseveration, visuospatial deficits (copying and topographical orientation), incontinence, and ataxia. Confabulation, dysprosody, unilateral spatial neglect, and eye movement disorders may also be present. Frontal release signs (root, snout, suck, and palmomental reflexes; glabellar tap; and Hoffman's sign) may appear late. Sensitivity and specificity of a CT scan of the brain are greater than 95%.

IX. Hepatolenticular degeneration (Wilson disease).
Deposition of copper in the liver and brain may present

with mental illness indistinguishable from major depression, bipolar affective disorder, or schizophrenia long before there is clinical evidence of liver disease. Diagnosis requires a serum ceruloplasmin level of less than 20 mg/dL and either the demonstration of copper deposits in Descemet membrane (Kayser-Fleischer rings) by slit-lamp examination or abnormal liver biopsy results >250 μg copper per gram of dry weight). The absence of Kayser-Fleischer rings in a patient with frank neuropsychiatric disease usually excludes the diagnosis of Wilson disease.

X. **Seizure disorders: interictal mental status.** Behavioral manifestations associated with seizure disorders are usually seen in the context of well-established disease. There are little consistent data correlating specific personality traits with specific types of seizures. Nevertheless, depression is common and may result in suicide (especially in patients with complex partial seizures).

A clinical syndrome indistinguishable from schizophrenia appears to be more common in patients with left-sided seizure foci. Notably absent are the family and premorbid histories usually seen in schizophrenics. The psychosis usually begins over 14 years after onset of seizures and is not responsive to anticonvulsant medication.

Temporal lobe epilepsy may be associated with interictal hyper-religiosity or an exaggerated preoccupation with philosophic issues. Also seen are inappropriately intense affective responses, obsessiveness, circumstantial speech, hypergraphia, and hypersexuality or hyposexuality.

XI. **Chronic CNS infection.** The CNS is vulnerable to bacterial, viral, fungal, and parasitic infections. The frequent association of fever and signs of meningeal irritation (headaches, nuchal rigidity, and Brudzinski and Kernig signs) with clinical delirium makes the diagnosis straightforward. Chronic infection may proceed with few or none of these signs, however, and generate a syndrome similar to that described under brain tumors (v. supra). Patients more commonly present with dementia than with subtle personality changes; the early subtleties are not appreciated by clinicians and often are not seen in perspective by those living with the patient.

A. **Neurosyphilis.** General paresis of the insane may present as a dementia or a psychosis. Gradual onset of altered judgment, memory, and intellect may lead to deterioration of personal hygiene, speech, sensation, and gait. Frank hallucinations and delusions may or may not appear. Focal neurologic signs may or may not be found; the psychosis may take any form. In any case, progressive deterioration of intellect and motor function leads to paralysis and death within 5 years. Diagnosis of neurosyphilis requires clinical suspicion and positive serology; confirmation is by positive cerebrospinal spinal fluid (CSF) VDRL. Frequent false-positive results render the more sensitive fluorescent treponemal antibody absorption test (FTA-ABS) of no value in CSF testing.

B. **Human immunodeficiency virus (HIV) and human T-cell lymphotropic virus III.** The acquired immunodeficiency syndrome (AIDS) virus may cause CNS infection with or without systemic manifestations of immunodeficiency. Diagnosis requires positive CSF serology or culture.

Malignancy (CNS lymphoma, Kaposi sarcoma) and opportunistic infections (cytomegalovirus, toxoplasmosis, cryptosporidium, herpes simplex virus (HSV), tuberculosis (TB), and atypical mycobacterium) may follow the immunosuppression of AIDS. Depression, personality change, etc., may be present without other neurologic dysfunction. This neurotropic virus may cause a rapidly progressive dementia; such patients are not infrequently thought simply to be depressed. Azidothymidine (AZT) may be effective in slowing progression of chronic HIV encephalomyelitis.

We expect to see depression in response to any life-threatening diagnosis; nevertheless, any change in mental status—cognitive or emotional—should trigger a search for CNS complications of AIDS.

C. **Progressive multifocal leukoencephalopathy.** A unique papovavirus infection, seen almost exclusively in patients with chronic malignancy (Hodgkin disease, lymphosarcoma, and myeloproliferative) or AIDS, and less frequently with tuberculosis, sarcoidosis, or immunosuppressive therapy. It may present with frontal/temporal lobe syndrome, with death 3 to 6 months after onset.

XII. **Adult metachromatic leukodystrophy (MLD).** Perhaps 25% of MLD patients have their first symptoms after the age of 21 years. This autosomal recessive metabolic disorder is more common in men (2:1) and may begin with memory dysfunction, irrationality, delusions, and bizarre behavior. There is no known therapy for this illness; progression leads to cerebellar ataxia, pyramidal dysfunction, and bizarre postures before death. Diagnosis: Decreased arylsulfatase A level in white blood cells, serum, and urine, or elevated urinary sulfatide levels; nerve conduction is slowed, and nerve biopsy specimen shows metachromatic deposits.

XIII. **Collagen vascular disease.**

A. **SLE.** Mania, depression, and psychosis are well-known complications of SLE and may respond to steroids; bizarre, atypical behavioral disorders may also be seen. The clinical differentiation of lupus encephalopathy from steroid-induced psychosis is often challenging and resolved only by withdrawal (rock) or increase (hard place) of steroid therapy. Inflammation of brain parenchyma or vasculature is not consistently present in patients with SLE-associated mental status changes that improve with increased steroid therapy. Several vasculitides involve CNS structures; patients most commonly present with stroke. Ten percent of patients with *periarteritis nodosa* may develop mental status changes at some time. *Wegener granulomatosis, meningovascular syphilis,* and *granulomatous angiitis* may present with encephalopathy, including somnolence and confusion. There are rare reports of psychosis in mixed connective tissue disease as well.

XIV. **Intoxications, excluding alcohol.**

A. **Amphetamines.** Chronic amphetamine use may lead to full-blown psychosis, marked by anxiety, belligerence, psychomotor agitation, and delusions of reference; rapid onset usually follows recent use of a sympathomimetic substance in the context of chronic abuse.

B. **Cocaine and cocaine withdrawal, PCP, and MDMA ("Ecstasy").**

C. **Hallucinogens.** Chronic abuse of hallucinogens may lead to episodic recurrences of prior hallucinatory experiences (usually visual but also may be somatic, delusional, or emotional reactions): Persistent hallucinatory psychosis develops in a few individuals and is distinguished from typical schizophrenia by the predominance of intense visual hallucinations that are resistant to standard neuroleptic therapy. Anticonvulsant therapy may be effective in such cases; abstinence is essential.

D. **Iatrogenic.** A large number of frequently prescribed drugs (especially the antihypertensives) may cause psychiatric syndromes, including psychoses, depression, mania, agitation, and a range of alterations of consciousness (confusion, delirium, drowsiness, and sleep disturbances, including nightmares). Central nervous system side effects are common. Such reactions may be typical or entirely idiosyncratic, e.g., steroid-induced psychosis or an acute confusional state induced by quinine given for leg cramps. When in doubt, check the *Physicians' Desk Reference,* or a textbook of pharmacology.

1. **Possible drug side effects.**

a. **Psychosis.**

(i) Hallucinogens (acute or chronic use).

(ii) Antidepressants (tricyclic antidepressants [TCAs] or monoamine oxidase inhibitors [MAOIs]).

(iii) Antihistamines.

(iv) Anticholinergics, atropine.

(v) Antibiotics.

(a) Cephalosporins (paranoia).

(b) Metronidazole (hallucinations).

(c) Aminoglycosides (hallucinations).

(d) Trimethoprim-sulfamethoxazole.

(vi) Antiarrhythmics.

(vii) Corticosteroids.

(viii) Narcotics, meperidine, pentazocine.

(ix) β-Blockers, other antihypertensives.

(x) L-dopa.

(xi) Amantadine.

(xii) Digoxin.

(xiii) Isoniazid (INH).

b. **Manic states.**

(i) Sympathomimetics.

(ii) Corticosteroids.

(iii) Antidepressants (TCAs or MAOIs).

(iv) L-dopa.

c. **Depression.**

(i) Antihypertensives, especially centrally acting chemotherapy.

(ii) Oral contraceptives.

(iii) Withdrawal of sympathomimetics, cocaine, amphetamines.

(iv) Barbiturates.

(v) Nonsteroidal anti-inflammatory agents.

d. **Sleep disturbance.**

(i) MAOIs.

(ii) L-dopa.

(iii) Antihypertensives, especially β-blockers.

(iv) Sympathomimetics.

XV. **Porphyria.** Deficiency of uroporphyrinogen I synthase is an autosomal dominant trait with variable expression, resulting in acute intermittent porphyria (AIP). One third of patients with AIP have psychiatric symptoms, including acute psychosis, severe anxiety, and affective lability with emotional outbursts that may resemble conversion reactions. The chronic remitting course may lead to suspicion of conversion disorder.

Gastrointestinal complaints (pain, vomiting, and/or constipation) may be severe; peripheral, autonomic, and cranial neuropathies may be present as well. Concurrent hyponatremia (syndrome of inappropriate secretion of antidiuretic hormone?) is common and renders the picture even more confusing. Attacks may be precipitated by drugs (especially barbiturates), alcohol, menses, pregnancy, parturition, fasting, or infection.

Diagnosis requires primarily *suspicion*: Urine must be tested *during attacks* for elevated aminolevulinic acid and porphobilinogen. Medical treatment is supportive, intravenous (IV) glucose may help, as may IV hematin. Consult a textbook of medicine.

Phenothiazines and oxazepam may be used in the treatment of mental disorders due to AIP.

XVI. **Pheochromocytoma.** Anxiety, fear, trembling, and panic may accompany the episodic release of cate-

TABLE 2–1.

Nondiscriminatory Findings: Signs and Symptoms Common to Both Organic and Psychiatric Illness*

Vegetative Signs	Cortical Signs
Insomnia	Diminished memory
Hypersomnia†	Diminished attention
Reversed sleep/wake cycle	Psychomotor retardation
Decreased appetite	Abulia, apathy
Increased appetite†	Dissociative states, especially brief
Increased libido‡	Irritability
Decreased libido	Perseveration
Diarrhea (<600 cc/day)	Confabulation
Enuresis, incontinence of urine†	Verbigeration
Encopresis†	Emotional lability
Palpitations	
Other	
Rage reactions, e.g., suspiciousness‡, impulsivity‡	

*In isolation, most of these suggest medical illness; all suggest a need for more history.
†More commonly medical.
‡More commonly psychiatric.

---

cholamines responsible for the more commonly seen headache, perspiration, and hypertension. Twenty-four-hour urine collection during at attack reveals increased vanillylmandelic acid, metanephrines, and free catecholamines.

XVII. **Multiple sclerosis.** Personality changes and mood swings may accompany the widespread neurologic deficits of MS. Depression is the most common psychiatric symptom; euphoria signifies widespread cortical involvement and is generally seen with dementia and pseudobulbar palsy. The early phases of MS may be taken for hysteria or conversion disorder. Clinical diagnosis is aided by magnetic resonance imaging.

XVIII. **Pancreatic carcinoma.** The diagnosis of carcinoma of the pancreas may be preceded by many months

TABLE 2–2.
Mental Status Examination of OBS vs. Psychiatric Illness*

Suggest OBS
  Decreased or fluctuating sensorium
  Visual hallucinations
  Disorientation
  Confusion
  Incoherence
  Olfactory hallucinations
  Gustatory hallucinations
  Any abnormality of cortical function not due to diminished attention
  Anosognosia
Suggest Psychiatric Illness
  Coherent auditory hallucinations, especially blaming, persecutory, suicidal
  Bizarre notions with intact sensorium, e.g., delusions of reference, delusions of influence, hyperacusis
Possibly Either
  Delusions
  Depression
  Apathy

OBS = organic brain syndrome.

---

of depression marked by a sense of doom. The loss of drive and interest in life is thought to be more marked than with other terminal illness.

XVIX. **Malnutrition and refeeding.**

XX. **Other neurologic diseases.** A variety of primary neurologic diseases may present with psychiatric symptoms. See Chapter 9.

3 Psychological Testing

When requesting psychological testing, specify the purpose and what specific information is being sought. The various purposes of testing include (1) to describe a cluster of symptoms, (2) to aid in diagnosis, (3) to investigate etiology, (4) to suggest prognosis, (5) to assess deficits and assets, and (6) to help plan treatment.

I. **Intelligence testing.**

A. **Stanford-Binet.** The test comprises a large variety of specific tasks that assess eye-hand coordination, perceptual abilities, naming objects, memory, interpretation of pictures, practical judgment, language functions, common information, and problem solving, with the tasks roughly ordered in terms of difficulty. Performance is quantitated to an age equivalent, which would be the age at which children, on average, perform at the same level. This is the child's *mental age*.

The intelligence quotient (IQ) was the mental age divided by the actual chronological age of the subject, with this ratio multiplied by 100. In the most recent revisions, the Stanford-Binet IQ scores are derived on a statistical basis.

The age range for the test is from a mental age of 2 years to adulthood. This test is better for assessing mental retardation than the Wechsler test, which tends to overestimate the IQ of retarded persons.

Problems: The test is not good in testing adults, is difficult to administer, does not break down the score into subscale scores, and places heavy emphasis on verbal skills.

B. Wechsler adult intelligence scale. The most recent (1981) version is the Wechsler Adult Intelligence Scale, revised (WAIS-R). It is designed for people aged 16 years or older. It consists of 11 subtests, administered and scored separately, that are divided into verbal skills and those that reflect *performance* (primarily nonverbal skills). The verbal subtests are labeled: Information, Comprehension, Arithmetic, Similarities, Digit Span, and Vocabulary. The performance subtests are: Digit Symbol, Picture Completion, Block Design, Picture Arrangement, and Object Assembly. Within each subtest, the items are ordered by difficulty. Performance is tested until failure is manifest.

1. **Scoring.** The IQ is a standardized score with a population mean of 100 and an SD of 15. Thus, 67% of the population have an IQ between 85 and 115, and 95% have an IQ between 70 and 130. The average IQ for high school graduates is 105, for college graduates 110, and for people with doctoral degrees 130. An IQ is reported for the verbal subtests (VIQ) and the performed subtests (PIQ), as well as for the full-scale IQ, which includes all the scales (Table 3-1).

2. **An interpretive approach.**

a. Examine the full-scale IQ, which is a global estimate of the person's mental abilities.

b. Compare the VIQ with the PIQ. The PIQ can be regarded as an estimate of perceptual organizational ability. A difference of more than 15 points is significant, although for individuals with high IQ, the VIQ may routinely be 15 points higher than the PIQ. The VIQ may reflect a person's academic achievement. The lower VIQ may be seen in underachievers. Learning disabled persons may do particularly poorly on tests that require sequencing (Digit Span, Digit Symbol, and

TABLE 3–1.
IQ Classification*

Score Range	Label	If Cutoffs IQ	If Cutoffs SD	Then This Represents This % of Population
>145	Very superior		>+3	Upper 0.14
>130	Very superior	>130	>+2	Upper 2.3
120–130	Superior	>120		Upper 10
110–120	Bright normal	>110	>+1	Upper 16
90–110	Normal	90–110		Upper 25 / Middle 50
80–90	Dull normal	<90	<−1	Lower 25 / Lower 16
70–80	Borderline retardation	<85 / <80		Lower 10
55–70	Mild retardation	<70	<−2	Lower 2.3
40–54	Moderate retardation	<65 / <55		Lower 1
25–39	Severe retardation		<−3	Lower 0.14
<25	Profound retardation			

*IQ = intelligence quotient.

Picture Arrangement). Whether VIQ-PIQ differences can indicate the presence of lateralized brain damage is controversial.

c. Look at the scatter within the verbal and performance subtests. In comparing two subtest scores, they must differ by 3 to 4 points to be regarded as significantly different.

d. Look at intrasubtest scatter. The items in each subtest are arranged to be progressively more difficult. If the testee misses some earlier items and passes later ones, this may indicate a problem with attention, memory loss, or anxiety.

e. While the WAIS is primarily regarded as a quantitative test, the qualitative features of the subject's answers may be informative. The content may reflect important aspects of the person's intellectual functioning and emotional processes. The WAIS may reveal psychodynamic issues in the same manner as a projective test. The *behavior* of the subject with the tester, and with the challenge of the test, may demonstrate major aspects of the person's functioning.

3. **Diagnostic uses.** The WAIS is used primarily to assess intelligence and aptitude. In this regard, IQ is correlated .70 with years of education attained, .50 with grade point average, .50 with level of occupational attainment, and .20 with success on the job.

While it was hoped that the WAIS could be used to diagnose psychopathologic and neuropathologic conditions, it has not proved to be a very reliable indicator. While the WAIS is not accurate in diagnosing the presence and location of brain damage, the subtest differences and patterns can serve as a source for localization hypotheses. In neuropsychology, there are patterns that are associated with various lesion locations. The WAIS data are most meaningful only as they contribute to a fuller neuropsychiatric examination.

4. **General assessment.** The WAIS is the most

widely used intelligence test. It has the best-established norms, and it provides a breakdown in terms of subscale performance. The *problems* with it are as follows: it may be biased against minorities and subjects with impaired English language skills, it does not include a good test of memory functions or aphasic disabilities, and it is not as accurate as the Stanford-Binet test in assessing the IQ of mentally retarded persons.

The WAIS is designed for people aged 16 years and older. For children aged 5 to 15 years, there is a modified version: Wechsler Intelligence Scale for Children, revised. There also is the Wechsler Preschool and Primary Scale of Intelligence for children aged $4^{1}/_{2}$ to $6^{1}/_{2}$ years.

II. **Objective personality testing: The Minnesota Multiphasic Personality Inventory (MMPI).** Tests of personality are divided into "projective" and "objective" tests. The latter are distinguished by the structured and standardized nature of the test stimuli, response options, and scoring. The MMPI is a commonly used objective test.

The MMPI consists of 566 true/false questions. First published in 1943, the test was empirically derived. The authors started with 1,000 statements about personality. They retained those questions that statistically discriminated between psychiatric patients with various diagnoses and normal people. Because the items were chosen on statistical grounds, it is not always obvious why a specific item is scored as contributing to a certain scale.

The patient groups that they used were variously pure cases of hypochondriasis, depression, hysteria, psychopathy, homosexuality, paranoia, psychasthenia, schizophrenia, and hypomania. The original attempt was to use the MMPI to help with the diagnosis, with each diagnostic group represented by a scale on the test report. The test did not prove to be good for this, because any one group tended to have elevations on a number of scales. This also was a result of the fact that the items of the test were chosen to discriminate patients from normal subjects, not to discriminate the different diagnostic groups from each other. Because the scales cannot individually be used for diagnosis, the labels on the scales can be misleading. A better approach is to identify each scale by its number rather than its label, with an awareness of the underlying traits and features that the scale assesses (Table 3–2).

While the results of the MMPI do not directly provide a diagnosis, the test provides a picture of the person's traits, behavior, symptoms, attitudes, underlying dynamics, and adjustment. From this information, supplemented by all other information known about the person, a formulation of diagnosis, prognosis, future behavior, and treatment recommendations can be attempted.

The MMPI interpretation is complicated. The person's sex, age, race, cultural background, and socioeconomic status can all affect the MMPI. For example, the schizophrenia, psychasthenia, and psychopathic deviate scales tend to be elevated in adolescents, such that norms for them should be consulted rather than using the adult norms. Similarly, because of racial group differences, test results from black subjects need to be interpreted with caution. Scale score elevations may have many interpretations.

A. **Interpretation.** The test takes around an hour and a half. If it takes more than 2 hours, this may suggest major disturbance, obsessiveness, organic brain disease, low IQ, or poor reading skills. Completion times under 1 hour suggest impulsivity and an invalid test.

The raw score is for each scale plotted on a graph. From the graph, a T score equivalent can be derived. The T score is a standard score, with a mean of 50 and an SD of 10. Thus, a value of 70 is 2 SD above the norm and is usually regarded as clinically significant.

One then looks at the overall profile, including the

TABLE 3–2.

MMPI Scales*

The MMPI consists of ten clinical scales (numbered 0-9) and three validity scales (L, F, and K). They will be summarized below in the following format: scale No. (scale symbol) scale label: a capsular description of what the scale assesses.

Clinical scales:
1. (Hs) Hypochondriasis: Exaggerated concern with physical symptoms.
2. (D) Depression: Includes low mood, low self-esteem, and apathy.
3. (Hy) Hysteria: Reflects the conversion of emotional pain into physical pain.
4. (Pd) Psychopathic Deviate: Measures potential for amoral and unsocialized behavior.
5. (Mf) Masculinity-Femininity: Reflects the balance of a person's interests and traits between what would conventionally be termed feminine vs. masculine.
6. (Pa) Paranoia: Reflects characteristics, such as suspiciousness, oversensitivity, moral rigidity, aloofness, and guardedness.
7. (Pt) Psychasthenia: Measures anxiety, phobias, worrying, guilt, obsessive-compulsive behavior, and narcissism.
8. (Sc) Schizophrenia: High scorers have unconventional, schizoid life-styles. They are moody, feel confused, have unusual ideas, and underlying negative self-attitudes.
9. (Ma) Hypomania: High scores reflect energetic, expansive, egotistical, impulsive characteristics, with elevated mood.

(Continued.)

TABLE 3–2 (cont.)

10. (Si) Social introversion: High scorers show shyness, withdrawal, overcontrol, lethargy, tension, and guilt proneness.

Validity scales:

(?) The ? Scale: This is the number of unanswered items. If over 30 items are left unanswered, it suggests defensiveness, uncooperativeness, and an invalid test.

(L) Lie: This consists of 15 items referring to socially desirable but rather unlikely behaviors. High scores reflect a tendency to present an overly favorable self-image.

(F) Deviant response: Measures the tendency to endorse rare or unusual attributes. High scores may suggest confusion, not understanding the directions, responding without reading the questions, markedly unconventional thinking, a wish to present themselves in a bad light (malingering), unwarranted self-criticalness, disorganization, or severe disturbance. This is meant to detect random or otherwise invalid records.

(K) Defensiveness: High scores reflect defensiveness or the individual's unrealistic view of himself/herself. The defensiveness reflected in this scale is expected to have limited the subject's endorsement of items on the other scales that suggest pathology. To correct for this, various empirically derived proportions of the K value are added to the raw scale scores on some of the other scales.

Some special scales (nonstandard, but commonly presented):

(A) Anxiety: This scale measures anxiety or general maladjustment.

(Continued.)

TABLE 3–2 (cont.)

(R) Repression: This scale measures the tendency to use repression and overcontrol to deal with anxiety.

(Es) Ego Strength: This scale attempts to measure the ability to withstand stress and to deal effectively with problems.

(Mac, AMac, or MAC) MacAndrew Alcoholism Scale: This scale measures an individual's proneness to becoming a substance abuser.

F-K Index: This ratio has been used as an indication of faking. When it is positive and greater than 11, it suggests a conscious attempt to look bad or call for help. When it is negative and greater than 12, it suggests an effort to look good and to deny emotional problems.

Goldberg Neurotic-Psychotic Index is constructed by the sum $(L + Pa + Sc - Hy - Pt)$. If the index value is greater than 45, this suggests psychosis.

MMPI = Minnesota Multiphasic Personality Inventory.

---

peaks and valleys. One should not consider the scales in isolation. There are systems of interpretation that focus on profiles. For example, interpretation may make use of two-point codes that focus on the two highest scales and what personality features are correlated with this pattern. Also, some of the items are regarded as particularly important in assessing the presence of a psychopathologic condition, and these critical items may be reported.

B. **Problems and advantages of the MMPI.** There are many problems with the MMPI: the reliability (repeatability of scores) has not been proved to be robust, there are high intercorrelations between the scales, the test is long, and some of the items dealing with religion or sex may be offensive. The test is problematic for subjects of differing cultural backgrounds. It is designed to evaluate for pathologic conditions, and is not appropriate for the assessment of normal people. On the other hand, the test is widely known, easy to administer, has extensive supporting validity studies, and numerous studies on the meaning of the scales and associations between scale scores and behavior.

III. **Projective testing.** In projective tests, the subject interprets ambiguous stimuli or fantasy scenarios. All projective tests are based on the hypothesis that an individual, presented with an understructured stimulus, attempts to impose his/her own structure and, in so doing, reveals personality characteristics, including emotional needs, moods, conflicts, defense mechanisms, and interpersonal style.

The *disadvantages* of projective tests are as follows: they usually cannot be objectively scored, interpretation relies heavily on the expertise of the scorer, and reliability and validity are nearly impossible to determine. There have been severe challenges to the reliability and validity of projective tests. The results obtained from different examiners with the same projective test data can often vary enormously. As a result, the utility of projective tests is in generating hypotheses that then need to be assessed in terms of other information and test results available from the subject.

A. **The Rorschach test.**

1. **Introduction and overview.** The Rorschach test involves ten ink blots: five are in shades of black and gray, two also have areas of red, and three are multicolored. The subject reports what he/she sees in the formless blots, or what it suggests to him/her. A verbatim record is kept of what the testee says, the time until the initial response is given, the total time spent on each card, as well as notes on the subject's behavior. This is the "free-association" phase. The subject can give any number of responses to the same card. In the following "inquiry" phase, the cards are again reviewed. The tester asks the subject what specifically in

the card led him/her to see what was reported. The testee explains and physically points to the parts of the card that contributed to the percept. The features that lead to the percept are called *determinants* and include categories of *form, color, shading,* and *perceived movement*.

The overall goal of the technique is to assess the subject's personality structure, with particular emphasis on the unconscious manner in which he/she responds and organizes the environment. In telling what he/she sees, the subject reveals information pertinent to his/her attitudes, feelings, conflicts, and aspects of his/her personality, such as mechanisms of defense, impulses, rigidity, strengths, and adaptive tendencies.

The Rorschach test may be seen as involving two tasks. First, it is a *perceptual-cognitive* problem in which the subject has to organize an ambiguous stimulus. This will reveal general (also termed "formal") aspects of the subject's perceptual processing. A second aspect is as a *stimulus to fantasy* in which it is presumed that the subject projects onto the stimuli dynamically relevant percepts that can be taken as symbolic of internal dynamics.

Therefore, the Rorschach protocol provides three sources of data: (1) the *formal* aspects of the perceptual responses; (2) the *content* of the responses and their sequence, interpreted psychodynamically; and (3) the subject's *behavior* in the test situation.

2. **Scoring the responses.** There are several scoring systems for the Rorschach test. The most widely used is Exner's Comprehensive System, aspects of which are described below. The scales have become associated with personality attributes. However, elevations on any scale may have a number of possible interpretive possibilities. It is inappropriate to draw conclusions from single-scale elevations. Below are presented some of the common attributes that are scored (with their associated symbol in parentheses).

a. **Location**—Location is correlated with what can

be regarded as the person's intellectual approach: the disposition to generalize, to be concretely practical, or to be pedantically preoccupied with trifling details.

b. **Determinants**—The determinant of each response reflects what there was about the blot that made it look the way the patient thought it looked. Determinants include *form* (F), the degree the response is determined by the shape or configuration of the blot, use or nonuse of *color* (C or c), and the perception of *movement* (M or m).

Various combinations of these determinants with varying emphasis can be designated. Thus, an FC response is determined primarily by form and secondarily by color; a CF response is primarily determined by color and secondarily by form. One can compare the number of FC percepts (form-dominated color, such as "a red butterfly") with CF and C percepts (color-dominated form or pure color, such as "a blazing fire" or "blood"). An FC response is associated with well-mediated affective responding and an ability to delay responding, and CF and C responses with less well-controlled displays of affect. Adult nonpatients typically have about twice as much FC as CF and C responses.

c. **Content areas**—Responses are also scored in terms of the content reflected in the responses, i.e., human, animal, anatomy, food, etc. In general, content areas indicate the emphasis and range of the person's needs, interests, preoccupations, and social interactions. Human content responses imply interest in and awareness of others; few such responses suggest limited empathy and withdrawal from relationships. In excess, animal responses reflect a stereotyped manner of approaching the world, immaturity in thought, or lack of cultural breadth.

d. **Popular responses (P)**—The P score represents the degree to which the subject gave common responses. Lists of common responses are available. The number of P responses is related to the ability to think along usual, conventional lines. When high, it may reflect anxious self-consciousness with overconforming and guarded responses. A low P score can be seen in psychosis, psychopathy, and in creative individuals.

3. **Examples.** By way of example, some of the Rorschach test features that are seen in schizophrenia can be summarized as follows: poor accuracy in form perception, fusing two separate responses to the same area into a single percept, paucity of conventional responses (less than five P responses), violation of ordinary rules of logic and language, highly personalized and idiosyncratic responses, clang associations, neologisms, reacting to the card as if it were (nearly) real, blots perceived as changing in front of the observer's eyes, seeing sexual responses in atypical areas, a limited number of whole human percepts, the presence of unmodulated color (C as opposed to CF or FC).

Borderlines may show thinking disturbances on the Rorschach test similar to schizophrenics, while performing entirely normally on objective psychological tests like the WAIS.

B. **Thematic apperception test (TAT).** This test was devised by Henry Murray in the mid-1930s. It involves presenting to subjects up to 20 pictures of people in dramatic but ambiguous situations. In practice, usually less than eight pictures are presented. The pictures are numbered 1 to 20. Some of the pictures have alternative versions for males (M), females (F), boys (B), and girls (G), in which case the number of the card is followed by the letter symbolizing the group for which it is intended, e.g., 3BM, 12M, or 13MF.

1. **Instructions.** The subject is to make up as dramatic a story as he/she can for each picture shown, which is to include who the characters are, what is happening to them, the thoughts and feelings of the characters, preceding events, and the outcome. About 5 minutes is to be used for each card.

2. **Interpretation.** The subject usually identifies

himself/herself with one of the characters (termed the "hero"), who presumably becomes a target of projection for the subject's own internal dynamics and external stresses. Other figures may also be viewed as targets on which projections are made, possibly with figures least like the subject receiving the least acceptable traits of the subject.

The experimenter records the time it takes for the subject to start the story, a verbatim record of the story, and any notable behaviors of the subject.

One strength of the TAT scenes is their ability to tap the patient's pattern of interaction with other significant figures. However, the interpersonal scenes described by the subject cannot be taken at face value necessarily to indicate the subject's actual relationships. If they do have a bearing on the subject it may be as wishes, fears, anticipations, or defensive covers for other issues.

Quantitative analysis is difficult. Although several scoring systems have been developed, they are rarely used clinically. One approach to interpretation is to note: who is the hero; the personality of the hero and his/her relation to the outside world with particular attention to the needs and strivings of the hero, as well as the obstacles encountered; the theme of the story; the outcome; and the overall emotional tone. Consistent themes across the stories are sought. The material may also be used to evaluate for evidence of thought disorder.

There are a number of variants of the TAT. One is the Make-a-Picture Story test by Edwin Schneidman, in which the subject is given various cutout figures and various backgrounds from which to formulate a story.

C. **Projective drawing tests.** There are several projective drawing tests, such as the Draw-a-Person (DAP) test, the House-Tree-Person test, and the Draw-a-Family test. As an example, the DAP test will be described more fully.

The subject is first asked to draw a person. The sex of the figure is noted, and usually is the same as the subject. The subject is then asked to draw a person of the opposite sex. The examiner may ask certain questions about the personal characteristics of the people drawn and even request a story about them. Interpretive principles rest largely on the assumed functional significance of each body part, as well as associations that are reputed to exist between personality features and aspects of pictorial rendition. An example would be the association of small figures with poor self-concept, depression, withdrawal, or anxiety.

D. **Sentence completion test.** There are many versions of this test. The subject is to finish various incomplete sentences. Typically, 75 to 100 sentences are presented. Various areas of life and attitudes of the subject about himself/herself and others are explored, including fears, worries, aspirations, and regrets. This test elicits more conscious associations to areas of functioning than the other projective tests. While numerous scoring systems have been devised, most psychologists simply inspect the answers looking for replies that are notable because they express strong affect, are repeated, are unusual or informative, or because of the affect of the subject. An analogous kind of test that has proved to be less useful because of greater difficulty in interpretation is word-association tests.

IV. **Neuropsychological testing.** The purpose of neuropsychological testing is to assess cognitive impairments due to organic causes. It is used to assist in establishing the diagnosis, helping in localization, planning rehabilitation, monitoring progress, and assessing prognosis.

There are two main approaches to neuropsychological testing. One involves the administration of comprehensive test batteries, of which the most widely used are the *Halstead-Reitan* and the *Luria-Nebraska*. A second approach is to individualize the specific tests used with each patient, with the choice depending on the referral question, clinical history, presenting symptoms, and the patient's ability to comply with examination procedures.

As with other testing, the following other explanations for defective performance need to be ruled out: lack of cooperation possibly due to psychiatric problems; inattention or performance problems associated with anxiety; lack of energy due to depression or illness; poor understanding of the task (e.g., illiteracy, retardation, or aphasia); malingering and simulation; or major psychiatric ("functional") impairments, such as psychosis (this last factor is particularly troublesome for many neuropsychological tests). These tests can be sensitive to cognitive dysfunction but not be able to discriminate whether it is on an organic basis or functional basis (particularly from chronic schizophrenia).

A. **Comprehensive test batteries.**

1. **Halstead-Reitan neuropsychological battery.** The standard battery consists of nine subtests. The battery requires certain equipment and, thus, generally cannot be administered at bedside. It takes 6 to 8 hours. There are several different scoring systems, and often several things are scored on each test (e.g., speed and accuracy). The scores on the subtests can be converted to standard scores and profiled. Profile analyses can be used to attempt to give a clinical correlation. Reitan has produced a large amount of empirical data relating specific lesions to test performance.

This is the most widely used comprehensive battery. The problems with the test are its length, there is no official manual on administering the test, the subtests are themselves complex and do not isolate specific skills, and no good test of memory is included.

2. **Luria-Nebraska test battery.** Luria was a prominent Russian neuropsychologist. Charles Golden tried to systematize, quantify, and standardize many of Luria's tests. The battery contains 269 items. Each item is administered separately and represents a specific as-

pect of functioning. The items vary along such dimensions as complexity, mode of stimulus input, mode of answering (e.g., motor, speech, multiple choice, or open ended), speed tested or not, and amount of information available. Eleven major areas of performance are examined.

Each item is scored in one or more ways (e.g., accuracy, speed, quality of response, time, trials to criterion, and/or number of responses). The raw score for each item is then translated to a scale score from 0 (normal) to 2 (clear abnormality) on the basis of instructions in the manual. Within each of the 11 major areas of performance, the item scale scores can be tallied. Three additional derivative summary scales are left hemisphere (sum of items implicating this hemisphere), right hemisphere, and pathognomonic (31 items that are especially sensitive to brain damage). For each summary index, the scores are transformed into T scores with a mean of 50 and an SD of 10. These can then be displayed in a profile. The criterion for a significantly abnormal T score is 60 in an otherwise normal person or 70 in a patient with a psychiatric history. However, different cutoffs can be used to correct for age and education differences. In general, differences of ten points separating the T scores of total score, IQ, memory quotient (MQ), or left vs. right are significant.

The test takes $2^{1}/_{2}$ hours. It is not as widely used or as thoroughly validated as the Halstead-Reitan battery, but this is due to the newness of the Luria-Nebraska battery. As with the Halstead-Reitan battery, this test is inadequate as a test for aphasia or memory problems.

B. **Specialized approach.** Using one of the standard comprehensive neuropsychological batteries is somewhat like using a shotgun, as a wide variety of cognitive functions are tested, at least superficially. An alternative approach (or an addition) is to select from a wide variety of possible measures a set of tests particularly appropriate to address the issues relevant to a particular patient.

There are literally hundreds of possible clinical tests and measures available. They differ not only in what they assess, but also in the quality of their construction (quantification, standardization, proven validity, and available research on the test). Two specialized tests that deserve separate description follow:

1. The *Wechsler memory scale* has seven subtests. The sum of all the scores can be transformed into an age-corrected MQ similar to an IQ. If the MQ is 15 points less than the IQ, an impairment is suggested. The limitations of the test are that it emphasizes verbal memory and immediate memory with little testing of recent or remote memory.

2. The *Bender visual motor gestalt test* (Bender-Gestalt) is a classic test assembled by Lauretta Bender. Each of nine simple geometric figures is presented individually on a card. The subject is to copy the figures onto a page. There are many variants to the testing procedure, including reproduction of the figures after a delay, possibly on paper with distracting wavy lines. There are several scoring systems, but none is uniformly embraced. The scoring systems give particular attention to lack of closure, rotations, simplifications, and perseverations. The test has been purported to discriminate subjects with brain damage, but the sensitivity of the test has been challenged. It has also been used as a test of developmental maturation. The quality of the reproduction is taken to reflect a child's cognitive maturity and perceptual fine-motor coordination. Scoring systems and norms have been devised. Additionally, the test has been used as a projective test. Here, various features in the reproduction may be associated with certain types of psychodynamic interpretations. As a projective test, there is no accepted manner to administer, score, and interpret the test.

4. Psychiatric Rating Scales

I. **Introduction.** Psychiatric rating scales can be useful to both the clinician and researcher. For the clinician, rating scales can be an aid to clinical judgment in establishing a diagnosis, determining a disposition, or evaluating the effectiveness of treatment. For the researcher, rating scales provide objective data that can be reproducible and reliable. Moreover, rating scales allow clinicians and researchers of different backgrounds to work from the same frame of reference. Rating scales supplement, but do not replace, clinical judgment. All rating scales are reproduced at the end of this chapter.

II. **Rating scales.**

A. **Grave disability/psychosis.**

1. **Global Assessment Scale:** Useful for consultation-liaison or disability evaluations. Variations are used to assess Axis V in *DSM III-R*. Scale ranges from 1 to 100, with 100 being without symptoms; hospitalization is necessary.

2. **Folstein Mini-Mental State Examination:** Evaluates organic, cognitive, and perceptual impairment. Rated scale totals 30 points; <25 = organicity.

3. **Brief Psychiatric Rating Scale:** Oriented for inpatients to evaluate thought and mood disorder; 18 items are rated on scale from 1 = not present to 7 = extremely severe.

4. **Schedule for Affective Disorders and Schizophrenia (SADS):** An interview that records information on functioning and symptoms that meet Research Diagnostic Criteria criteria and correlates with *DSM III*.

5. **Structured Clinical Interview for DSM-III (SCID) II:** A yes/no format to assess personality disorders that takes 45 to 60 minutes to administer; based on *DSM III-R*.

B. **Affective disorder.**

1. **Beck Depression Inventory:** A self-rated scale that covers 21 depressive symptoms and attitudes, including suicidal ideation; critical score >18 indicates clinical depression.

2. **Hamilton Depression Scale:** Twenty-one items each, with a 3- to 5-point scale that covers signs and symptoms of depression. This scale is primarily used for research (>18 is a common cutoff in research protocols requiring patients with major depression).

3. **Visual Analog Scale:** A self-rated assessment of present mood that is useful in assessing a change in subjective mood over time, such as in response to treatment. This is a very limited, but useful, indicator of the patient's mood.

4. **SADS:** See I./A./4.

C. **Anxiety disorders.**

1. **State-trait anxiety scale:** Self-rated or administered in a diagnostic interview, with 40 items and a four-point scale.

   a. A-State (A stands for anxiety) measures present status.

   b. A-Trait measures general character style.

D. **Organic brain syndromes.**

1. Folstein Mini-Mental State Examination (see I./A./2.)

E. **Personality disorders.**

1. **Minnesota Multiphasic Personality Inventory:** A self-report based on nine clinical scales (see Psychologic Testing Chapter 3 for further details).

2. **SCIDS-II:** Follows *DSM III-R* criteria. Answer format is yes/no; it takes 45 to 60 minutes to administer.

III. **Clinically Useful Mnemonics.**

A. **Suicide Scale: S.A.D. P.E.R.S.O.N.S.**

*S*ex: men kill themselves three times more frequently than women.

*A*ge: people 19 years or younger and 45 years or older are at greater risk for suicide.

*D*epressed people have a suicide rate 30 times more than nondepressed people.

*P*revious attempters have a suicide rate up to 64 times that of the general population.

*E*thanol abusers: An estimated 15% of alcoholics commit suicide.

*R*ational thinking loss, e.g., psychosis, mania, depression, or organic brain syndrome.

*S*ocial supports lacking, especially if there has been a recent loss of support.

*O*rganized plan, whether by direct or indirect communications.

*N*o spouse, e.g., single, divorced, widowed, or separated.

*S*ickness: Severe, chronic, or debilitating.

One point is given for each factor; scores from 0 to 2 allows for a home disposition with follow-up, 3 to 6 warrants consideration of hospitalization depending on confidence in follow-up, and 7 to 10 suggests either hospitalization or commitment. This scale is most useful in evaluating a potential suicide case. The clinician's own judgment is more reliable than the resulting scores.

B. **Homicide/violence scale: D.A.N.G.E.R.O.U.S.**

*D*iagnosis, as in paranoid schizophrenic, manic-depressive, organic brain syndrome, and antisocial/borderline personality disorders.

*A*ge: 16- to 30-year-old males are at greatest risk.

*N*othing to lose; Homeless, history of being abused, and/or history of abuse, assault, or murder.

*G*roup dynamics, e.g., quality of staff interactions with patient.

*E*xplicit threats against something or someone, particularly family members. (Remember Tarasoff vs. V. C. Regents.)

*R*ational thinking loss, e.g., psychosis, mania, depression, and/or organic brain syndrome.

*O*bservable behavior, e.g., pacing, tightening of jaw and fists, throwing back of shoulders, moving in a jerky or brisk manner, raising voice, and/or widening of eyes.

U: As in You and Your reaction to the patient; if you are frightened, act accordingly with the support of other staff or security personnel present and let the patient know he/she seems to be threatening.

*S*ubstance abuse, intoxication or withdrawal from alcohol, phencyclidine, heroin, cocaine, etc.

D.A.N.G.E.R.O.U.S. has not been assessed for its clinical effectiveness, but like S.A.D. P.E.R.S.O.N.S., it is based on epidemiologic factors and will be useful in at least organizing the clinician's evaluation of the violent patient.

C. **Alcoholism: C.A.G.E.**

   C-Have you ever felt the need to *cut* down drinking?

   A-Have you ever been *annoyed* by criticism of drinking?

   G-Have you had *guilt* feelings about drinking?

   E-Ever take a morning *eye-opener*?

Each criteria earns one point; a score of 3 to 4 suggests alcoholism. Even one point should arouse suspicion and further evaluation.

IV. **Appendix of rating scales.**

60 *Evaluation and Diagnosis*

APPENDIX 4-1

Global Assessment Scale (GAS)
Robert L. Spitzer, M.D., Miriam Gibbon, M.S.W., Jean Endicott, Ph.D.

Rate the subject's lowest level of functioning in the last week by selecting the lowest range which describes his functioning on a hypothetical continuum of mental health-illness. For example, a subject whose "behavior is considerably influenced by delusions" (range 21–30), should be given a rating in that range even though he has "major impairment in several areas" (range 31–40). *Use intermediary levels when appropriate* (e.g., 35, 58, 62). Rate actual functioning independent of whether or not subject is receiving and may be helped by medication or some other form of treatment.

Name of Patient _____ ID No. _____ Group Code _____
Admission Date _____ Date of Rating _____ Rater _____
GAS Rating: _____

100
—   Superior functioning in a wide range of activities, life's problems never seem to get out of hand, is
91   sought out by others because of his warmth and integrity. No symptoms.

90
—   Good functioning in all areas, many interests, socially effective, generally satisfied with life. There
81   may or may not be transient symptoms and "everyday" worries that only occasionally get out of
     hand.

80–71	No more than slight impairment in functioning, varying degrees of "everyday" worries and problems that sometimes get out of hand. Minimal symptoms may or may not be present.
70–61	Some mild symptoms (e.g., depressive mood and mild insomnia) OR some difficulty in several areas of functioning, but generally functioning pretty well, has some meaningful interpersonal relationships and most untrained people would not consider him "sick."
60–51	Moderate symptoms OR generally functioning with some difficulty (e.g., few friends and flat affect, depressed mood and pathological self-doubt, euphoric mood and pressure of speech, moderately severe antisocial behavior).
50–41	Any serious symptomatology or impairment in functioning that most clinicians would think obviously requires treatment or attention (e.g., suicidal preoccupation or gesture, severe obsessional rituals, frequent anxiety attacks, serious antisocial behavior, compulsive drinking, mild but definite manic syndrome).
40–31	Major impairment in several areas, such as work, family relations, judgment, thinking or mood (e.g., depressed woman avoids friends, neglects family, unable to do housework), OR some impairment in reality testing or communication (e.g., speech is at times obscure, illogical or irrelevant), OR single suicide attempt.

(Continued.)

30–21	Unable to function in almost all areas (e.g., stays in bed all day) OR behavior is considerably influenced by either delusions or hallucinations OR serious impairment in communication (e.g., sometimes incoherent or unresponsive) or judgment (e.g., acts grossly inappropriately).
20–11	Needs some supervision to prevent hurting self or others, or to maintain minimal personal hygiene (e.g., repeated suicide attempts, frequently violent, manic excitement, smears feces), OR gross impairment in communication (e.g., largely incoherent or mute).
10–1	Needs constant supervision for several days to prevent hurting self or others (e.g., requires an intensive care unit with special observation by staff), makes no attempt to maintain minimal personal hygiene, or serious suicide act with clear intent and expectation of death.

APPENDIX 4-2

Feelings Rating Scales

NAME _____

Please rate how you feel today, at this moment, by placing an (x) in the appropriate circles.

Saddest Ever	OOOOOOOOOOOOOOO	Happiest Ever	Date:
Least Anxious Ever	OOOOOOOOOOOOOOO	Most Anxious Ever	
Most Tired Ever	OOOOOOOOOOOOOOO	Least Tired Ever	Time:
Worst I Have Ever Felt	OOOOOOOOOOOOOOO	Best I Have Ever Felt	
Least Energetic Ever	OOOOOOOOOOOOOOO	Most Energetic Ever	
Saddest Ever	OOOOOOOOOOOOOOO	Happiest Ever	Date:
Least Anxious Ever	OOOOOOOOOOOOOOO	Most Anxious Ever	
Most Tired Ever	OOOOOOOOOOOOOOO	Least Tired Ever	Time:
Worst I Have Ever Felt	OOOOOOOOOOOOOOO	Best I Have Ever Felt	
Least Energetic Ever	OOOOOOOOOOOOOOO	Most Energetic Ever	
Saddest Ever	OOOOOOOOOOOOOOO	Happiest Ever	Date:
Least Anxious Ever	OOOOOOOOOOOOOOO	Most Anxious Ever	
Most Tired Ever	OOOOOOOOOOOOOOO	Least Tired Ever	Time:
Worst I Have Ever Felt	OOOOOOOOOOOOOOO	Best I Have Ever Felt	
Least Energetic Ever	OOOOOOOOOOOOOOO	Most Energetic Ever	
Saddest Ever	OOOOOOOOOOOOOOO	Happiest Ever	Date:
Least Anxious Ever	OOOOOOOOOOOOOOO	Most Anxious Ever	
Most Tired Ever	OOOOOOOOOOOOOOO	Least Tired Ever	Time:
Worst I Have Ever Felt	OOOOOOOOOOOOOOO	Best I Have Ever Felt	
Least Energetic Ever	OOOOOOOOOOOOOOO	Most Energetic Ever	

64 *Evaluation and Diagnosis*

APPENDIX 4–3

Brief Psychiatric Rating Scale
Overall and Gorham

DIRECTIONS: Place an X in the appropriate box to represent level of severity of each symptom.

PATIENT _____
RATER _____
NO. _____
DATE _____

	Symptom	Not Present	Very Mild	Mild	Moderate
1.	Somatic concern—preoccupation with physical health, fear of physical illness, hypochondriases.	☐	☐	☐	☐
2.	Anxiety—worry, fear, over-concern for present or future.	☐	☐	☐	☐
3.	Emotional withdrawal—lack of spontaneous interaction, isolation, deficiency in relating to others.	☐	☐	☐	☐
4.	Conceptual disorganization—thought processes confused, disconnected, disorganized, disrupted.	☐	☐	☐	☐
5.	Guilt feelings—self-blame, shame, remorse for past behavior.	☐	☐	☐	☐
6.	Tension—physical and motor manifestations or nervousness, overactivation, tension.	☐	☐	☐	☐

☐	☐	☐☐☐	☐	☐	☐☐☐	☐☐	
☐	☐	☐☐☐	☐	☐	☐☐☐	☐☐	
☐	☐	☐☐☐	☐	☐	☐☐☐	☐☐	
☐	☐	☐☐☐	☐	☐	☐☐☐	☐☐	

7. Mannerisms and posturing—peculiar, bizarre unnatural motor behavior (not including tic).
8. Grandiosity—exaggerated self-opinion, arrogance, conviction of unusual power or abilities.
9. Depressive mood—sorrow, sadness, despondency, pessimism.
10. Hostility—animosity, contempt, belligerence, disdain for others.
11. Suspiciousness—mistrust, belief that others harbour malicious or discriminatory intent.
12. Hallucinatory behavior—perceptions without normal external stimulus correspondence.
13. Motor retardation—slowed weakened movements or speech, reduced body tone.
14. Uncooperativeness—resistance, guardedness, rejection of authority.
15. Unusual thought content—unusual, odd, strange, bizarre thought content.
16. Blunted affect—reduced emotional tone, reduction in normal intensity of feelings, flatness.
17. Excitement—heightened emotional tone, agitation, increased reactivity.
18. Disorientation—confusion or lack of proper association for person, place, or time.

*From Overall JE, Gorham DR: Psychol Rep 1962; 10:799–812. Used with permission.

66 *Evaluation and Diagnosis*

APPENDIX 4–4

Mini-Mental State
by M.F. Folstein, S.E. Folstein and P.R. McHugh

Tester Name _____ Month _____ Day _____ Year _____

SCORE 1 = CORRECT   ≤15 = dementia
                    24-30 = normal

I. *Orientation* (10 pts)

Ask, "What is today's date?"
Then ask specifically for parts omitted; e.g., "Can you also tell me what season it is?"

Date (e.g., Jan. 21)	1
Year	2
Month	3
Day (e.g., Monday)	4
Season	5

Ask, "Can you tell me the name of this hospital?"
"What floor are we on?"
"What town (or city) are we in?"
"What country are we in?"
"What state are we in?"

Hospital	6
Floor	7
Town	8
County	9
State	10

II. *Registration* (3 pts)

Ask the subject if you may test his/her memory. Then say "ball," "flag," "tree" clearly and slowly, about one second for each. After you have said all 3, ask him/her

"Ball"	11
"Flag"	12
"Tree"	13
Number of trials	14

to repeat them. This first repetition
determines his/her score (0-3) but keep
saying them until he/she can repeat all 3,
up to 6 trials. If he/she does not eventually
learn all 3, recall cannot be meaningfully
tested.

III. *Attention and Calculation* (5 pts)
Ask the subject to begin with 100 and
count backwards by 7. Stop after 5
subtractions (93, 86, 79, 72, 65). Score the
total number of correct answers. If the
subject cannot or will not perform this task,
ask him/her to spell the word "world"
backwards. The score is the number of
letters in correct order. For example, dlrow
= 5, dlorw = 3.

"93" 15
"86" 16
"79" 17
"72" 18
"65" 19

Record how subject spelled "World" backwards

d	l	r	o	w

Number of letters in correct order ......20 _____

(Continued.)

68 *Evaluation and Diagnosis*

IV. *Recall* (3 pts)

Ask the subject to recall the 3 words you previously asked him/her to remember. Score 0-3.

"Ball" 21
"Flag" 22
"Tree" 23

V. *Language* (9 pts)

naming: Show the subject a wristwatch and ask him/her what it is. Repeat for pencil.

Watch 24
Pencil 25

repetition: Ask the subject to repeat, "No ifs, ands, or buts."

Repetition 26

3-stage command: Give the subject a piece of plain blank paper and say, "Take the paper in your right hand, fold it in half and put it on the floor."

Takes paper in right 27
Folds paper in half 28
Puts paper on floor 29

reading: On a blank piece of paper print the sentence, "Close your eyes," in letters large enough for the subject to see clearly. Ask him/her to read it and do what it says. Score correct only if he/she actually closes his/her eyes.

Closes eyes 30

writing: Give the subject a blank piece of paper and ask him/her to write a sentence. It is to be written spontaneously. It must contain a subject and a verb and be sensible. Correct grammar and punctuation are not necessary.

Writes sentence 31

copying: On a clean piece of paper, draw intersecting pentagons, each side about 1 inch, and ask subject to copy it exactly as it is. All 10 angles must be present and two must intersect to score 1 point. Tremor and rotation are ignored.

e.g.

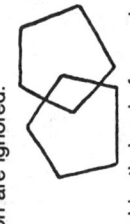

Draws pentagons 32

Rate subject's level of consciousness:
(Circle)

(a) Coma
(b) Stupor
(c) Drowsy
(d) Alert

TOTAL SCORE:
(Maximum score = 30)

APPENDIX 4-5
Depression Inventory

NAME _____
DATE _____

- 3 I am so sad or unhappy that I can't stand it.
- 2 I am blue or sad all the time and I can't snap out of it.
- 1 I feel sad or blue.
- 0 I do not feel sad.

- 3 I feel that the future is hopeless and that things cannot improve.
- 2 I feel I have nothing to look forward to.
- 1 I feel discouraged about the future.
- 0 I am not particularly pessimistic or discouraged about the future.

- 3 I feel I am a complete failure as a person (parent, husband, wife).
- 2 As I look back on my life, all I can see is a lot of failures.
- 1 I feel I have failed more than the average person.
- 0 I do not feel like a failure.

- 3 I am dissatisfied with everything.
- 2 I don't get satisfaction out of anything anymore.
- 1 I don't enjoy things the way I used to.
- 0 I am not particularly dissatisfied.

3	I feel as though I am very bad or worthless.
2	I feel quite guilty.
1	I feel bad or unworthy a good part of the time.
0	I don't feel particularly guilty.
3	I hate myself.
2	I am disgusted with myself.
1	I am disappointed in myself.
0	I don't feel disappointed in myself.
3	I would kill myself if I had the chance.
2	I have definite plans about committing suicide.
1	I feel I would be better off dead.
0	I don't have any thoughts of harming myself.
3	I have lost all my interest in other people and don't care about them at all.
2	I have lost most of my interest in other people and have little feeling for them.
1	I am less interested in other people than I used to be.
0	I have not lost interest in other people.
3	I can't make any decisions at all any more.
2	I have great difficulty in making decisions.
1	I try to put off making decisions.
0	I make decisions about as well as ever.

(Continued.)

3   I feel that I am ugly or repulsive looking.
2   I feel that there are permanent changes in my appearance and they make me look unattractive.
1   I am worried that I am looking old or unattractive.
0   I don't feel I look any worse than I used to.

3   I can't do any work at all.
2   I have to push myself very hard to do anything.
1   I get tired more easily than I used to.
0   I don't get any more tired than usual.

3   I get too tired to do anything.
2   I get tired from doing anything.
1   I get tired more easily than I used to.
0   I don't get any more tired than usual.

3   I have no appetite at all anymore.
2   My appetite is much worse now.
1   My appetite is not as good as it used to be.
0   My appetite is no worse than usual.

APPENDIX 4–6

Hamilton Depression Scale

For each item write the correct number in the box (only one response).

1. DEPRESSED MOOD *(Sadness, hopeless, helpless, worthless)*
   - 0 = Absent
   - 1 = These feelings states indicated only on questioning
   - 2 = These feeling states spontaneously reported verbally
   - 3 = Communicates feeling states non-verbally—i.e., through facial expression, posture, voice, and tendency to weep
   - 4 = Patient reports VIRTUALLY ONLY these feeling states in his spontaneous verbal and non-verbal communication

   1. ☐

2. FEELINGS OF GUILT
   - 0 = Absent
   - 1 = Self reproach, feels he has let people down
   - 2 = Ideas of guilt or rumination over past errors or sinful deeds
   - 3 = Present illness is a punishment. Delusions of guilt
   - 4 = Hears accusatory or denunciatory voices and/or experiences threatening visual hallucinations

   2. ☐

(Continued.)

74 *Evaluation and Diagnosis*

3. SUICIDE
 0 = Absent
 1 = Feels life is not worth living
 2 = Wishes he were dead or any thoughts of possible death to self
 3 = Suicide ideas or gesture
 4 = Attempts at suicide *(any serious attempt rates 4)*

 ☐ 3.

4. INSOMNIA EARLY
 0 = No difficulty falling asleep
 1 = Complains of occasional difficulty falling asleep—i.e., more than 1/2 hour
 2 = Complains of nightly difficulty falling asleep

 ☐ 4.

5. INSOMNIA MIDDLE
 0 = No difficulty
 1 = Patient complains of being restless and disturbed during the night
 2 = Waking during the night—any getting out of bed rates 2 *(except for purposes of voiding)*

 ☐ 5.

6. INSOMNIA LATE
 0 = No difficulty
 1 = Waking in early hours of the morning but goes back to sleep
 2 = Unable to fall asleep again if he gets out of bed

 ☐ 6.

7. WORK AND ACTIVITIES
0 = No difficulty
1 = Thoughts and feelings of incapacity, fatigue or weakness related to activities: work or hobbies
2 = Loss of interest in activity: hobbies or work—either directly reported by patient, or indirect in listlessness, indecision and vacillation *(feels he has to push self to work or activities)*
3 = Decrease in actual time spent in activities or decrease in productivity. In hospital, rate 3 if patient does not spend at least three hours a day in activities *(hospital job or hobbies)* exclusive of ward chores
4 = Stopped working because of present illness. In hospital, rate 4 if patient engages in no activities except ward chores, or if patient fails to perform ward chores unassisted

7. ☐

8. RETARDATION *(Slowness of thought and speech; impaired ability to concentrate; decreased motor activity)*
0 = Normal speech and thought
1 = Slight retardation at interview
2 = Obvious retardation at interview
3 = Interview difficult
4 = Complete stupor

8. ☐

(Continued.)

76 Evaluation and Diagnosis

9. AGITATION
 0 = None
 1 = "Playing with" hands, hair, etc.
 2 = Hand wringing, nail-biting, hair pulling, biting of lips

9. ☐

10. ANXIETY PSYCHIC
 0 = No difficulty
 1 = Subjective tension and irritability
 2 = Worrying about minor matters
 3 = Apprehensive attitude apparent in face or speech
 4 = Fears expressed without questioning

10. ☐

11. ANXIETY SOMATIC
 0 = Absent   Physiological concomitants of anxiety, such as
 1 = Mild   Gastrointestinal—*dry mouth*, *wind*, *indigestion*, *diarrhea*, *cramps*, *belching*
                   Cardiovascular—*palpitations*, *headaches*
 2 = Moderate
 3 = Severe   Respiratory—*hyperventilation*, *sighing*
                   Urinary frequency
 4 = Incapacitating Sweating

11. ☐

12. SOMATIC SYMPTOMS GASTROINTESTINAL
   0 = None
   1 = Loss of appetite but eating without staff encouragement. Heavy feelings in abdomen.
   2 = Difficulty eating without staff urging. Requests or requires laxatives or medication for bowels or medication for GI symptoms

   ☐ 12.

13. SOMATIC SYMPTOMS GENERAL
   0 = None
   1 = Heaviness in limbs, back or head. Backaches, headache, muscle aches. Loss of energy and fatigability
   2 = Any clear-cut symptom rates 2

   ☐ 13.

14. GENITAL SYMPTOMS   Symptoms such as: *Loss of libido*
   0 = Absent   *Menstrual*
   1 = Mild   *disturbances*
   2 = Severe

   ☐ 14.

15. HYPOCHONDRIASIS
   0 = Not present
   1 = Self-absorption (bodily)
   2 = Preoccupation with health
   3 = Frequent complaints, requests for help, etc.
   4 = Hypochondriacal delusions

   ☐ 15.

(Continued.)

78 Evaluation and Diagnosis

16. LOSS OF WEIGHT *Rate either A or B*
   A. When Rating By History:
      0 = No weight loss
      1 = Probable weight loss associated with present illness
      2 = Definite (according to patient) weight loss
   B. On Weekly Rating By Ward Psychiatrist. When Actual Weight Changes are Measured:
      0 = Less than or equal to 1 lb. weight loss in week
      1 = Greater than 1 lb. but less than or equal to 2 lb. weight loss in week
      2 = Greater than 2 lb. weight loss in week

   ☐ 16.

17. INSIGHT
   0 = Acknowledges being depressed and ill
   1 = Acknowledges illness but attributes cause to bad food, climate, overwork, virus, need for rest, etc.
   2 = Denies being ill at all

   ☐ 17.

18. DIURNAL VARIATION *Rate both A and B, but ADD 18B ONLY into total score*
   A. Note whether symptoms are worse in morning or evening, if NO diurnal variation, mark none
      0 = No variation
      1 = Worse in A.M.
      2 = Worse in P.M.

   ☐ 18A

Psychiatric Rating Scales

B. When present, mark the severity of the variation. Mark "None" if NO variation
   0 = None
   1 = Mild
   2 = Severe

   18B ONLY [ ]

19. DEPERSONALIZATION AND DEREALIZATION   Such as: *Feelings of unreality*
    0 = Absent
    1 = Mild
    2 = Moderate
    3 = Severe
    4 = Incapacitating

    19. [ ]

20. PARANOID SYMPTOMS
    0 = None
    1 = Suspicious
    2 = Ideas of reference
    3 = Delusions of reference and persecution

    20. [ ]

21. OBSESSIONAL AND COMPULSIVE SYMPTOMS
    0 = Absent
    1 = Mild
    2 = Severe

    21. [ ]

TOTAL HAMILTON SCORE [ ]

REFERENCES

1. Carr AC: Psychological testing of personality, in Kaplan HI, Sadock BJ (eds): *Comprehensive Textbook of Psychiatry*, ed 4. Baltimore, Williams & Wilkins, 1985, pp 533–535.
2. Ewing JA: Detecting alcoholism: The CAGE questionnaire. *JAMA* 1984; 252:1905–1907.
3. Patterson WM, et al: Evaluation of suicidal patients: The SAD PERSONS scale. *Psychosomatics* 1983; 24:343–349.
4. Spielberger, et al: *STAI Manual for the State-Trait Anxiety Inventory*. Palo Alto, Calif., Consulting Psychologists Press, 1970.
5. Spitzer RL, Williams JBW, Gibson M: *Instruction Manual for Structured Clinical Interview for DSM III-R*. New York, Biometrics Research Department, 1987.

5

The Use of EEG in Psychiatry

I. **Introduction.** The primary role of the electroencephalogram (EEG) in psychiatry is in helping to discriminate between functional and organic etiologies for abnormal mental states. Striking examples include distinguishing the potentially treatable dementia syndrome of depression ("pseudodementia") from less treatable degenerative dementias, and separating conversion symptoms (i.e., pseudocoma) from organic symptoms (i.e., true coma) and hysterical "pseudoseizures" or dissociative states from genuine seizure phenomena. In most such cases, especially where there is a history of abrupt onset, a normal EEG is consistent with a functional illness, whereas an abnormal EEG indicates organicity. It should always be remembered that an abnormal EEG demonstrates an organic pathologic condition, whereas a normal EEG is inconclusive and may suggest further workup. The major uses of an EEG are in (1) suspected organic mental disorders, (2) suspected seizure disorders and psychiatric disorders that mimic seizure disorders, and (3) characterization of sleep disorders. Table 5–1 outlines the basic EEG wave/rhythm patterns, and some basic definitions, on page 82.

TABLE 5–1.
Normal EEG Patterns*

Basic Types of EEG Activity
1. Rhythm—fairly continuous pattern of a particular frequency (i.e., beta rhythm).
2. Transient forms—brief discharges that interrupt the underlying pattern (i.e., spikes, sharp waves).
3. Background activity—the underlying activity on which transient and rhythmic activity is superimposed.

Basic Wave/Rhythm Frequencies in Normal Adult Subjects

Delta: Less than 4 Hz—seen in normal stage 3 and 4 sleep.

Theta: 4 Hz to less than 8 Hz—seen in earlier stage 1 and 2 sleep.

Alpha: 8 Hz to 13 Hz—alpha rhythm is a bilateral posterior rhythm in the alpha range. It is the pattern seen in normal adults under standard conditions (relaxed with eyes closed).

Beta: Greater than 13 Hz—seen randomly in waking, alert state. Also in various psychotropic drug states (sedative/hypnotics).

Slow waves: When dominant frequency is below the alpha range.

Fast waves: When dominant frequency is above the alpha range.

Normal Sleep EEG Patterns

Awake: (eyes open)	Low voltage, random, fast.
Relaxed-drowsy: (eyes closed)	Alpha waves predominate.

(Continued.)

TABLE 5–1 (cont.)

Stage 1: Theta waves (4–8 cps) replace alpha waves.
Stage 2: Progressively higher and slower waves in the theta range with bursts of sleep spindles (12–14 cps) and K complexes (high-voltage transient waves).
Stage 3: Increasing delta activity (20%–50%) with occasional spindle and K complex activity.
Stage 4: Generalized high-voltage delta activity comprising more than 50% of the record.
NOTE: Stage 3 and 4 together, are call "delta sleep."
REM: Low-voltage, random-fast wave similar to waking pattern. Includes occasional "sawtooth" waves. REM comprises 20%–25% of total sleep time in normal adult.

EEG = electroencephalographic; REM = rapid eye movement.

II. **Organic mental disorders.** The *DSM III-R* lists three broad categories of organic mental disorders: (1) dementias arising in the senium and presenium, (2) psychoactive substance-induced organic mental disorders, and (3) organic mental disorders associated with Axis III physical disorders or whose etiology is unknown. The latter two categories include syndromes that mimic other "functional" psychotic disorders but are thought to originate from separate, identifiable organic etiologies. These include secondary dementias, deliria, organic amnestic disorders, delusional disorders, hallucinoses, mood disorders, anxiety disorders, and personality disorders.

A. **Delirium.** The EEG changes associated with organic brain mental disorders are typically nonspecific and most commonly reveal generalized regular and irregular slowing. *Delirium* from almost all causes is accompanied by diffuse EEG slowing that corresponds to the degree of symptom severity, and clinical resolution is well correlated with normalization of the EEG. *Delirium tremens* is a notable exception in which there is minimal slowing even in the presence of profound mental status changes. *Anticholinergic delirium* has an atypical pattern with reduced slow-wave activity and desynchronization. *Neuroleptic malignant syndromes* have a variable alteration in mental status, but usually present with a fluctuating stuporous state. The EEG abnormalities are usually mild and nonspecific.

B. **Dementia.** Progressive degenerative dementia is the most common type of organic mental disorder encountered in clinical practice. The primary EEG findings are those of generalized slowing and the disappearance of fast activity. The presence and extent of these features correlate well with the degree of cognitive deterioration and, to some degree, with the rate of decline. Thus, the EEG is normal in the early course of Alzheimer disease, but becomes abnormal in later stages, making the EEG a helpful staging tool. Generally, demented and elderly normal patients can be distinguished by EEG studies; however, individual exceptions are not uncommon, and therefore, the EEG results alone are not diagnostic. The EEG studies may be particularly helpful in identifying underlying toxic or metabolic conditions through the presence of uncharacteristically marked EEG changes early in the clinical course of dementia, or assisting in the discrimination between organic and functional etiologies (i.e., depressive "pseudodementia"), a situation where a normal EEG is recorded in the presence of marked cognitive loss. The EEG findings in other dementing illnesses are listed in Table 5–2.

C. **Toxic/metabolic disorders.** Toxic and metabolic disorders are not uncommon causes of delirium, dementia, or other specific organic mental disorders. Generally, prominent EEG changes are discernible early in the clinical course. This is important, since many of these disorders are potentially reversible. The predominant states found with metabolic disorders is generalized regular or irregular slowing. Specific findings for a variety of toxic, metabolic, nutritional, and endocrinological abnormalities are found in Table 5–3.

III. **Seizure disorders, pseudoseizures, and dissociative states.**

A. **Seizure disorders.** Seizure disorders may lead to a full range of organic mental disorders. Postictal delirium is not uncommon and shows generalized slowing. Patients with chronic uncontrolled seizures may develop a dementia with EEG findings similar to multi-infarct dementia. This dementia is thought to be secondary to recurrent anoxia. Mesial temporal lobe foci may occasionally present as an organic amnestic syndrome, organic hallucinosis, an organic personality syndrome, or even a schizophrenia-like syndrome. Temporal lobe epilepsy is sometimes associated with interictal behavioral changes that may include personality changes, deepening of affect, decreased libido, hyper-religiosity, and hypergraphia. Abnormal sexual behavior and disorders of impulse control may also suggest a previously undiagnosed partial complex seizure disorder. In any case, careful history taking, as well as EEG studies, will be important data for proper diagnosis and treatment.

B. **Conversion disorders and hysterical "seizures."** Conversion disorders are psychiatric syndromes in which the predominant disturbance is a loss or alteration in physical function that suggests a physical disorder but which is instead an expression or resolution of intrapsychic conflict. Classic conversion symptoms include those that suggest neurological disease, such as blindness, paralysis, coma, and seizures. In these cases, EEG studies are usually normal. The separation of true from hysterical attacks can be difficult as studies can be contaminated by muscle movements (false-positive result), and genuine temporal lobe seizures may occur without detectable EEG changes (false-negative

TABLE 5–2.
EEG Findings in Dementia*

Disease	Incidence of Abnormal EEG (%)	Findings
Alzheimer (DAT)	Early-low, late-near 100	Generalized, irregular slowing (decreased alpha activity), EEG abnormality may predict rate of progression but not necessarily severity
Multi-infarct (MID)	80	Generalized slowing similar to DAT, may have focal abnormalities due to cerebral infarction
Pick disease	<30	Normal to minimal changes (minimal generalized slowing as in DAT but less marked)
Huntington chorea	90	Frequently abnormal with markedly low voltage and irregular theta and delta activity
Normal-pressure hydrocephalus	60	Variably abnormal with diffuse focal slowing, primarily delta waves
Parkinson disease	35	Diffuse slow activity (primarily theta but occasional delta patterns)
Wilson disease	50	General or paroxysmal slowing
Multiple sclerosis	50	Focal or generalized slowing, primarily theta range

		Normal EEG findings
Dementia syndrome of depression	...	
Chronic subdural hematoma	90	Decreased amplitude, variable changes with generalized and focal slowing
Alcoholic dementia	>75	Fast activity with diffuse theta and delta activity
Neurosyphilis dementia	>80	Diffuse slowing of basic alpha rhythm, with increased theta
Dialysis dementia	...	Slowing of background rhythms with frontal abnormalities of predominant delta activity with occasional sharp waves and triphasic complexes

*EEG = electroencephalographic; DAT = dementia of the Alzheimer type; and MID = multi-infarct dementia.

TABLE 5–3.

EEG Findings for Toxic, Metabolic, Endocrinologic, and Nutritional States*

	EEG Findings
Toxic/drug states	
Sedative-hypnotics	Increase in fast activity (20–30 Hz range), marked individual differences in amount of change
Neuroleptics	Generalized decrease in fast activity and increase in slow activity, more so at higher dosages
Tricyclic antidepressants	Similar to slower activity seen in neuroleptics
Lithium carbonate	Minimal changes at therapeutic dosage, generalized diffuse slowing at toxic levels
Anticonvulsants	Little or no effect at therapeutic doses, toxic levels show increasing theta activity
Analgesics/narcotics	Little or no effect at therapeutic doses, serious overdoses show diffuse slowing with decreased amplitude
Stimulants	Decreased alpha activity and increased low-voltage fast activity
Hallucinogens	Little or no effect
Toxic/metabolic states	
Heavy metal poisoning	Diffuse theta or delta activity

(Continued.)

TABLE 5–3 (cont.)

Renal failure/uremia	Normal until significant clinical signs of failure, then random theta activity to generalized delta activity
Hepatic encephalopathy	Progressive generalized slowing as clnical condition deteriorates, may become diffuse low-amplitude beta and finally isoelectric in end stages
Basic electrolyte abnormalities	Generally normal EEG findings even in extreme cases
Toxic/drug states	
Dehydration	Normal EEG findings
Water intoxication	Generalized slowing
Acidosis	Normal EEG findings
Alkalosis	High-voltage waves of generalized delta activity against background of faster activity
Hyperthermia	Normal EEG findings
Hypothermia	Slowing and attenuation of background activity
Endocrine disorders	
Hyperthyroidism	Decreased alpha activity and increased beta (15–30 Hz) in central regions
Thyrotoxic encephalopathy	Diffuse bilateral theta and delta activity
Hypothyroidism (mild)	Normal EEG findings to mild slowing
Myxedema	Low voltage with decreased alpha and random theta and delta activity

(Continued.)

TABLE 5–3 (cont.)

Myxedema coma	Very low-amplitude slow activity to virtual isoelectric
Diabetic coma	Generalized theta and delta activity progressing to delta dominance in frank coma
Hypoglycemia (insulin shock)	Progressive slowing paralleling drop in glucose with extensive bilateral delta activity in coma
Vitamin deficiencies	
Thiamine (B_1) (Wernicke encephalopathy)	Mild—slowed alpha to theta predominant, severe-generalized delta activity
Nicotinic acid (associated delirium, depression, catatonia)	Generalized temporal slowing
B_{12} (pernicious anemia, associated organic brain syndrome with paranoia and depression common)	Generalized slowing—with theta predominance being most common

EEG = electroencephalographic.

result). Multiple recordings and careful clinical judgment are usually needed to confirm the correct diagnosis (particularly multiple-personality disorder). For this reason, EEG studies—usually multiple testings under a variety of laboratory conditions—are necessary for diagnosis.

IV. **Sleep disorders.** Our knowledge of the nature and architecture of brain electrical activity in sleep is based on EEG studies. Thus, it is not surprising that the EEG is the primary means of studying sleep disorders. This work is generally conducted in a sleep laboratory where continuous EEG monitoring can be done. For a review of sleep disorders, their diagnosis and treatment, see Chapter 16.

II
Psychiatric Disorders

6
Affective Disorders

I. **Introduction.** The affective disorders are disorders of mood defined in the *DSM III* glossary as "pervasive and sustained emotion that, in the extreme, markedly colors the person's perception of the world." These disorders are divided into three major groupings:

1. Major affective disorders
2. Other specific affective disorders
3. Atypical affective disorders

The following is a brief overview of the major issues to be considered in the assessment of affective disorders; please see *DSM III* for a complete description of symptoms.

II. **Major affective disorders.**

A. **Bipolar disorder.**

1. **Mixed.** A person presents with an episode that involves both manic and depressive elements. The depressive elements last at least 1 full day. The manic and depressive episodes may be alternating or intermixed.

2. **Manic.** The person presents in a manic episode.

3. **Depressed.** The patient has had at least one manic episode but currently has a major depressive episode.

B. **Major depression.**

1. Single Episode
2. Recurrent

The primary fact is that the person has never had a manic episode, but has had at least one major depressive episode.

III. Other specific affective disorders.

A. **Cyclothymic disorder.** This is a chronic (at least 2 years' duration) cyclic mood disorder in which the person has several episodes of depressive and hypomanic symptoms that are not severe enough to meet criteria for either a full manic or depressive episode. These episodes may alternate, be intermixed, or have periods of normal mood.

B. **Dysthymic disorder.** This is also a chronic disorder (adults, 2 years' duration; children, 1 year's duration) with features of depressed mood and anhedonia not severe enough to meet criteria for a major depressive episode.

IV. Atypical affective disorders.

A. **Atypical bipolar disorder (bipolar II).** At least one major depressive episode and episodes of hypomania but not mania.

B. **Atypical depression.** Individuals who manifest depressive symptoms while they have a mixed or unusual picture that precludes the diagnosis of a major depressive episode. The following examples are given in *DSM III*:

1. Individuals with schizophrenia, residual type, who have a depressive episode that develops without activation of psychotic symptoms.

2. Disturbances that meet the criteria for dysthymic

disorder, with periods of normal mood lasting longer than a few months.

3. A brief episode of depression that does not meet criteria for either major affective disorder or adjustment disorder.

V. Etiologies of affective disorders. The etiology of the affective disorders is not fully known. However, a number of important theories have been proposed. It is possible that these theories each detail different aspects of a multifactored etiology.

A. Psychologic factors. Psychologic factors may be more important among the cyclothymic and atypical depressives.

1. **Psychodynamics.** The hostility that was directed at an object that has been lost is now turned against the self.

a. The lost object is introjected. Anger toward the object (including for being lost) is aimed at the ego and leads to depression.

b. If the ego overcomes the "hostile" superego, the resulting release of energy manifests as manic symptoms.

c. There appears to be a vulnerability to loss and a lack of adaptive resources to cope with a given level of challenge, both for acute stressors and chronic "hassles." The quality and availability of family and social support are also important.

d. Early loss of a parent (before the age of 20 years) is associated with an increased incidence of depression.

e. Personality styles:

Higher Risk	Lower Risk
Dependent	Antisocial
Obsessive-compulsive	Paranoid
Hysterical	

f. Low-risk individuals may use projection and externalizing defenses.

2. **Psychosocial.** Recent major life difficulties may be triggers.

3. **Behavior.** The environment may "teach" helpless or dependent behavior. The "learned helplessness theory" arose from studies, such as if two animals are subjected to the same painful stimulus and one has some control while the other does not, then the "helpless" one will "give up" and appear to be withdrawn and hypoactive. Interestingly, tricyclic antidepressants (TCAs) effectively reverse the learned helplessness response.

4. **Cognitive.** Patients learn a negative view of the self. From negative past experiences, patients develop a negative view of the world and the future. This is reinforced by errors in logical thinking, such as overgeneralization of negative experiences and immunization of positive experiences.

B. **Biologic factors.**

1. **Symptoms.** Factor analysis of symptoms reveals that the presence of the following symptoms is independent of precipitating events and highly predictive of reaction to electroconvulsive therapy (ECT) or TCAs:

Early-morning awakening

Anhedonia

Decreased appetite

Increased weight

Psychomotor changes

2. **Genetics.** Monozygotic twins, reared apart, have an approximate 65% concordance for affective disorder (bipolar and unipolar tend to breed true within families). X-linkage is suggested by marker studies, but is doubtful considering the frequency of illness in father-son pairs.

3. **Neurotransmitters.**

a. **Catecholamines.** A relative decrease in brain catecholamines or activity of catecholamine systems causes or contributes to depression. This is supported by following observations:

(i) Amphetamines, TCAs, and monoamine oxidase inhibitors (MAOIs) potentiate brain catecholamines and also decrease depression.

(ii) Reserpine, methyldopa, and propranolol deplete or inactivate catecholamines and can increase or cause depression.

(iii) 3-Methoxy-4-hydroxyphenylglycol (MHPG) (a catecholamine metabolite) has been reported in some studies to be decreased in the cerebrospinal fluid (CSF) and urine of depressed patients and increased in the CSF and urine of manic patients. (This finding is still controversial.)

b. **Acetylcholine.** An increase in cholinergic activity may be a causal factor in depression. Supporting evidence includes:

(i) Cholinesterase inhibitors induce depressive symptoms (seen in insecticide poisonings).

(ii) Physostigmine (a centrally active cholinesterase inhibitor) causes a dramatic, brief decrease of manic symptoms.

(iii) Rapid eye movement (REM) latency is decreased by acetylcholine and increased by adrenergic agents. In depressed patients, REM latency is decreased.

c. **Serotonin.** A deficit in serotoninergic systems may be a causal factor in depression.

(i) Trazodone and some TCAs that decrease depression also potentiate brain serotonin activity.

(ii) Low levels of the serotonin metabolite 5-hydroxyindoleacetic acid have been found in the CSF of depressed and suicidal patients. Low levels are also seen in the brains of suicide patients at autopsy. (This decrease may relate more to aggressiveness than depression.)

(iii) Reserpine, which can cause depression, also depletes serotonin.

4. Endocrine. Mood disturbances are associated with endocrine disturbances, including Cushing disease, hypothyroidism and hyperthyroidism, exogenous estrogen therapy, and the postpartum period.

a. **Association with growth hormone (GH).**

(i) An insulin challenge induces a decreased GH response in unipolar patients and an increased response or no change in bipolar patients.

(ii) Human infants with "failure to thrive" and rat pups with maternal deprivation show a decreased secretion of GH. This is reversed in rat pups with a return to their mother.

(iii) Growth hormone secretion increases with dopaminergic stimulation.

b. **Association with cortisol.**

(i) Many depressed patients have hypersecretion of cortisol. This may be secondary to increased corticotropin releasing factor (CRF), which is caused by decreased norepinephrine (NE) activity. (NE activity inhibits CRF release.)

(ii) Fifty percent of depressed patients have a positive dexamethasone suppression test (DST). Conditions, such as anorexia, bulimia, and dementia, may increase the rate of positive DSTs.

c. **Association with thyroid hormone.**

(i) Affective symptoms are common with hypothyroidism or hyperthyroidism.

(ii) The thyroid-stimulating hormone (TSH) response to thyrotropin-releasing hormone challenge is decreased in 30% to 40% of depressed patients (and in 10% of controls). The TSH response is also increased in other conditions, such as bulimia.

5. **Chronobiology.** Disturbances of circadian rhythms are a feature of affective disorders.

a. Sleep patterns are altered, including early awakenings, decreased total sleep, decreased REM latency, and an overall shift in REM so that a larger portion occurs earlier in the night.

b. Manipulations of sleep (sleep deprivation, REM deprivation, and phase advancing) all appear to decrease depressive symptoms, at least temporarily.

c. Phase shifts have been found in the cycles of some depressed patients for temperature, cortisol secretion, and urinary MHPG excretion.

d. Some patients appear to have an annual cycle of depression (seasonal affective disorder). Such patients may respond to extension of the length of "daylight" hours by using bright, artificial lights.

6. **Summary.** Many of the studies that support an etiologic factor are not conclusive. Depression may result from a complex interaction of a number of these factors. Depression may also represent a similar clinical picture for a number of different syndromes.

VI. **Treatment of affective illness.**

A. **Manic episode (manic phase of bipolar affective illness).**

1. **Priority considerations.**

a. Danger to self/to others with purposeful or random excessive motor activity.

b. Poor judgment: Expansiveness and psychosis.

c. Rapid cyclers may quickly change to depression (observe for suicidal ideation).

d. Rule out exogenous/medical etiologies before assuming primary mania.

2. **Somatic interventions.**

a. Acute primary manic episode: Neuroleptics (rapid onset of action); lithium or novel antimanic agents (carbamazepine [Tegretol], intravenous lorazepam [Ativan], and clonazepan).

b. ECT: Controversial.

c. Prophylaxis: Lithium for maintenance; consider alternate of Tegretol for lithium intolerance.

3. **Psychosocial treatment.**

a. Acute psychotic phase: Supportive, avoid overstimulation or uncovering.

b. Postmanic phase: Patients are often demoralized and confused. Watch for depression and "relative dysphoria" compared with expansive manic state.

c. Patients, during acute phase, may need to avoid family and group treatment situations. One-to-one care important during acute phase.

4. **Miscellaneous.**

a. Patients may require seclusion and restraint, to prevent self-injury, especially during a psychotic phase.

B. **Major depressive episode: unipolar or bipolar.**

1. **Priority considerations.**

a. Rule out medical/exogenous causes.

b. Suicide precautions, especially during recovery phase.

c. Evaluate for psychotic features.

d. Past effective therapies for that patient may help determine current therapy.

2. **Somatic interventions.**

a. **Pharmacotherapy.**

(i) TCAs: This first-line therapy is for primary unipolar depression; it may require 3 to 6 weeks for resolution of neurovegetative signs. Watch for induction of increased frequency of cycling in bipolar patients.

(ii) MAOIs: These may be especially useful in patients with atypical depression. They require the avoidance of certain foods (tyramine) and drugs (sympathomimetics).

(iii) Second-generation antidepressants (e.g., amoxapine, maprotiline, trazodone): These may have fewer anticholinergic side effects.

(iv) Lithium: This prophylactic may be used against depression in bipolar illness.

(v) Neuroleptics: These may be indicated in treating patients with depression with psychotic features.

(vi) Triiodothyronine (T_3): This may be used in combination with other therapy; in treating refractory depression, this may require combinations of above therapy (e.g., use of TCA and lithium, or T_3 and TCA).

b. **ECT.** Long-standing proved efficacy. ECT remains a treatment of choice *after* pharmacotherapy.

3. **Psychosocial treatment.**

a. Psychodynamic therapy: Often long-term therapy with emphasis on intrapsychic conflict resolution and uncovering.

b. Interpersonal therapy: Relative short-term intervention that focuses on the role of grief, interpersonal disputes, deficits, and nature of role transitions.

c. Behavioral treatment: Highly structured, short-term treatment based on reinforcement of positive interactions and the subsequent change in patients' thoughts and feelings.

d. Cognitive behavioral therapy: Short-term therapy wherein patient is "educated" to identify and modify negative cognitions.

e. Family and marital therapy: Long-term treatment that focuses on clarification and changing of dysfunctional interaction patterns; it is used as an adjunct and not a primary form of treatment.

f. Supportive therapy: A good relationship with advice, counseling, and a focus on practical problem solving.

g. Miscellaneous:

(i) Combinations of pharmacotherapy and psychosocial intervention have been shown to be more effective than one type of intervention alone in many cases.

(ii) During euthymic periods, patients may require continuing psychosocial intervention, as well as possible prophylactic pharmacotherapy.

(iii) Patients with dysthymic disorder may have Axis II (characterologic) features that require more long-term psychosocial intervention.

C. **Other affect states.**

1. **"Mixed state."** Patients with bipolar illness may present with depressive and manic features. Treatment often requires somatic interventions with neuroleptics/lithium. Often, ECT is responsive; it may overlap with catatonia.

2. **Schizoaffective illness.** Psychosis with affective symptoms often requires neuroleptic therapy and antidepressant therapy. Antimanic agents (especially lithium, Tegretol) may be effective.

3. **"Atypical depression."** Intervention requires attention to affective and characterologic components, especially in chronic cases. Somatic and psychosocial therapies are described above.

D. **Cyclothymic.**

1. **Priority considerations.**

a. May be considered "characterologic" or a mild form of bipolar illness.

2. Somatic interventions.

a. Depression: Lithium may be helpful. Use antidepressants with caution (to avoid inducing rapid cycling).

b. Hypomanic episodes: These often do NOT require pharmacologic intervention. Lithium may be helpful.

3. Psychosocial interventions.

a. Supportive therapy: This can help an individual to cope with shifts in mood states.

b. Long-term insight oriented: This should be considered for characterologic features.

c. Family/marital: This may be helpful to improve coping.

d. Self-help and support groups for patients and families.

4. Miscellaneous.

a. May be chronic, with milder forms leading to maladaptive coping styles.

b. May adversely effect occupational and social aspects of individual.

E. Dysthymia.

1. Priority considerations.

a. Evaluate extent of dysphoria and disability.

b. Careful evaluation of characterologic features is essential.

2. Somatic interventions.

a. May respond to antidepressant therapy.

b. ECT not indicated.

3. Interpersonal intervention.

a. See "Major Depression" section.

b. May require long-term psychotherapy.

c. Self-help and support groups for patient and family.

F. **Family therapy.**

1. May be a useful adjunct for all affective disorders.

2. **Advantages.**

a. Educate family to early symptoms and nature of the patient's problems. The resulting alliance will improve patient compliance.

7 | Schizophrenic Disorders and Other Nonaffective Psychoses

I. **Schizophrenic disorders.**

A. **Diagnosis.**

1. Schizophrenia is not a single disease entity but rather refers to a group of disorders of differing etiologies with the following common features: the presence of certain psychotic features during the acute phase of the illness (at least one from the list below), duration of at least 6 months including prodromal symptoms, initial onset before the age of 45 years, deterioration from a previous level of functioning, a characteristic-associated psychologic disruption in the affected individual, and the absence of certain organic disorders and distinct affective mental disorders that also result in the above symptoms.

2. Psychosis is defined as a gross distortion or disorganization of a person's mental capacity, i.e., an inability to communicate or recognize reality leading to difficulty in the person's ability to perform adequately in everyday life.

3. Mental status abnormalities commonly seen in schizophrenia and other psychotic states include the following:

   a. Auditory hallucinations, i.e., clearly audible voices

that appear to arise from outside of one's head; these must consist of more than whispers, unintelligible mumbling, or single words. Often, these voices comment on or direct the patient's action.

b. Bizarre or absurd delusions without any possible basis for truth; these are often of a grandiose, somatic, or religious nature.

c. Paranoid ideas and/or persecutory delusions when accompanied by hallucinations of any type.

d. Delusions of one's thoughts, feelings, and actions as not one's own but instead under the control of an external force.

e. Thought broadcasting, i.e., the sense that one's thoughts are escaping out loud or are being transmitted from one's head.

f. Thought insertion, i.e., the sense that another's thoughts are being inserted into or transmitted to the patient.

g. Incoherence, i.e., markedly illogical thinking or loosening or associations (stream of thought that is vague, unfocused, and illogical), when associated with any of the following: flat or inappropriate affect, delusions, hallucinations, grossly disorganized behavior, or catatonia.

h. Associated features sometimes seen as follows:

(i) Gross psychomotor overactivity or underactivity.

(ii) Poverty in content of speech.

(iii) Rituals or other behavior done secondary to magical-thinking dysphoric mood.

(iv) Ideas of reference, when one falsely feels that one is being talked about by others.

(v) Eccentric or disheveled appearance.

(vi) Little to no rapport with others.

(vii) Mannerisms or grimacing.

4. It is important to note that psychosis does not equal schizophrenia. Psychotic features are not uncommon in the affective disorders (manic-depressive and depressive illness) and in drug-induced states, in addition to being reported in Axis II (personality) disorders. Usually, when psychotic symptoms appear in an affective or personality disorder, they appear afterward and/or are brief in comparison with the primary disorder. Indeed, one cannot absolutely diagnose a first-break psychotic patient as a schizophrenic, as the clinical course of the illness bears much on the definitive diagnostic label and prognosis. An equivalent schizophrenic-like presentation that does not meet the time requirement of 6 months is termed a schizophreniform disorder.

5. Regardless of the etiology, schizophrenia may be further categorized on the basis of clinical syndromes into the following types:

a. *Disorganized type (DSM III code: 295.10)*: This is marked by frequent incoherence, silly, or inappropriate affect and by the absence of systematized delusions.

b. *Catatonic type (DSM III code: 295.20)*: The primary feature is of a pronounced psychomotor disturbance that possibly involves stupor, negativism, rigidity, excitement, or posturing. There may be movement between these states. Associated symptoms include waxy flexibility and mannerisms.

c. *Paranoid type (DSM III code: 295.30)*: This schizophrenic syndrome is characterized by persecutory or grandiose delusions. Hallucinations along these lines are common, as well as a delusional jealousy. This type is not to be confused with paranoid personality disorder or trait which are nonpsychotic clinical syndromes in which the paranoid delusion is less fixed and global in nature.

d. *Undifferentiated type (DSM III code: 295.90)*: These are prominent delusions, hallucinations, incoherence, or grossly disorganized behavior.

e. **Residual type** (*DSM III* code: 295.60): This term is useful in a clinic situation in which there are no current psychotic symptoms in a patient known to have suffered from schizophrenic episodes.

B. Epidemiology. The current prevalence rate in the United States and worldwide is 1% of the population. For diagnostic purposes, one must be aware of cultural beliefs and rituals, but it has been shown that schizophrenic disorders exist worldwide and that current diagnostic criteria are reliable even across sharply different cultures. The current economic cost of schizophrenia in the United States is thought to be $10 to $20 billion annually, with two thirds of this being lost wages (and placing an economic value on the pain and suffering borne by the patients and their families).

C. Postulated etiologies of schizophrenia. As stated above, schizophrenia is not thought of as a single disease but rather as a group of illnesses with common clinical features. A number of important theories have been proposed about the etiology and expression of these disorders.

1. **Biologic and genetic theory.** Family studies (including twin and adoption studies) strongly support the theory that genetic factors play a major role in the transmission of schizophrenia, or at least impart a psychobiologic vulnerability and may also account for the increased incidence of schizophrenic-like syndromes (schizoaffective, schizotypal personality disorder, and others) that occur in families.

2. **Neurotransmitter hypothesis.** Current research centers around various neurotransmitter abnormalities found in schizophrenics and has focused on the dopaminergic system as the responsible "chemical imbalance" or lesion, and recent studies have shown an excess of dopaminergic receptors in the central nervous system (CNS) of schizophrenic patients. Indeed, neuroleptics are thought to be effective because of their ability to block dopaminergic receptors. Studies of un-

treated schizophrenics also reveal an excess of dopaminergic receptors that directly contradict the theory that these findings were instead related to the neuroleptic administration.

3. **Psychosocial precipitants.** Socioenvironmental stressors are often correlated temporally to the initial break and to relapses and can be thought of as breaking through protective forces, keeping the psychobiologic vulnerability in check. Increased relapse rates are significantly related to three measures of expressed emotion (EE) in the home environment: critical comments, hostility, and emotional over involvement. Studies have shown that separation of the patients from their high EE families (or even a decrease in the amount of contact) improved the relapse rate.

D. **Treatment of schizophrenia.**

1. **First break.**

a. Workup and differential diagnosis.

b. History and physical examination.

c. Routine chemistry studies, toxicology screening, VDRL, and thyroid function tests.

d. Special studies as indicated by findings from history and physical examination.

e. Electroencephalogram (to rule out temporal lobe epilepsy, neoplasms) and psychologic testing.

2. For all acute occurrences, outpatient care vs. a need for hospitalization is dependent on:

a. Presence of a danger to self or others and/or inability to care for one's basic needs. (See forensic section, Chapter 40, for details on involuntary hospitalization and treatment.)

b. Severity of symptoms (agitation, psychologic distress, disorientation, etc.).

c. Presence or absence of social supports.

d. Ability to understand and comply with medications.

e. Education of the patient and of significant others: investigate patient's support system and environment; determine if socioenvironmental stressors may have contributed and, if so, how these may be minimized or abolished.

f. Emphasize need for long-term follow-up, preferably with a single physician or clinic.

g. Evaluate need for social skills training.

h. Address all current medical problems.

i. Medication: Primarily, neuroleptics are used. One cannot overemphasize the need for a simple outpatient regimen (every day or every evening at bedtime). Amantadine (Symmetrel) or anticholinergics, such as benztropine (Artane) or trihexyphenidyl (Cogentin), are used to prevent and treat extrapyramidal symptoms (EPS). One should refer to separate sections on neuroleptics and medications used to treat EPS for further details, and bear in mind that neuroleptics do not have immediate effects and may require readjustment periodically. If the patient is violent or in distress, some practitioners use rapid-acting intramuscular neuroleptics given relatively frequently and titrated to the current symptoms and behavior.

j. Explanation of the need for medication(s), their benefits and side effects including the possibility of EPS and/or tardive dyskinesia (TD), and what the treatment options would be in the event that these occurred is very important. Note: Some states require that before initiating neuroleptics in the inpatient psychiatric setting, written informed consent be obtained from the patient (or conservator if one exists) or parent if the patient is a minor.

3. Nonacute management consists primarily of medication at the lowest possible doses, supportive encouragement, and ensuring social supports and reha-

bilitative opportunities. Long-acting intramuscular depot neuroleptics (with a schedule as infrequent as every 4 weeks) are particularly useful in patients who have difficulties with daily medications. Specialized types of psychotherapy for schizophrenics are used by some practitioners.

4. Refractory psychosis may be a signal that there is an untreated affective component to the illness or that this is a nonschizophrenic organic condition (e.g., alcoholic hallucinosis, encephalopathy, Korsakoff psychosis, heavy metal intoxication, uremia, porphyria, CNS infections, seizure disorders, lupus cerebritis, cranial neoplasms, dementia, and thyroid or adrenal gland dysfunction). Often, antidepressants, antimanic agents, or electroconvulsive therapy (ECT) is quite useful in treating schizophrenics with an affective component to their episode.

5. Statistical outcomes, as with all chronic illnesses, vary across individuals and over time. One may see a steady baseline of functioning with falls into dysfunction with each recurrence or a progressively deteriorating course with exacerbations during acute recurrences. The majority of schizophrenics "do well" in the sense of few to no acute recurrences with a fair to good socioeconomic status. Ten percent to 30% do not do as well suffering a chronic impairment (thought disorder, delusions, hallucinations, and social withdrawal distractibility) and disability (poor self-care, work incapacity and unemployment, and homelessness).

6. The EPS are a variety of involuntary bizarre movements induced by the use of neuroleptics. They are thought to be secondary to the blockade of dopaminergic receptors in the basal ganglia. These movements include acute dystonia, akasthisia (inability to sit still), and a triad of resting tremor, akinesia, and rigidity resembling parkinsonism. Symptoms may be reduced, abolished, or guarded against with anticholinergic medication, by reducing the dosage of the neuroleptic or by switching to a different class of neuroleptic whenever clinically possible.

7. TD appears in a minority of patients who have received long-term neuroleptic treatment, and TD consists of:

a. Facial-lingual hyperkinesias.

b. Lip smacking, licking of the lips, tongue movements, and protrusion sucking movements.

c. Bizarre expressions and spastic facial movements.

d. Blinking.

e. Neck and trunk movements.

f. Spastic torticollis.

g. Hip rocking.

h. Choreoathetoid movements of the extremities. The symptoms of TD may be reduced or abolished, in some cases, by reducing or discontinuing the neuroleptic whenever clinically feasible.

8. Neuroleptic malignant syndrome is a rare but serious potentially life-threatening illness that consists of generalized muscular hypertonicity with moderate to severe fever, along with altered mental status and autonomic instability. Neuroleptics must be discontinued immediately. Hospitalization and supportive care are usually indicated. (See neuroleptics section in Chapter 18 for further details.)

II. Atypical psychotic disorders.

A. **Brief reactive psychosis.** This is seen immediately following a profoundly upsetting environmental event. It may require hospitalization and/or medication. Duration is more than a few hours but less than a week. Follow-up evaluation and psychotherapy may be indicated to sort out any underlying conditions and to deal with the consequences of the stressful event.

B. **Drug-induced psychosis.** This is seen frequently with many classes of both legitimate and illicit drugs, particularly with the stimulants phencyclidine and cocaine. Toxicology screening and specific drug levels should be obtained for diagnostic purposes. Caution must be exercised, as occasionally patients do harm themselves or others during a drug-induced psychosis. It is not uncommon for schizophrenic and other psychiatric patients to abuse these drugs and to have an acute psychosis superimposed over a baseline condition. Many substance abusers have a treatable psychiatric disorder apart from the abuse, but they must abstain from the substance if they are to participate in an effective treatment program for that particular disorder.

C. **Postpartum psychosis.** This is a rare phenomenon that usually manifests itself soon after parturition, but it may occur up to 1 year after childbearing and may be a component of the more common syndrome, postpartum depression. Indeed, there is a professional debate over whether postpartum psychosis is a distinct entity. Current postulated etiologies center around either the hormonal changes of the peripartum period or intrapsychic conflicts involved in assuming motherhood. Besides the usual psychotic symptoms, the following may be present in postpartum psychosis:

1. Inability to sleep for days at a time even when the infant is quiet.

2. Crying spells for more than 3 consecutive days.

3. Unusual fear of household utensils, food, medicine, and water. Continued feeling of not wanting the baby.

4. Fearing the baby as an evil object, threat, or danger (generalized fear or anxiety).

The most commonly used treatment modalities include antidepressant medications and ECT. Lithium has been effective when there appears to be a manic component to the illness. Hospitalization and brief use of neuroleptics may be indicated. While this syndrome is rare, recurrence rates following further childbearing are significant and signal the need for psychiatric involvement and possibly even prophylactic treatment.

D. **Nonpsychotic disorders.** These occur in the differential diagnosis of psychotic symptoms.

1. Factitious disorder and malingering must be considered appropriate. They differ in that the goal is usually recognizable in malingering.

2. Post-traumatic stress disorder is a nonpsychotic disorder that often contains auditory and visual hallucinations clearly related to the stressor. Special attention should be paid to patients in selected groups, such as victims of catastrophe, rape, or assault, combat veterans, and witnesses to violent acts.

8
Psychiatric Aspects of Alcohol Abuse

I. **Introduction.**

A. **General facts.**

1. Alcohol is the major substance of abuse.

2. Sixty-eight percent of Americans drink.

3. Twelve percent of Americans are heavy drinkers (male-female ratio, 2:1).

4. Approximately 10 million Americans have alcohol abuse problems.

5. Fifty percent of homicides and automobile deaths are alcohol related.

6. Twenty-five percent of suicide deaths are alcohol related.

7. All social statuses are affected; less than 5% are "skid row" types.

B. **Definitions.**

1. **Alcohol abuse.**

a. Pattern of pathologic alcohol use, i.e., binges, blackouts.

b. Inability to abstain from drinking or to stop drinking once started.

c. Impairment of social or occupational functioning for at least 1 month.

2. **Alcohol dependence.**

a. Two of the above two criteria.

b. Evidence of tolerance or history of abstinence symptoms during alcohol withdrawal.

3. **Tolerance.**

a. Definition: Demonstrated by higher blood levels required to produce same level of intoxication.

b. Two types of tolerance.

II. **Recognition of alcoholism.**

A. **Principle.** A majority of alcoholics go undiagnosed until they present with physical complications or marked impairment in occupational or social functioning. It is important to keep a high index of suspicion while taking a history.

1. **Presenting psychiatric symptoms may include:**

a. Insomnia.

b. Chronic anxiety.

c. Depressed mood.

d. Mood swings.

e. Personality change.

f. Hallucinations, usually visual.

g. Blackouts, anterograde amnesia for events that occurred during acute intoxication.

h. Suicidal ideation, attempts.

i. Poor memory.

j. Decreased libido.

k. Aggressive behavior.

2. **Medical history may include:**

a. Tremors ("jitters").

b. Seizures ("rum fits").

c. Delirium tremors (DTs).

d. Hypertension.

e. Cardiac arrhythmia, tachycardia.

f. Congestive heart failure.

g. Hypoglycemia.

h. Pneumonia.

i. Frequent falls, trauma.

j. Multiple fractures, especially ribs.

k. Peptic ulcer disease.

l. Hepatitis.

m. Pancreatitis.

n. Impotence.

o. Hemorrhoids.

3. **Investigate social and occupational impairment.**

a. Occupational.

(i) Absenteeism.

(ii) Job loss.

(iii) Frequent job changes.

(iv) Personality problems on the job.

b. Social.

(i) Marital conflicts.

(ii) Divorce.

(iii) Deteriorating relationship with children.

c. Legal.

(i) Citation for driving while intoxicated ("DWI," "502").

(ii) Arrests for:

(a) Disorderly conduct.

(b) Reckless driving.

(iii) Disturbing the peace.

(iv) Assault.

4. Define specific drinking pattern.

a. Binge vs. continuous.

b. Amount (check size of glass or container).

c. Duration.

d. Time of last drink.

e. Drink alone vs. with "buddies" from bar.

5. Interview relatives and friends.

a. Denial is a prominent defense mechanism in alcoholism.

6. Michigan Alcoholism Screening Test: a brief screening questionnaire (Table 8–1).

a. Score of 6 or more may indicate alcoholism.

7. Physical signs.

a. Tremulousness.

b. Mild hypertension.

c. Tachycardia.

d. Multiple bruises, different colors.

e. Cigarette burns on body and clothing.

f. Poor hygiene.

g. Dull eyes.

h. Erythematous face.

i. Cushingoid facies.

j. Palmar erythema.

l. Caput medusae.

m. Ascites.

n. Pedal and ankle edema.

TABLE 8–1.
Brief MAST for Screening Alcoholism*

Questions	Circle Correct Answers	
1. Do you feel you are a normal drinker?	Yes (0)	No (2)
2. Do friends or relatives think you are a normal drinker?	Yes (0)	No (2)
3. Have you ever attended a meeting of Alcoholics Anonymous?	Yes (0)	No (2)
4. Have you ever lost friends or girlfriends/boyfriends because of drinking?	Yes (0)	No (2)
5. Have you ever gotten in trouble at work because of drinking?	Yes (0)	No (2)
6. Have you ever neglected your obligations, your family, or your work for 2 or more days in a row because you were drinking?	Yes (0)	No (2)
7. Have you ever had DTs, severe shaking, heard voices, or seen things that were not there after heavy drinking?	Yes (0)	No (2)
8. Have you ever gone to anyone for help about your drinking?	Yes (0)	No (2)
9. Have you ever been in a hospital because of drinking?	Yes (0)	No (2)
10. Have you ever been arrested for drunk driving or driving after drinking?	Yes (0)	No (2)

*From Pokorny AD, Miller BA, Kaplan HB: The brief MAST: A shortened version of the Michigan Alcoholism Screening Test. Am J Psychiatry 1972; 129:342–345.

o. Diminished sensation in distant extremities (vibration sense is first to deteriorate).

8. **Laboratory abnormalities.**

a. Anemia.

(i) Normocytic, normochromic, e.g., blood loss.

(ii) Microcytic, hypochromic, e.g., iron deficiency.

(iii) Megaloblastic, e.g., folate or vitamin B_{12} deficiency.

b. Thrombocytopenia.

c. Blood urea nitrogen/creatinine ratio greater than 3, e.g., dehydration.

d. Elevated serum glutamic oxaloacetic transaminase, serum glutamic pyruvic transaminase, alkaline phosphatase, and total bilirubin levels.

e. Elevated amylase level.

f. Hyperuricemia.

g. Elevated triglyceride levels.

h. Elevated creatine phosphokinase level, e.g., skeletal myopathy, trauma.

i. Low magnesium level.

j. Folate deficiency.

B. **Neurologic syndromes associated with chronic alcohol use.**

1. **Wernicke encephalopathy.**

a. Alcohol-induced thiamine B deficiency.

b. Clinical manifestations:

(i) Nystagmus.

(ii) Bilateral sixth cranial nerve palsies leading to paralysis of conjugate gaze.

(iii) Ataxia.

(iv) Mental status changes.

(a) Apathy.

(b) Lassitude.

(c) Disorientation.

(d) Drowsiness.

c. Treatment.

(i) Thiamine, 50 mg intravenously (IV) and 50 mg intramuscularly (IM), now.

(ii) Then, thiamine, 100 mg orally every day.

(iii) Note: Always give thiamine before IV glucose or oral food intake. Thiamine is a cofactor in the metabolism of glucose. Metabolism of IV glucose may precipitate Wernicke disease by depleting already preexisting low thiamine stores.

2. **Korsakoff psychosis (alcohol amnestic disorder).**

a. Confabulation.

b. Severe anterograde and retrograde amnesia.

c. Severe learning impairment.

d. Found often in conjunction with Wernicke encephalopathy.

e. Lesion in mammillary bodies in postmortem brain examination.

3. **Polyneuropathy.**

a. Secondary to alcohol-induced vitamin deficiency and/or direct toxic effect of alcohol.

b. Clinical manifestations.

(i) Symmetric loss of sensation in distal extremities (vibratory sensation is first to deteriorate).

(ii) Reduced or absent ankle tendon reflex.

4. **Alcohol amblyopia (rare).**

a. Associated with nutritional deficiency.

b. Clinical manifestations:

(i) Blurred vision.

(ii) Inflammation or pallor of optic discs.

5. Cerebellar degeneration.

6. Marchiafava-Bignami disease (degeneration of the corpus callosum).

7. Pontomyelinolysis.

8. Cerebral atrophy.

9. Laminar corticosclerosis (Morell disease).

C. **Medical complications of chronic alcohol use.**

1. **Cardiovascular.**

a. Hypertension.

b. Cardiomyopathy.

2. **Gastrointestinal.**

a. Mallory-Weiss tears.

b. Gastritis.

c. Peptic ulcer disease.

d. Hepatitis.

e. Pancreatitis.

f. Upper or lower gastrointestinal (GI) tract bleeding.

g. Diarrhea.

h. Constipation.

i. Hemorrhoids.

3. **Hematologic.**

a. Megaloblastic anemia, e.g., folate or vitamin B_{12} deficiency.

b. Iron deficiency anemia, e.g., blood loss, diet.

c. Hemolytic anemia.

d. Thrombocytopenia.

4. **Plasma lipids.**

a. Increased triglyceride levels.

b. Increased very-low-density lipoprotein levels.

c. Increased high-density lipoprotein levels.

d. Increased lipoprotein and chylomicron levels.

5. **Carcinoma.**

a. Mouth.

b. Oropharynx.

c. Esophagus.

d. Lung.

e. Breast.

f. Pancreas.

g. Liver.

6. **Skeletal muscle.**

a. Skeletal myopathy.

III. Fetal alcohol syndrome.

A. Ethanol is one of the most frequent causes of teratogenically induced mental deficiency in the Western World. Amount of alcohol exposure required to produce the syndrome is unknown.

B. Congenital abnormalities may include:

1. Facial abnormalities.

a. Short palpebral fissures.

b. Epicanthic folds.

c. Small chin.

d. Maxillary hypoplasia (narrow upper lip).

e. Strabismus.

f. Short nose.

2. Mental retardation.

3. Low birth weight.

4. Microcephaly.

5. Abnormal palmar creases.

6. Joint abnormalities.

7. Cardiac anomalies.

a. Septal defects.

8. Genital abnormalities.

9. Capillary hemangiomas.

10. Abnormal electroencephalogram (EEG).

11. Delayed postnatal growth.

C. Newborn behavior may include:

1. Irritability.

2. Weak sucking ability.

3. Tremulousness.

4. Hypotonicity.

D. These features may be due to a direct action of ethanol to inhibit cellular proliferation early in gestation.

IV. **Acute alcohol intoxication.**

A. Clinical manifestations (see Table 8–2).

B. Odor of breath is an unreliable indicator of level of intoxication.

C. Alcohol level, therefore, must be determined for medicolegal purposes via:

1. Breathalyzer test.

2. Blood level determination.

3. Urine screening.

D. Legal intoxication in most states is 100 mg/dL.

TABLE 8–2.

Relationship of Blood Ethanol Level in Clinical Manifestations*

Blood Ethanol Level (mg/dL)	Effect
100	Mild intoxication, judgment often impaired, reaction time diminished, relaxation, disinhibition; baseline for legal intoxication in most states
200	Mild to moderate intoxication, slurred speech, unsteady gait, may have flushed face or nystagmus, nausea, mood changes of loquacity and euphoria or irritability, may have hostility, and may have desire to fight
300	Marked intoxication, incoherent speech, stupor, markedly impaired judgment and motor skills, and vomiting may occur (all patients with a blood alcohol level of 300 mg/dL are alcoholic)
400	Stupor, deep sleep or coma, difficult or impossible to arouse with vigorous stimulation (some tolerant alcoholics are not so severely affected)
500	Death can occur at these and higher blood alcohol levels

*From Rund DA: Emergency Psychiatry. St Louis, CV Mosby Co, 1983.

E. Central nervous system (CNS) effects are more pronounced when blood alcohol level is rising than when it is falling.

V. **Idiosyncratic ("pathologic") intoxication.**

A. Small dose of alcohol may induce profound state of intoxication in few individuals.

B. Clinical manifestations include:

1. Confusion.

2. Disorientation.

3. Delusions.

4. Hallucinations, auditory or visual.

5. Aggressiveness.

6. Rage.

7. Violence.

8. Suicide attempts in patients with pre-existing depression.

C. Usually episode lasts 2 to 3 hours, but may persist for up to 24 to 48 hours.

D. Amnesia typically occurs for the event.

E. May be associated with EEG abnormalities.

1. Temporal lobe spikes after ingestion of small amounts of ethanol.

F. Coexisting history of brain trauma or encephalitis may be present.

VI. **Alcohol withdrawal syndromes.**

A. **Tremulousness due to withdrawal.**

1. Occurs 6 to 8 hours after cessation of drinking or diminished intake.

2. Clinical manifestations.

a. Tremulousness.

b. Muscle tension.

c. Blushing.

d. Sweating.

f. Vague sense of anxiety.

g. GI complaints.

(i) Nausea.

(ii) Vomiting.

(iii) Anorexia.

(iv) Abdominal cramps.

h. Hyperreflexia.

i. Easily startled.

3. Treatment.

a. Substitute with longer-acting cross-tolerant sedative.

B. **Alcoholic hallucinosis.**

1. Begins 24 to 48 hours after cessation of drinking or reduced intake.

2. Clinical manifestations.

a. Visual hallucinations.

b. Auditory hallucinations (less common).

c. Orientation to time, place, and person.

(i) There is no clouding of consciousness, unlike DTs.

d. Resting tremor.

3. Duration is a few hours to 1 week.

4. Ten percent of patients may continue to hallucinate for weeks or months.

5. A few patients develop a chronic form that may mimic schizophrenia.

6. Treatment.

a. Suggested regimen:

(i) Haloperidol (Haldol), 5 mg by mouth/IM every 2 hours, until a reduction in hallucinations occurs.

(ii) Benztropine (Cogentin), 2 mg by mouth/IM every 2 hours, as needed for extrapyramidal symptoms, not to exceed 8 to 10 mg/24 hr.

C. **Alcohol withdrawal seizures.**

1. Begin 8 to 48 hours after cessation of drinking or reduced intake.

2. Occur in up to 10% of withdrawing alcohols.

3. Clinical manifestations.

a. Generalized type (grand mal).

(i) If focal, suspect underlying CNS lesion.

(ii) Typically occur in rapid succession over several hours and are self limited.

4. Progression to status epilepticus rarely occurs.

a. Patients with pre-existing seizure disorders are at a greater risk of developing status epilepticus.

5. One third of patients with alcohol withdrawal seizures progress to DTs.

6. Treatment.

a. Diazepam (Valium), 2- to 10-mg slow (5-mg/min) IV push every 5 to 15 minutes for immediate control. Do not exceed 20 mg.

b. Prophylactic use of antiseizure medication is controversial.

(i) Indicated only in patients with concomitant seizure disorder.

(ii) Suggested phenytoin (Dilantin) regimen.

(a) Loading dose of 400, 300, and 300 mg at 2-hour intervals.

(b) Maintenance dose of 100 mg by mouth three times daily.

(iii) Follow blood level closely.

D. **Alcohol withdrawal delirium (DTs).**

1. Seventy-two to 96 hours after cessation of drinking or diminished intake.

2. Clinical manifestations.

a. Clouding of consciousness (disorientation).

b. Autonomic hyperactivity.

(i) Tachycardia.

(ii) Hypertension.

(iii) Diaphoresis.

(iv) Vomiting.

c. Tremulousness.

d. Hallucinations.

(i) Visual, at times frightening.

(ii) Tactile, e.g., insects crawling on skin.

(iii) Auditory.

(iv) Olfactory.

3. Medical Complications.

(i) Hypoglycemia.

(ii) Dehydration.

(iii) Electrolyte imbalance.

(iv) Seizures.

(v) Aspiration pneumonia.

4. Ten percent mortality if untreated (Table 8–3).

5. Management of alcohol withdrawal syndromes.

a. Principles.

(i) Suppress withdrawal with a longer-acting cross-tolerant drug.

(ii) Alcohol withdrawal can be fatal.

(iii) If patient is also addicted to drugs associated with less medically serious withdrawal syndrome, always treat the alcohol withdrawal first.

TABLE 8-3.

Alcohol Withdrawal Syndromes in Relationship With Time After Cessation of Drinking or Reduced Intake*

Time of Last Drink, hr	Symptom
0	Tremulousness
24	Hallucinations
48	Seizures ("rum fits")
72-96	Delirium tremens

*This is a general pattern of alcohol withdrawal. Clinically, the patient may present with one or more symptoms during an earlier or later time period.

b. Monitor vital signs every 4 hours for at least 72 hours.

c. Most commonly used sedative regimens.

(i) Chlordiazepoxide (Librium).

(a) Begin with 50 to 200 mg and half the dose every day, if tolerated.

(b) Example: 50 mg by mouth every 6 hours for 24 hours, then 50 mg by mouth every 8 hours, then 25 mg by mouth every 6 hours, then 25 mg by mouth twice daily, and then 25 mg by mouth every day, then discontinue.

(ii) Phenobarbital.

(a) Average initial dose is 100 mg.

(b) Example: 50 mg by mouth every 6 hours for 24 hours, then taper by half the dose every day.

(iii) Short-acting benzodiazepines.

(a) Consider as the first choice if patient has history of liver disease.

(b) Examples:

(1) Lorazepam (Ativan), 2 mg by mouth every 6 hours for 24 hours, then taper.

(2) Oxazepam (Serax), 30 to 60 mg by mouth every 6 hours; then 15 to 30 mg by mouth every 6 hours, then discontinue.

(c) Note: Many other sedatives, including alcohol, may be used.

(1) Examples: chloral hydrate, diazepam, and paraldehyde.

d. Avoid drugs that are not true sedatives.

(i) Hydroxyzine (Atarax, Vistaril).

(ii) Diphenhydramine (Bendadryl).

(iii) Neuroleptics, i.e., chlorpromazine (Thorazine), haloperidol (Haldol).

(a) Neuroleptics lower seizure threshold.

(b) Patients in alcohol withdrawal are at risk for seizures.

(c) Low-potency neuroleptics (e.g., chlorpromazine) have greater tendency to lower seizure threshold and induce hypotension than high-potency neuroleptic agents (e.g., haloperidol).

e. Treat nutritional deficiencies.

(i) "Alcoholic cocktail."

(a) Thiamine, 100 mg IM, then 100 mg by mouth every day.

(b) Folate, 1 mg by mouth every day.

(c) Magnesium sulfate, 1 cc IM, each buttock one time.

f. Hallucinosis may be treated with a high-potency neuroleptic.

(i) Suggested regimen.

(a) Haloperidol (Haldol), 5 to 10 mg by mouth/IM every 2 hours until a reduction in hallucinations occurs.

(b) Benztropine (Cogentin), 2 mg by mouth/IM every 2 hours, as needed for extrapyramidal symptoms, not to exceed 8 to 10 mg in 24 hours.

g. Prophylactic use of antiseizure medication is controversial.

(i) Indicated only in patients with concomitant seizure disorder.

(ii) Suggested phenytoin (Dilantin) regimen.

(a) Loading dose, 400 and 300 mg, by mouth every 2 hours.

(b) Maintenance dose of 100 mg by mouth t.i.e.

6. Treatment of DTs.

a. Ten percent mortality in untreated cases.

b. Monitor vital signs closely.

c. In case of active delirium.

(i) Diazepam (Valium), 5-mg slow (5-mg/min) IV push every 5 to 15 minutes until patient is calm.

(a) Do not exceed 20-mg diazepam.

(b) Avoid small veins, intra-arterial injection, and extravasation because diluent is a local irritant.

(c) Diazepam is long-acting benzodiazepine with half-life of 20 to 100 hours.

(d) Do not mix or dilute diazepam with other solutions.

(e) Avoid IM form because of erratic absorption.

d. Chlordiazepoxide (Librium), 50 to 100 mg by mouth every 1 hour, until patient is calm.

(i) Do not exceed 400 to 600 mg in 24 hours.

(ii) Titrate to clinical symptoms.

(iii) Avoid IM form because erratically absorbed.

e. If the patient does not respond to the above regimen and/or has underlying psychosis.

(i) Haloperidol (Haldol), 5 to 10 mg by mouth /IM, until there is a decrease in the thought disorder.

f. Thiamine, 100 mg IV, before IV glucose, then every day.

g. Magnesium sulfate, 1 gm in 5% sterile solution IV every day.

h. Supportive measures.

(i) Intravenous fluids.

(ii) Seizure precautions.

(iii) Monitor electrolytes, renal function, glucose, and liver function.

VII. Treatment of alcoholism: A multidisciplinary approach.

A. Alcoholics Anonymous.

1. Defines alcoholism as a disease.

2. Abstinence is a goal of treatment.

3. Provides strong support system, including individual sponsors within the group.

4. Local chapters are numerous and accessible.

5. Twelve steps to promote sobriety (Table 8–4).

B. Al-Anon.

1. Support group for family members of alcoholics.

C. Alcoholism treatment programs may include:

1. Detoxification (if indicated).

2. Individual and group therapy.

3. Education.

4. Family therapy.

5. Participation in Alcoholics Anonymous.

D. **Disulfiram (Antabuse).**

1. Adjunctive treatment of chronic alcoholism.

2. Disulfiram is not a cure for alcoholism.

3. Irreversibly inhibits acetaldehyde dehydrogenase.

a. Raises blood acetaldehyde level 5 to 10 times the amount found in untreated individuals.

4. "Antabuse reaction" (acetaldehyde syndrome).

a. Symptoms.

(i) Flushing.

(ii) Headache (may be pulsating).

(iii) Nausea.

(iv) Vomiting.

(v) Diaphoresis.

(vi) Thirst.

(vii) Chest pain.

(viii) Shortness of breath.

(ix) Hypotension.

(x) Syncope.

(xi) Weakness.

(xii) Blurred vision.

(xiii) Vertigo.

b. Lasts 30 minutes to several hours.

c. Sensitization to alcohol may last for up to 6 to 12 hours.

d. Few patients may not experience a reaction when they drink while they are being treated with Antabuse.

5. Relative contraindications.

a. Psychiatric.

TABLE 8–4.

Twelve-Step Program of Recovery in Alcoholics Anonymous

1. We admitted we were powerless over alcohol—that our lives had become unmanageable.
2. Came to believe that a Power greater than ourselves could restore us to sanity.
3. Made a decision to turn our will and our lives over to the care of God as we understood Him.
4. Made a searching and fearless moral inventory of ourselves.
5. Admitted to God, to ourselves, and to another human being the exact nature of our wrongs.
6. Were entirely ready to have God remove all these defects of character.
7. Humbly asked Him to remove our shortcomings.
8. Made a list of all persons we had harmed, and became willing to make amends to them all.
9. Made direct amends to such people wherever possible, except when to do so would injure them or others.
10. Continued to take personal inventory, and when we were wrong, promptly admitted it.
11. Sought through prayer and meditation to improve our conscious contact with God as we understood Him, praying only for knowledge of His will for us and the power to carry that out.
12. Having had a spiritual awakening from the rest of these steps, we tried to carry this message to alcoholics, and to practice these principles in our affairs.

(i) Active psychosis.

(ii) Delirium.

(iii) Depression with suicidal ideation.

(iv) Poor impulse control.

(v) History of noncompliance with medication and/or periodic monitoring.

b. Medical.

(i) Myocardial disease.

(ii) Hypertension.

(iii) Severe pulmonary insufficiency.

(iv) Advanced liver disease.

(v) Diabetes mellitus.

(vi) Thyroid disease.

(vii) Neuropathy.

c. In combination with drugs that:

(i) Impair blood pressure regulation.

(a) Adrenergic antagonists.

(b) Vasodilators.

(ii) Inhibit same enzymes as disulfiram.

(a) Monoamine oxidase inhibitors.

(iii) Affect CNS catecholamines.

(a) Sympathomimetic amines.

(b) Tricyclic antidepressants.

(c) Neuroleptics.

(iv) Have metabolism inhibited by disulfiram.

(a) Phenytoin (Dilantin).

(b) Warfarin (Coumadin).

(c) Benzodiazepine.

TABLE 8–5.

Schedule of Monitoring During Disulfiram Treatment*

Procedure†	Monthly	Every 3 mo	Every 6 mo
Drug, alcohol abuse	X		
Mental status	X		
Psychosocial assessment	X		
Review of systems	X		
CBC count		X	
Alkaline phosphatase		X	
Glutamyl transpeptidase or aspartate aminotransferase		X	
Urinalysis			X
Cholesterol			X
Triglycerides			X
Electrolytes			X
BUN/creatinine			X
Total protein, albumin			X
T_3, T_4			X
ECG			X

*From Gorelick DA: Unpublished data. UCLA School of Medicine, Los Angeles, and West Los Angeles Veterans Administration Medical Center.
†CBC = complete blood cell; BUN = blood urea nitrogen; T_3 = triiodothyronine; and T_4 thyroxine.

(d) Isoniazid.

6. Absolute contraindication.

a. First-trimester pregnancy.

7. Monitoring is essential during disulfiram treatment (see Table 8-5).

REFERENCE

1. *Alcoholics Anonymous*, ed 3. New York, Alcoholics Anonymous World Services, Inc, 1976, pp 59–60.

9 Organic Brain Syndromes

I. **Introduction.** *DSM III-R* has established two subclassifications to describe the psychologic and behavioral abnormalities that may be associated with brain dysfunction: (1) organic brain syndromes (noted above) and (2) organic mental disorders (such as primary degenerative dementia of the Alzheimer type, multi-infarct dementia, and psychoactive substance-induced organic mental disorders). This chapter will address the syndromes of dementia and delirium, organic mood, organic personality seizure disorders, and amnestic disorders.

II. **Dementia.**

A. **Definition.** Dementia is an acquired deficit in intellectual functioning, including disturbances of language, cognition (calculation, judgment, and abstraction), personality (including mood and behavior), visuospatial skills, and memory. Its onset may be abrupt but is more often gradual, its time course is protracted (characteristically measured in months to years), and its outcome is temporary or permanent.

B. **Major clinical features.** Dementia differs from aphasic or other isolated cognitive disorders, such as amnesia, and by its involvement of several areas of mental functioning. Furthermore, dementia typically progresses through clinical stages of increasing severity.

1. **Early stage.** The presentation may be very vague. Patients may demonstrate somewhat less concern with their physical appearance or social manners. They may demonstrate very subtle forgetfulness or preoccupations with seemingly uncharacteristic reactions to routine stresses. In addition, routine tasks become more difficult, and patients rely more on schedules and lists to stay abreast of their life activities. Some patients may show vaguely described personality alterations, such as an uncharacteristic decrease in concern for others, or suspiciousness.

2. **Middle stage.** It is generally in this stage that the patient, his/her family, and the physician are aware of obvious cognitive dilapidation that involves several spheres. Memory impairment is especially striking. Recent or short-term recall is most clearly compromised, with such deficits giving rise to orientation difficulties. Deficits in long-term memory may also be apparent, usually evident as lost detail when recalling past events. The second- or middle-stage victim of dementia demonstrates impaired calculation, abstracting ability, and judgment. Furthermore, the patient's fund of information becomes exceedingly impoverished. Aphasic difficulties and disorders of thought process, including tangentiality, circumstantiality, and perserveration, are manifest.

3. **Final stage.** There is a profound impairment of memory, often resulting in disorientation and misidentification of relatives or caretakers. Immediate recall, previously preserved, may now be compromised. The patient's personality has been lost with suspiciousness typically replaced by unsystematized paranoid delusions. Such patients also demonstrate bradykinesia, stereotyped behaviors, and fecal and urinary incontinence. Fixed postures with rigidity may eventually result. Spontaneous speech is impoverished with verbal output often limited to echolalia, palilalia, and occa-

sionaly, mutism. Apraxias (inability to perform, on command, activities that can be done spontaneously), agnosias (inability to identify familiar objects or persons), and aphasias render the late-stage demented patient unable to attend to even the most basic activities of daily living. Death of the end-stage demented patient is often the result of aspiration pneumonia or urinary tract infection that results in sepsis. Such patients also typically die of pre-existing cardiac disease.

C. **Cortical vs. subcortical dementias.** On the basis of neuroanatomic involvement and clinical features, dementia has been subdivided into two essential types: (1) cortical and (2) subcortical. Those functions especially mediated by the cerebral cortex include language, praxis, visuospatial perception, and learning. Consequently, disease processes that involve the cerebral cortex will manifest as deficits in these areas. Alternatively, involvement of the subcortical structures (thalamus, basal ganglia, and rostral brain stem) clinically gives rise to deficits in alertness, attention, motivation, and speed of performance. As a result of the above, the following generalizations can be made:

1. **Cortical dementias.**

   a. Alzheimer disease (AD), Pick disease.

   b. Anatomic involvement of neocortical association areas and hippocampus.

   c. Intellectual impairment characterized by aphasia, apraxia, agnosia, acalculia, diminished abstraction ability, amnesia, and visual perception deficits.

   d. Personality characterized by indifference.

   e. Motor system intact until late stages of illness.

   f. Speech is unaffected until late stages of illness.

2. **Subcortical dementias.**

   a. Extrapyramidal diseases, such as Parkinson disease, Huntington disease, Wilson disease, progressive supranuclear palsy, and Fahr disease (idiopathic basal ganglia calcification).

b. Anatomic involvement of basal ganglia, thalamus, and rostral brain stem.

c. Impairment characterized by psychomotor retardation, poor insight, forgetfulness, and general cognitive decline with poor strategy formulation.

d. Personality characterized by depressed mood with saddened or blunted affect.

e. Motor systems clearly abnormal (chorea, tremor, rigidity, dystonia, etc.).

f. Speech is dysarthric.

3. **Mixed features (cortical and subcortical).**

a. Multi-infarct dementias.

b. Infectious dementias.

c. Traumatic dementias.

d. Toxic and metabolic dementias.

e. Neoplastic dementias.

f. Hydrocephalic dementias.

g. Pseudodementia (dementia syndrome of depression).

D. **Etiologies.**

1. **AD.** This is single most common cause for dementia, accounting for nearly 55% of all cases.

a. **Common histopathologic findings.**

(i) Grossly, the brain is atrophic with widened sulci, shrunken cortical convolutions, and enlarged ventricles.

(ii) Histologic findings include neurofibrillary tangles, senile plaques, granulovacuolar degeneration, and neuronal loss. While these findings are common to other dementing illnesses and the normal aging process, it is the increased quantity and characteristic anatomic distribution of these changes that are specific for AD.

There is a correlation between the degree of postmortem brain pathology detected and the severity of the clinically observed dementing illness. The neurochemical deficit in this disorder involves cholinergic systems, specifically decreases in brain choline acetyltransferase, an enzyme responsible for acetylcholine synthesis, and deficits in acetylcholinesterase, an acetylcholine degradation enzyme. In the nucleus basalis of the inferior medial forebrain, a loss of cholinergic neurons correlates with decreased cholinergic innervation of the cerebral cortex.

b. **Etiologic factors.**

(i) **Genetic factors.** In 20% of cases, the disease is inherited as autosomal dominant. In the remaining 80%, there appears to be an increased familial incidence. There appears to be a relationship between Down syndrome and AD. Individuals afflicted with the former, who survive into their third decade, seem to develop the latter uniformly. Also, there is an increased incidence of Down syndrome in relatives of patients with AD.

(ii) **Aluminum.** In animal models, aluminum has been found to cause dementia with neurofibrillary degeneration. Also, in patients affected with AD, elevated brain concentrations of aluminum have been detected.

(iii) **Other factors.** Although data remain scarce, viral and autoimmune etiologies have been entertained.

2. **Multi-infarct dementia.** This accounts for 10% to 15% of dementias. Because timely intervention may impact on the course of this illness, it is essential that clinical manifestations be recognized. The following characteristics are still felt by many authors to be useful.

a. **Characteristics.**

(i) Onset is abrupt with stepwise and paroxysmal deterioration over time. Coarse may be fluctuating.

(ii) Clinically, patients demonstrate signs of cortical (aphasia, apraxia, amnesia, and agnosia), as well as subcortical (depression, psychomotor slowing, forgetfulness, and cognitive dilapidation) dementia.

(iii) Focal neurologic deficits are present (hyper-reflexia, pathologic reflexes, gait disturbance, extremity weakness, and pseudobulbar palsy).

(iv) Personality is relatively preserved with insight comparatively intact.

(v) Patient has history of hypertension, arteriosclerosis, transient ischemic attacks, myocardial infarction, cardiac arrhythmia, or other cardiovascular disease.

(vi) An electroencephalogram (EEG) may show multifocal slowing. A computed tomographic (CT) scan may show multiple asymmetric areas of lucency.

b. **Pathogenesis.** The exact pathogenesis of this disorder is unknown. Persistent hypertension may cause fibrinoid necrosis of cerebral arterioles, leading to vascular occlusion. The most common type of multi-infarct dementia may be the lacunar state; this is characterized by multiple, small infarcts located in the basal ganglia, thalamus, and internal capsule. Other etiologies, some of which are extracranial in origin, may be:

(i) The occurrence of multiple emboli from the neck vessels or heart.

(ii) Nonhypertension-related atherosclerosis of the peripheral vasculature.

(iii) Inflammatory disorders.

(iv) Hematologic abnormalities.

3. **Extrapyramidal syndromes.**

a. **Parkinson disease.** Parkinson disease results from a loss of dopamine-containing cells in the nigrostriatal pathway and ventral tegmentum. Clinically, it is characterized by bradykinesia, tremor, rigidity, decreased facial expression, and shuffling gait and, in approximately 60% of afflicted patients, a subcortical dementia. Subtle neuropsychologic deficits may be present in as many as 90% of such patients. The dementia is poorly correlated with the tremor of this disorder, but seems to vary with the severity of bradykinesia present. Some clinical improvement in the dementia is evident with levodopa pharmacotherapy. In approximately 50% of patients, depression is also found. Although not responsive to levodopa or anticholinergic therapy, patients do show some improvement with tricyclic antidepressants or electroconvulsive therapy.

b. **Huntington disease.** Huntington disease is inherited as an autosomal dominant disorder. Subcortical dementia is a common manifestation of this illness that is characterized by a choreiform movement disorder and a slowly progressive course. The dementia of Huntington usually follows, but may precede the appearance of the movement disorder, or exist alone, as the sole manifestation of this illness. Other psychiatric sequelae of this disorder involve depression and/or a psychosis with hallucinations and delusions that resemble schizophrenia. The rate of suicide in these patients is significantly increased. Pathologically, the illness is distinguished by marked neuronal loss in the caudate nucleus and putamen. The thalamus is involved to a somewhat lesser extent. Atrophy of the caudate nucleus is frequently evident on a CT scan of the basal ganglia. Selective deficit in the neurotransmitter γ-aminobutyric acid (GABA) has been implicated in this disorder. The psychiatric manifestations are treated using the same modalities as their idiopathic counterparts.

c. **Progressive supranuclear palsy.** Progressive supranuclear palsy is characterized by a mild subcortical dementia, supranuclear gaze palsy, axial rigidity, and a pseudobulbar palsy (inappropriate affect in degree and/or direction, dysphagia, and dysarthria). In the initial and middle phases, depression is occasionally found.

d. **Miscellaneous.** Other diseases of the extrapyramidal system that may involve a subcortical dementia are as follows.

(i) **Wilson disease.** The neuropsychiatric manifestations include mania, a schizophrenia-like psychosis, depression, and a subcortical dementia.

(ii) **Fahr disease.** The neuropsychiatric manifestations include a schizophrenia-like psychosis and a subcortical dementia.

(iii) **Spinocerebellar degeneration.** The neuropsychiatric manifestations include depression, a schizophrenia-like psychosis, and a subcortical dementia.

e. **Infectious causes.**

(i) **Jakob-Creutzfeldt disease.** This condition is a rapidly progressive viral infection of the nervous system that usually culminates in death within 6 months of onset. Its features include:

(a.) Clinically diverse presentation, begins in fifth or sixth decades.

(b.) Several different regions of the nervous system are involved (cerebellum, basal ganglia, spinal cord, etc.).

(c.) Myoclonus is usually evident.

(d.) The EEG shows background slowing with superimposed polyphasic sharp wave discharges.

(e.) Inactivation is resistant and transmitted by unknown route.

(f.) No antibody response is elicited.

(g.) No available treatment.

(ii) **Acquired immunodeficiency syndrome (AIDS) dementia complex.** This dementia results from a direct central nervous sytem (CNS) infection of the human immunodeficiency virus (HIV). Clinical features include:

(a.) Presence of risk factors for AIDS.

(b.) Progressive dementia with apathy, psychomotor retardation, dilapidated cognition, and forgetfulness.

(c.) A CT scan may show atrophy and periventricular lucencies.

(d.) Headache is common.

(e.) Opportunistic CNS infections may occur, such as toxoplasmosis (apathy, dementia, seizures, and frontal lobe dysfunction).

(iii) **Bacterial dementias.** Syphilitic general paresis, although no longer common, is the most important of these. Dementia may be accompanied by psychosis with the onset typically 15 to 30 years after the initial infection. Treatment is with penicillin. Whipple disease is another bacterial cause of dementia, treated with antibiotics. Chronic meningitis secondary to bacterial, parasitic, or fungal infection may also result in dementia.

f. **Nutritional deficiencies.** The most common vitamin deficiencies to produce dementia include B_{12}, folate, and niacin. Thiamine deficiency produces an amnesia in the context of the Wernicke-Korsakoff syndrome, with little intellectual impairment.

g. **Endocrinologic abnormalities.** The following endocrinologic conditions may include dementia in their clinical presentation: hypothyroidism, hyperthyroidism, hypoparathyroidism, hyperparathyroidism, hypoadrenocorticism (Addison disease), and hyperadrenocorticism (Cushing disease).

h. **Electrolyte disturbances.** These must be considered in patients with pre-existing renal or gastrointestinal illnesses, as well as patients receiving medication.

i. **Hypoxia.** Several conditions can contribute to cerebral anoxia, including disturbances in cardiac and respiratory function, and anemia.

j. **Dialysis dementia and uremia.** The following two conditions are most clinically important:

(i) Progressive uremic encephalopathy (dialysis dementia).

(a.) This is evident in chronically uremic patients treated with hemodialysis for greater than 3 years.

(b.) Dementia usually follows speech abnormalities that are characterized by stuttering, dysarthria, and dysphasia. Myoclonus and seizures are present.

(c.) This may be a consequence of aluminum toxicity and, thus, may respond to decreased aluminum in the dialysate.

(d.) Abnormal EEG.

(ii) **Chronic uremic encephalopathy.**

(a) Dementia progresses slowly in context of slowly developing renal failure.

(b) Changes in levels of consciousness are characteristic.

(c.) Correction of uremia improves dementia.

(d.) Abnormal EEG.

k. **Drugs, metals, and industrial chemical exposure.** Several of these agents can give rise to reversible dementias. The list of drugs, metals, and volatile and industrial agents is extensive.

l. **Hepatic encephalopathy.** Chronic progressive hepatic encephalopathy is characterized by:

(i) Usual presence in long-term, severe liver disease.

(ii) Slowly progressive dementia that may precede overt liver disease.

m. **Porphyria.** This is actually a group of clinically diverse conditions manifested by defects in heme biosynthesis. It is thought that the neuropsychiatric manifestations of these conditions are limited by that group of porphyrias characterized by overproduction of the porphyrin precursors porphobilinogen and aminolevulinic acid (ALA).

n. **Pseudodementia.** This is a loss in intellectual abilities, resulting from depression. Particularly in the elderly, pseudodementia may be difficult to distinguish from other dementias. The following clinical features of pseudodementia help to distinguish it from other dementias:

(i) Onset rapid with symptoms of short duration.

(ii) Patients frequently complain of distress. They exaggerate cognitive and memory difficulties.

(iii) Patients highlight difficulties with frequent "I don't know" answers on mental status examination.

(iv) Patients make little effort to perform on tasks of ability.

(v) Variable performance on similar tests of difficulty.

(vi) Frequent preoccupation with self-reproach or self-derogatory statements.

(vii) Depressed mood, constricted affect.

(viii) Preserved attention and concentration.

(ix) History of affective illness.

(x) Symptoms rarely worsen at night. Patients with pseudodementia typically respond to treatment of their underlying depression with significant improvement of their cognitive and memory deficits. Pseudodementia may also coexist with other dementias.

o. **Hydrocephalic dementias.** Hydrocephalus refers to an excessive amount of cerebrospinal fluid in the CNS. It is characterized by enlarged ventricles. The many causes for this condition are divided into three categories: (1) nonobstructive hydrocephalus, (2) obstructive hydrocephalus, and (3) communicating (normal-pressure) hydrocephalus. The clinical characteristics of hydrocephalus include gait disturbance, incontinence, and dementia.

The dementia of hydrocephalus is characterized by impaired memory, inattention, apathy or indifference, poor judgment, and excessive concreteness.

p. **Traumatic and neoplastic dementias.** Any trauma to the brain can produce disruption of cerebral function and, thus, a dementing illness. This is a particularly common cause of dementia in the younger age groups. Traumatic dementias can coexist with alterations in personality and may be characterized by aphasia, amnesia, concreteness, and apraxia. Aside from contusion or shearing of brain tissue, subdural hematoma formation is also a consequence of trauma. Elderly patients are particularly susceptible to this, and may not give a history of significant trauma.

Neoplastic involvement of the CNS can also result in intellectual deterioration, excessive concreteness, and poor judgment. This is particularly characteristic of frontal lobe tumors that may not produce focal neurologic findings.

q. **Myelin disease–associated dementias.** Myelin disorders of the nervous system may include dementia in their clinical presentations. The most common disorders in which this may occur are multiple sclerosis, adrenoleukodystrophy, and metachromatic leukodystrophy.

r. **Diagnostic workup of dementia.**

(i) The differential diagnosis of dementia includes isolated aphasia, thought disorder secondary to functional psychiatric illness or intoxication, hearing impairment, factitious disorder, and delirium.

(ii) The following diagnostic evaluation is indicated in the workup of dementia:

(a) Thorough personal history of medical, neurologic, and psychiatric illness.

(b) Thorough family history.

(c) History of drug use, chemical exposure, trauma, prior transfusion, and homosexual practices.

(d) Thorough physical and neurologic examinations.

(e) Thorough mental status examination.

(f) Laboratory evaluation: complete blood cell (CBC) count; sedimentation rate; heavy metal screening (if possible exposure); serum glucose; electrolytes, including calcium and phosphorus; blood urea nitrogen (BUN); liver function tests; thyroid function tests; B_{12} and folate levels; VDRL; and if indicated, HIV determination.

(g) CT scan of the head.

(h) EEG.

(i) If specifically indicated, lumbar puncture (atypical presentation or evidence of CNS infection), chest x-ray film, electrocardiogram (ECG), and if nature of deficits is unclear, or baseline study is needed, more extensive neuropsychologic testing (Wechsler Adult Intelligence Scale, revised; Wechsler Memory Scale; Boston Diagnostic Aphasia Examination, etc.).

If the above workup is conducted in an appropriate fashion, the clinician should be able to answer the following questions:

1. Is the patient's illness a functional or organic condition?

2. If organic, is the disease process focal or diffuse?

3. If diffuse, is the process a dementia or delirium?

4. If dementia is diagnosed, does it have a reversible etiology?

s. **Treatment.** The treatment of dementia involves the following:

(i) Treat any reversible etiologies.

(ii) Manage behavioral problems (aggression, psychosis) with smallest possible doses of high-potency neuroleptics.

(iii) Treat any coexistent depression and concurrent medical problems.

(iv) Offer directive and supportive psychotherapy (especially in early stages).

(v) Help family to organize and coordinate care of patient, ensuring that all needs, including medical, psychiatric, and social, are met by the appropriate caregivers.

(vi) Educate, support, and be available to patient's family.

III. Delirium (acute confusional state).

A. Definition and major clinical features. Delirium (acute confusional state) is characterized by impaired alertness, attention, and concentration of acute onset and brief duration (hours to days). Its other features include:

1. Intellectual impairment involving:

a. Language (anomia, misnaming, agraphia, and comprehension difficulties).

b. Memory (disorientation).

c. Constructional ability.

d. Cognition (concreteness, dyscalculia).

2. Disturbances of perception:

a. Hallucinations (silent, visual, or tactile; less commonly auditory).

b. Illusions.

3. Autonomic disturbances:

a. Pallor, flushing, anhidrosis.

b. Miosis or mydriasis.

c. Tachycardia or bradycardia.

d. Hypertension or hypotension.

e. Constipation or diarrhea.

4. Motor system abnormalities:

a. Tremor, myoclonus, asterixis, dysarthria, hypoactivity, or hyperactivity (may alternate).

5. **Sleep-wake cycle abnormalities:**

a. Insomnia or hypersomnia.

6. **Thought content disturbances:**

a. Delusions (usually not self-referential, not systematized).

b. Confabulation with memory impairment.

7. **Mood alterations with labile affect.**

8. **Temporal variability (i.e., delirium waxes and wanes in severity):**

a. Diurnal variability (symptoms worse at night and early morning.

9. **Striking clinical variability (i.e., features vary considerably from one patient to another; symptoms may be very subtle or florid).**

10. **EEG shows diffuse slowing (theta or delta wave activity).**

B. **Etiologies.**

1. **Systemic disturbances.**

a. Hepatic abnormalities (hepatic encephalopathy).

b. Renal abnormalities (uremia).

c. Pulmonary abnormalities.

d. Cardiac abnormalities (arrhythmias, hypotension, and congestive heart failure).

e. Electrolyte disturbances and hypoglycemia.

f. Anemia.

g. Postoperative states (anoxia, medication side effects, sleep deprivation, sensory isolation, and pain).

2. **Endocrinologic dysfunction: pituitary, adrenal, thyroid, parathyroid, and pancreatic.**

3. **Infectious processes.** Sepsis and fever.

4. **Nutritional deficiencies.** Thiamine Wernicke encephalopathy (ataxia, delirium, ophthalmoplegia, folate, niacin, protein, and B_{12}).

5. **Intracranial processes.** Subarachnoid and subdural bleeding, trauma, infection (meningitis and encephalitis), stroke, migraine headache, tumor, epilepsy (ictal and postictal delirium), and hypertensive encephalopathy.

6. **Intoxicating.** Drugs and medications (especially anticholinergics), alcohol, poisons (metals, industrial agents, and carbon monoxide).

7. **Drug withdrawal.** Alcohol withdrawal delirium, benzodiazepine, and other withdrawal delirium.

8. **Psychiatric problems.** Catatonic stupor due to mania or schizophrenia.

9. **Miscellaneous causes.**

a. Heat stroke and hyperthermia.

b. Electrocution.

c. Radiation exposure.

C. **Delirium vs. dementia.** Delirium may be distinguished from dementia by the following:

1. Dementia persists for months to years; delirium persists hours or days to weeks.

2. Dementia has less attentional impairment.

3. Dementia has less frequent hallucinations, illusions, and delusions.

4. Dementia has an abnormal EEG less often.

5. Dementia usually has a less acute or abrupt onset and a slower progression.

6. Dementia has less disruption in the sleep-wake cycle.

7. Dementia has less autonomic dysfunction.

D. **Differential diagnosis and workup.**

1. **Differential diagnosis.** The differential diagnosis of delirium includes:

a. Dementia (see above).

b. Functional psychiatric disorders.

2. **Schizophrenic or manic psychosis.** This differs from delirium on the basis of:

a. Presence of premorbid history.

b. Less sleep-wake cycle problems.

c. No change in consciousness (arousal).

d. Alert and oriented.

e. Bizarre, self-referential content with more auditory hallucinations.

f. Less illusions.

g. Less intellectual and memory impairment.

h. More sustained and less labile effect.

i. No autonomic changes, myoclonus, or asterixis.

3. **Conversion and dissociative disorders.** These differ from delirium on the basis of:

a. No temporal variation.

b. Less sleep-wake cycle problems.

c. No change in awareness or alertness.

d. Well oriented.

e. Rare perceptual problems.

f. Preserved intellect.

g. No autonomic changes, myoclonus, or asterixis.

4. **Aphasia.** Differs from delirium on the basis of:

a. May have focal neurologic signs.

b. No change in awareness or alertness.

c. Neologisms more likely to be present.

5. **Workup and evaluation.** The workup of delirium must include:

a. Thorough medical history, including drug or medication use.

b. Thorough medical and neurologic examinations.

c. Blood chemistry evaluation, including CBC with differential cell count; serum glucose; BUN/creatinine; electrolyte profile; toxicology screening (urine or serum); sedimentation rate; liver function tests; arterial blood gas; and urine chemistry for glucose, ketones, cells, and protein.

d. ECG.

e. EEG.

f. Chest x-ray film.

g. If specifically indicated by examination or history, CT scan or magnetic resonance imaging of the head, and lumbar puncture (including cell counts, protein, glucose, VDRL, cultures, etc.).

E. **Treatment.** The treatment of delirium must incorporate the following:

1. Identifying and treating the underlying cause of the encephalopathy.

2. Offering supportive medical care that may involve:

a. Maintaining adequate nutrition, hydration, and electrolyte balance.

b. Treatment of insomnia.

c. Provision of appropriate amount of sensory stimulation (quiet well-lit room during day with some attenuated light at night, adequate verbal stimulation).

d. Frequent reassurance and reorienting by family or other caretakers.

3. Behavioral management that may involve:

a. Sedation as needed for disruptful agitation, typically with small doses (by mouth [PO] or intramuscularly [IM]), in frequent intervals, of neuroleptics (e.g., haloperidol, 1 mg PO/IM every 2 to 3 hours until stable) or benzodiazepines (e.g., lorazepam, 1 to 2 mg PO/IM every 3 to 4 hours). Doses to be tailored to degree of agitation and used sparingly, if possible, to avoid oversedation. After 24 hours, daily dose required of neuroleptic or benzodiazepine may be assessed, and standing order can be given.

Finally, one should remember that the metabolic milieu in the CNS may not correct as quickly as in the periphery. As a result, delirium may temporarily persist despite normalization and removal of offending systemic agents or processes. In a minority of patients, delirium may persist indefinitely, giving rise to a dementia, or may culminate in the patient's death, secondary to the underlying disease process.

IV. Psychiatric aspects of seizure disorders.

A. **Introduction.** Psychiatric symptoms occur with increased frequency in patients with seizures as a result of underlying brain tissue injury, side effects from anticonvulsant medications, or seizure-specific psychiatric disturbances. Psychosis, affective disturbances, and more enduring alterations in personality have been described in epileptics. Psychiatric symptoms may be preictal, ictal, interictal, or postictal manifestations of the underlying seizure disorder. Fear, dissociative experiences, intense affective experiences, and hallucinations have all been documented as seizure (ictal) phenomena.

B. **Complex partial seizures (psychomotor seizures, temporal lobe epilepsy).**

1. **Definition:** Brief, episodic, paroxysmal discharges of epileptic foci, usually located in limbic structures, particularly the temporal lobes.

2. **Clinical characteristics:**

a. Most common focal seizure disorder found in adults, 30% of all adult epilepsies.

b. May appear at any age, onset usually in adolescence.

c. Greater likelihood of psychiatric problems than any other type of seizure disorder.

d. Most common lesion responsible thought to be mesial temporal sclerosis (thought to be result of febrile seizures in infancy) or hamartomas of temporal lobe.

e. May result in long-term personality changes referred to as interictal behavior syndrome (see below).

f. Seizures may be triggered by bright lights, colors, noises, or heightened emotions.

g. Full-blown seizure often preceded by an aura (limbic involvement) with the following characteristics:

(i) Lasts seconds to hours.

(ii) May have abdominal discomfort.

(iii) May have olfactory (odors) or gustatory (tastes) hallucinations that are unpleasant.

(iv) May experience strange emotional state, such as déjà vu, intense fear, euphoria, dysphoria, or dissociative experiences.

h. As seizure begins, patient shows decreased spontaneous activity with diminished awareness of surroundings and vacant stare.

i. Patient may show motor automatisms that involve face and mouth (lip-smacking, chewing, swallowing, grimacing, etc.) and/or extremities (fidgeting with clothes, scratching, rubbing, etc.).

j. Patient may turn head or eyes or entire trunk to one side.

k. Seizure may progress to generalized motor seizure with loss of consciousness.

l. Patient may have autonomic symptoms.

m. Patient may occasionally have urinary incontinence, rarely fecal incontinence.

n. Duration of seizure is seconds to minutes.

o. EEG shows temporal area spikes with sphenoidal or nasopharyngeal leads. EEG findings not necessary for diagnosis.

C. **Pseudoseizures (pseudoepilepsy).** Pseudoseizures (false seizures) occur in approximately 20% of epileptics. They are characteristically found in other patients as well, most commonly those patients suffering from depression or those patients with pervasive personality disorders. Table 9–1 distinguishes pseudoseizures from true seizures, although differentiation may be difficult to even the most experienced examiner.

D. **Interictal psychiatric disorders.** Interictal conditions must be distinguished from aura, ictal, and postictal states. These disorders may actually worsen with better seizure control or improve. The interictal psychiatric disorders include:

1. **Depression (most common):**

a. Increased suicide rate in epileptics, especially those with complex partial seizures.

2. **Schizophreniform psychosis:**

a. More common in left-sided foci.

b. Begins an average of 14 years after the onset of seizures.

c. No family history of psychosis.

d. No premorbid history of psychiatric pathology.

e. Symptoms may include delusions, hallucinations

TABLE 9-1.

Differentiation of Pseudoseizures From Seizures

Distinguishing Feature	Pseudoseizures	Seizures
Onset	Often gradual	Abrupt
Movements	Struggling, asynchronous, thrashing, and flailing	Rigidity then tonic/clonic
Self-injury	Rare	Common
Biting	Lips, arms, and other areas	Tongue
Urination	Rare	Common
Defecation	Rare	Occasional
Cry	During ictus, quasipurposeful	At onset
Consciousness	Intact or partially retained	Lost
Affected by physician	Yes	No
Postictal confusion	Absent	Present
Duration	Several—many min	1/2 min—few min
EEG*		
Interictal	May be abnormal	May be abnormal
Ictal	Normal	Abnormal
Neuroendocrine effects	No change in prolactin level	Prolactin level increases 5-10 times
Anticonvulsant withdrawal	No increase in seizure frequency	Increase in seizure frequency

*EEG = electroencephalogram.

(auditory and visual), paranoia, and preservation of affective range.

f. Psychosis not usually responsive to anticonvulsants.

3. **Interictal behavior syndrome (personality alteration):**

a. Viscosity (inability to disengage during interpersonal communication).

b. Deepening of all affects with inappropriately intense reactions to events.

c. Passivity, obsessiveness, irritability, and humorlessness.

d. Increased concern for philosophic, moral, and ethical issues.

e. Hyper-religiosity.

f. Overinclusive, circumstantial, and repetitive speech.

g. Hypergraphia (diaries, journals, logs, and extensive notes).

h. Hyposexuality (sometimes hypersexuality).

i. Increased incidence of dissociation and phobic episodes.

E. **Evaluation and workup.** A complete evaluation is indicated for new-onset seizures or behavioral changes. The workup must include the following:

1. Thorough medical and neurologic examinations to evaluate for the presence of:

a. Intracranial masses.

b. CNS infection.

c. Metabolic/toxic abnormalities.

d. Post-traumatic processes (hematomas, brain contusion, etc.).

2. Laboratory evaluation, including CBC count;

electrolytes with glucose; BUN; liver function tests; toxicology screening; and VDRL.

3. EEG.

4. CT scan of head.

F. **Treatment.** The treatment of complex partial seizures involves treatment of the seizures themselves and treatment of any interictal psychiatric disorders.

1. **Seizure control:**

a. Pharmacotherapy:

(i) Carbamazepine (Tegretol).

(ii) Phenytoin (Dilantin).

(iii) Primidone (Mysoline).

b. Psychosurgery in seizures refractory to medication and resulting in significant disability (controversial).

2. **Treatment of Interictal Psychiatric Problems:**

a. Supportive psychotherapy (group and family therapy).

b. Pharmacotherapy.*

c. Neuroleptics for control of psychosis:

(i) Use those with lowest epileptogenicity (molindone, fluphenazine, thioridazine).

(ii) Use low doses, increasing dose slowly as needed (seizure resulting from lowered seizure threshold will usually occur within 10 days of starting psychotropic or changing dose).

It is important to remember that psychotropics and anticonvulsants interact to alter each other's blood levels during combined pharmacotherapy.

d. Antidepressants for control of depressive symptoms:

(i) Use desipramine or doxepin (lowest epileptogenicity).

(ii) Lithium can be used safely.

V. Other neuropsychiatric disorders.

A. **Organic mood syndrome.** This includes alterations in mood and affect caused by identifiable insults to the CNS. Careful study has revealed that abnormalities in specific neuroanatomic regions can be correlated with particular disturbances in mood and affect. Basal-limbic anatomy appears to be essential to the localization of mood. Mood disturbances have been observed in injury to cortical and subcortical structures. Disturbances in mood may be observed in systemic illnesses, drug intoxications (β-blockers, reserpine, etc.), endocrine disorders (thyroid, adrenal), vitamin deficiencies, and neurologic disorders. Neurologic disorders that produce mood or affect disturbances are as follows:

1. **Cerebrovascular disease.** Mood alterations following stroke have been well documented. Lesions that involve the frontal pole, particularly on the left side, are best correlated with depression. Patients appear to be most susceptible to an infarct-induced depression within 2 years of the initial vascular event. Treatment with antidepressants is often indicated. Mania has been reported as a consequence of lesions localized to the third ventricle and perithalamic regions and to right-sided hemispheric insults.

2. **Traumatic brain injury.** Damage localized to the frontal lobes is more likely to induce depression with the importance of laterality less clear. The localization of mania may be similar to that seen in stroke.

3. **Cerebral neoplasm.** Temporal lobe tumors often

present with depression. This is more common with left-sided temporal lesions. Frontal lobe tumors may also present with depression, but more commonly, present with manic symptoms.

4. **Multiple sclerosis.** Mood disturbances appear to be most common in those patients with cerebral plaques. Euphoria and depression have been well documented in these patients.

5. **CNS infections.** General paresis (syphilis) and viral encephalitis may present with depression or mania.

6. **Hydrocephalus.** Depression may be a feature, along with gait ataxia, urinary incontinence, and dementia.

7. **Epilepsy.** (See section IV on psychiatric manifestations of seizures).

8. **Extrapyramidal disorders.**

a. **Parkinson disease.**—Depression is very common, possibly present in 40% to 70% of cases (see section above).

b. **Progressive supranuclear palsy:**—Depression is often found in these patients and may be responsive to tricyclics.

c. **Huntington disease.**—Depression is a common manifestation, possibly occurring in up to 50% of patients (see section above).

d. **Wilson disease.**—Mania has been described as a symptom.

9. **Pseudobulbar palsy.** Typically, patients may exhibit a sudden, involuntary display of emotion (crying or laughing) that may be unrelated to the prevailing mood or exaggerated in degree. Disorders in which this may occur include:

a. Progressive supranuclear palsy.

b. Vascular disorders: Bilateral vascular infarction of the cortex or internal capsule arteriovenous malformation, cerebrovascular hemorrhage, and lacunar state. Trauma, amyotrophic lateral sclerosis, multiple sclerosis, brain-stem tumors, and CNS infections.

B. **Organic personality syndrome.** Definition: An acquired change in personality found to be etiologically related to an organic source, without evidence of delirium or dementia *(DSM III-R)*. Causes include neoplasms, infectious and inflammatory processes, head trauma, vascular accidents, seizure disorders, demyelinating disorders, and hydrocephalus.

The specific features of organically induced personality changes are varied and incompletely studied. Generally, a lack of premorbid psychiatric problems, and the onset of personality changes that follow a history of head trauma or illnesses with CNS involvement, are necessary to make the diagnosis. The following organic personality syndromes have received the most attention:

1. Interictal behavior syndrome (see above).

2. Frontal lobe syndrome: The clinical features of this condition are divided into three categories by region of anatomic involvement:

a. Orbitofrontal:

(i) Personality: Disinhibition (socially and sexually), inappropriate behavior, hyperactivity (manic-like), irritable, labile, jocular, mildly euphoric, facetious, diminished insight, and poor judgment.

(ii) Neuropsychologic findings: No predominant deficits, intact language, memory, and cognition.

(iii) Neurologic deficits: May have damage to olfactory nerve; may have grasp reflex, otherwise intact.

(iv) Treatment: No clearly effective pharmacologic treatment; neuroleptics, lithium, carbamazepine, propranolol, and benzodiazepines for disinhibition.

b. Frontal convexity:

(i) Personality: Apathetic, indifferent, diminished

initiative and motivation, psychomotor retarded, distractible, and appears to be depressed.

(ii) Neuropsychologic deficits: Perseveration (demonstrated in copying multiple loops or failure to change behavior when given new, specific commands or tasks); difficulty with motor programming and integration of verbal function with motor activity (demonstrated by deficits in following commands given by examiner, such as "fist-side-palm" test or reciprocal tapping tests); distractibility (poor performance on "A's" test); decreased abstracting ability (diminished performance on Wisconsin card sort test); decreased visuospatial ability (decreased performance on copying complex diagrams); and impaired word-list generation.

(iii) Neurologic deficits: Frequently intact.

(iv) Treatment: No clearly effective treatment. Trial of psychostimulants may be indicated, such as methylphenidate or amphetamine.

c. Medial-frontal:

(i) Personality: Akinetic; decreased verbalization or mutism; little response to environment, possibly catatonia.

(ii) Neuropsychologic deficits: Undetermined.

(iii) Neurologic deficits: May have incontinence (bilateral lesions); may have gait disturbance and lower-extremity sensory loss.

(iv) Treatment: Trial of dopamine agonists may be indicated, such as bromocriptine or levodopa.

Other features that may be present in the disease of the frontal lobes include confabulation, dysprosody, unilateral spatial neglect, mood disorders, callosal disconnection syndromes, eye movement disorders, and reduplicative paramnesia.

Most often, patients may present with elements of each of the different frontal lobe syndromes in a mixed presentation. Treatment must be directed at all reversible causes of frontal lobe syndromes and, when warranted, pharmacologic trials must be used to improve symptoms.

C. **Organic amnestic syndrome.** The organic amnestic syndrome is characterized by impairment in memory, with evidence of an organic source, but without evidence of delirium or dementia *(DSM III-R)*. The memory deficit may include short-term recall impairment and long-term and immediate recall spared.

The memory impairment may be further distinguished by both retrograde and the anterograde amnesia. Short-term memory is most affected.

Confabulation is present despite an absence of other deficits, such as decreased attention and consciousness, aphasia, apraxia, and agnosia.

The memory impairment is usually associated with bilateral pathology of limbic structures (mamillary bodies, perihippocampus, posterior hypothalamus, and thalamus). The causes of organic amnestic disorder are as follows:

1. Thiamine deficiency: This is found in chronic alcoholics, the elderly, and others with nutritional deficiencies, malabsorption problems, and deficiency of the transketolase enzyme, and in Wernicke-Korsakoff syndrome.

2. Cerebrovascular accidents: These occur especially in occlusion of the posterior cerebral artery bilaterally, basilar artery, or unilateral left cerebral artery (less often).

3. Head trauma: This is the most common cause of memory deficit, but rarely is it an isolated memory impairment. This may have both anterograde and retrograde components.

4. Infection (encephalitis): Viruses with particular infection of limbic system, especially herpes simplex encephalitis usually associated with other deficits.

5. Tumors: Especially those tumors in the region of the third ventricle and mesial temporal areas.

6. Anoxia: The hippocampus is especially sensitive to cerebral anoxia that may result from anesthesia complications, cardiopulmonary arrest, or carbon monoxide poisoning. Memory impairment may be permanent.

7. Acute hypoglycemia: Hippocampus is especially sensitive.

8. Electroconvulsive therapy.

In assessing amnesia, the organic amnestic syndrome is characterized by particular involvement of recent recall, and to a lesser extent, remote recall, with relative sparing of immediate recall. The differential diagnosis includes:

1. Transient global amnesia caused by intoxication, neoplasm, migraine headache, seizure, and cerebrovascular disturbances.

a. Characteristics:

(i) Lasts up to 24 hours.

(ii) Abrupt onset of disorientation to time and place.

(iii) Patient very distressed with frequent repetition of the same question.

(iv) Found mostly in older patients (age range, 50 to 70 years).

2. Psychogenic memory loss characteristics:

a. Lost remote recall.

b. Intact recent recall and ability to learn new information.

c. Lost information, especially related to personal information and disorientation to self.

d. History of prior or concurrent psychiatric illness (especially depression).

e. More common in younger patients (age range, 20 to 40 years).

D. **Organic hallucinosis.** This disorder includes the presence of any of the following types of hallucinations, with evidence of an organic source, but without evidence of dementia or delirium *(DSM III-R)*: visual, auditory, tactile, olfactory, and gustatory (Table 9–2).

TABLE 9–2.

Organic Hallucinations

Types	Causes
Visual	Ophthalmologic disorders
	CNS* disorders
	Optic nerve disease, brain-stem lesions, narcolepsy, migraine, hemispheric lesions, and epilepsy
	Acute confusional states
	Toxic causes
	Hallucinogens, antiparkinsonian agents, antibiotics, hormones, and antidepressants
Auditory	Peripheral auditory lesions, CNS disorders, epilepsy vascular insults, and neoplasms (frontal/temporal lobes)
	Acute confusional states
	Alcohol hallucinosis
Tactile	Toxic/metabolic derangement (cocaine)
	Withdrawal states
	CNS neoplasms (rare)
Olfactory	Epilepsy (ictal)
	Migraine
	Dementia (rarely)
Gustatory	Complex partial seizure

CNS = central nervous system.

E. **Organic delusional syndrome.** This includes the presence of delusions suspected to be secondary to an organic source, but without evidence of delirium or dementia *(DSM III-R)*. Possible etiologies include seizure disorders, degenerative disorders (AD, Huntington disease, etc.), cerebral infarction or tumors, and drug intoxication.

REFERENCES

1. American Psychiatric Association: *Diagnostic and Statistical Manual of Mental Disorders*, ed 3 (revised). Washington, DC, American Psychiatric Association, 1987, pp 97–163.
2. Murray GB: Confusion, delirium, and dementia, in Hackett TP, Cassem NH (eds): *Massachusetts General Hospital Handbook of General Hospital Psychiatry*, ed 2. Littleton, Mass, PSG Publishing Co Inc, 1987, pp 84–115.
3. Wells CE: Organic mental disorders, in Kaplan HI, Sadock BJ (eds): *Comprehensive Textbook of Psychiatry/IV*, ed 4. Baltimore, Williams & Wilkins, 1985, pp 834–882.
4. Cummings JL, Benson DF: *Dementia: A Clinical Approach*. Stoneham, Mass, Butterworth Publishers Inc, 1983.
5. Cummings JL: *Clinical Neuropsychiatry*. New York, Grune & Stratton, 1985.

10

Eating Disorders

I. *DSM III-R* classification of eating disorders.

A. **Diagnostic criteria for 307.10 anorexia nervosa.**

1. Refusal to maintain body weight over a minimal normal weight for age and height, e.g., weight loss leading to maintenance of body weight 15% below that expected, or failure to make expected weight gain during period of growth, leading to body weight 15% below that expected.

2. Intense fear of gaining weight or becoming fat, even though underweight.

3. Disturbance in the way in which one's body weight, size, or shape is experienced, e.g., the person claims to "feel fat" even when emaciated and believes that one area of the body is "too fat" even when obviously underweight.

4. In females, absence of at least three consecutive menstrual cycles when otherwise expected to occur (primary or secondary amenorrhea). (A woman is considered to have amenorrhea if her periods occur only following hormone, e.g., estrogen, administration.)

B. **Diagnostic criteria for 307.51 bulimia nervosa.**

1. Recurrent episodes of binge eating (rapid con-

sumption of a large amount of food in a discrete period of time).

2. A feeling of lack of control over eating behavior during the eating binges.

3. The person regularly engages in either self-induced vomiting, use of laxatives or diuretics, strict dieting or fasting, or vigorous exercise to prevent weight gain.

4. A minimum average of two binge-eating episodes a week for at least three months.

5. Persistent overconcern with body shape and weight.

II. Epidemiology.

A. Anorexia nervosa.

1. Incidence: 0.35/100,000 white females; age range, 15 to 24 years (upstate New York, 1960 to 1969); 0.64/100,000 (same population 1970 to 1976).

2. Prevalence: 0.5% to 1% British private school girls; age range, 12 to 18 years.

3. Sex: Approximately 95% are female.

4. Age at onset: Mainly age range, 13 to 25 years; peaks at 14 and 18 years.

5. Socioeconomic status: Predominantly upper and upper-middle classes.

6. Family history (FH): Increased incidence of eating disorders in first-degree relatives, increased alcoholism in parents, and 30% have positive (+) FH for major affective disorder.

B. Bulimia nervosa.

1. Incidence: Unknown.

2. Prevalence: 4% to 19% college females have bulimic symptoms; 1% to 3% meet *DSM-III-R* criteria.

3. Sex: Approximately 95% are female.

4. Age at onset: Mainly age range, 15 to 30 years, but occasionally older.

5. Socioeconomic status: Unknown.

6. FH: Increased alcoholism in parents, increased number of overweight first-degree relatives, and 60% have (+) FH for major affective disorder.

III. **Clinical presentation and evaluation.**

A. **Modes of presentation.**

1. Anorexia nervosa.

a. Adolescent brought to gynecologist with amenorrhea as chief complaint (20% have amenorrhea preceding weight loss).

b. Adolescent with isolated episode of weight loss associated with life stresses and/or depression.

c. Adolescent or young adult with progressive chronic anorexia nervosa, often with recurrent affective illness and medical complications of starvation, brought in by family with food restriction, dieting, and behavior out of control.

d. Presents to primary physician with multiple complaints, e.g., fatigue, abdominal discomfort, constipation, polyuria, cold intolerance, and sleep disturbance.

e. Most presentations associated with a high level of denial and resistance to treatment.

2. Bulimia nervosa.

a. Late adolescent or young adult presenting by herself or brought in by family with binge/purge behavior out of control.

b. Late adolescent or young adult presents with increasing symptoms of depression and bulimic behavior.

c. Presents with worsening substance abuse problem (opiates, cocaine, benzodiazepines, amphetamines, and alcohol) and bulimic behavior.

B. **Associated features.**

1. Anorexia nervosa.

    a. May have episodes of binge eating and vomiting.

    b. Often prepares elaborate meals for others.

    c. Food hoarding.

    d. Decreased libido.

    e. Ritualistic behaviors, e.g., hand washing and exercising.

    f. High frequency of depressive symptoms and concurrent major affective disorder.

    g. 40% to 60% have stressful life event that precedes onset of illness.

    h. Multiple medical complications (see Section V.).

2. Bulimia nervosa.

    a. 15% to 20% have history of being significantly overweight earlier in life.

    b. May be at slightly above or below normal weight for height and age at onset.

    c. Long history of dieting, food fads, and weight fluctuations.

    d. Binges defined as rapid consumption of usually high-calorie (mean = 3,500 calories), easily consumed foods, i.e., cakes, breads, candy, ice cream, etc.; mean duration of binge, approximately 1 hour.

    e. Purging: Vomiting is primary means of purging in 75%; chronic laxative abuse in 50%.

    f. High frequency of depressive symptoms and concurrent major affective disorder.

    g. 10% to 20% have concurrent substance abuse (alcohol, opiates, amphetamines, cocaine, and benzodiazepines).

    h. May resort to stealing food; significant association with kleptomania.

i. Diuretic abuse.

j. Mood state before binge, i.e., dysphoria, anxiety, irritability, and feeling of being out of control. Binges are often precipitated by anxiety, food-related thoughts, loneliness, rejection, and boredom.

k. During binge, patient may experience relief of anxiety. Following binge, patient often experiences guilt, shame, anger, abdominal pain, and fear of becoming fat. Vomiting reduces fear of becoming fat and may allow further bingeing.

l. Binge episode usually terminated by abdominal pain, vomiting, or sleep.

m. Multiple medical complications (see Section V.).

C. Risk factors in the development of eating disorders.

1. Premorbid obesity (especially for subsequent bulimia).

2. Diabetes mellitus.

3. Affective disturbance.

4. Poor impulse control, i.e., association with substance abuse, shoplifting, and borderline personality disorder.

5. Cultural pursuit of thinness, i.e., western ideal for beauty is thin; high frequency of anorexia nervosa and bulimia nervosa in models, dancers, etc.

IV. **Clinical evaluation.**

A. **History.**

1. Detailed history of specific eating behaviors, diet and weight history, and age at onset.

2. Specific purging behavior, i.e., vomiting, laxative abuse, and appetite suppressants.

3. History of depression, psychosis, current affective and anxiety (including somatic manifestations) symptoms, and suicidal ideation.

4. Substance abuse history.

5. Other ritualistic or compulsive behaviors, e.g., exercising, hand washing, etc.

6. Sexual history.

7. Degree of impulsivity, e.g., shoplifting, promiscuity, substance abuse, etc.

8. Trauma/abuse, e.g., physical, psychologic, and sexual.

9. Medical history.

10. Level of assertiveness.

11. Adjustment within and outside of family.

B. **Family history.**

1. Family psychiatric history, i.e., history of affective illness, psychosis, eating disorders, obesity, and substance abuse.

2. Assessment of family structure and boundaries.

a. Hierarchy and power sources.

b. Alliances and coalitions within family.

c. Level of protectiveness, intrusiveness, and rigidity.

d. Problem management.

e. Mechanisms of dealing with anxiety and anger.

C. **Mental status examination.**

D. **Careful physical examination,** regarding medical complications (see Section V.).

E. **Laboratory tests:** complete blood cell count with differential cell count; platelet count; sodium, potassium, chloride, bicarbonate, calcium, phosphate, magnesium, total protein, serum albumin, cholesterol, alanine and aspartate aminotransferase, alkaline phosphatase, bilirubin, amylase, triiodothyronine, thyroxine, and thyroid-stimulating hormone (TSH) levels; toxicology screening; and urinalysis.

F. Differential diagnosis of weight loss.

1. Psychiatric illnesses that may cause weight loss include anorexia nervosa, major affective illnesses, schizophrenia, obsessive-compulsive disorder, and stimulant dependency.

2. Endocrine disorders that cause weight loss include diabetes mellitus, hyperthyroidism, Addison disease, hyperparathyroidism, pancreatic insufficiency, and endocrine diarrheas related to hormone-secreting tumors.

3. Malignancy.

4. Gastrointestinal disorders, e.g., malabsorption and peptic ulcer disease (PUD).

G. Etiologies for binge eating other than bulimia nervosa.

1. Psychiatric illness (depression).

2. Obesity.

3. Central nervous system (CNS) lesions (hypothalamic lesions, tumor, Kleine-Levin syndrome, and epilepsy).

4. Endocrine disorders (diabetes mellitus and hypothyroidism).

H. Psychologic testing useful in evaluating patients with eating disorders.

1. Eating Attitude Test: 26-item questionnaire regarding dieting and weight, food preoccupation, and bulimia; normalizes with recovery.

2. Eating Disorder Inventory: 64-item questionnaire with eight subscales regarding drive for thinness, bulimia, body dissatisfaction, ineffectiveness, perfectionism, interpersonal distrust, interoceptive awareness, and maturity fears. (Patients with anorexia nervosa and bulimia nervosa differ on drive for thinness, ineffectiveness, and interoceptive awareness).

3. **Minnesota Multiphasic Personality Inventory:** Useful in evaluating personality factors, level of depression, and presence of psychosis.

4. Projective testing.

5. Neuropsychologic testing may be indicated following medical stabilization if the patient has persistent cognitive defects.

V. **Medical complications of eating disorders (Table 10–1).**

VI. **Neuroendocrine changes associated with eating disorders (Table 10–2).**

VII. **Neurotransmitter systems.**

A. **Monoamines.**

1. **Background.** Norepinephrine (NE) and serotonin (5-hydroxytryptamine [5-HT]) play important roles in the regulation of mood, appetite, and feeding behavior. Central monoamines also influence multiple neuroendocrine systems, including the hypothalamic-pituitary-adrenal (HPA) axis and the hypothalamic-pituitary-ovarian (HPO) axis. In rats, starvation reduces NE turnover in the medial basal hypothalamus and reduces postsynaptic NE receptor-binding affinity. Norepinephrine induces feeding through stimulation of α-adrenergic receptors in the paraventricular nucleus. In rats, NE also acts as a key excitatory neurotransmitter that mediates luteinizing hormone-releasing hormone release and, thus, regulates luteinizing hormone (LH) secretion by the pituitary gland. The 5-HT antagonizes NE-induced feeding and reduces meal size and duration without disturbing the latency to initiation of feeding, suggesting that 5-HT acts as a satiety factor.

2. **Disturbances of monoamines in anorexia nervosa and bulimia nervosa.** Underweight patients with anorexia nervosa have weight-dependent diminished plasma NE, urinary 3-methoxy-4-hydroxyphenylglycol (MHPG), cerebrospinal fluid (CSF), homovanillic acid, and CSF 5-hydroxyindoleacetic acid levels. Patients with

TABLE 10–1.
Medical Complications of Eating Disorders*

Organ/System	Anorexia Nervosa	Bulimia Nervosa
Dermatologic	Dry, pale, or yellow-tinged skin, hair loss, and lanugo	Calluses on dorsum of hand
HEENT	Dry mucous membranes if dehydrated	Painless parotid gland enlargement, dental caries, and erosion of dental enamel (due to acidity of stomach contents)
Pulmonary	...	Rare: aspiration pneumonia
Cardiovascular	ECG-low voltage, +/− NSSTT changes, bradycardia arrhythmias (SVT, AV blocks, and PVCs), LV atrophy (+/− decreased cardiac output), and orthostatic hypotension	ECG abnormalities and arrhythmias due to electrolyte disturbances, emetine-induced cardiomyopathy in ipecac abusers, and orthostatic hypotension
GI	Delayed gastric emptying (bloating), reduced intestinal motility (constipation), and elevated hepatic transaminase levels	Variable GI symptoms and signs (pain, constipation, diarrhea, hematemesis, rectal bleeding, rectal prolapse, rare gastric rupture, and esophagitis)

(Continued.)

TABLE 10-1 (cont.)

Renal	Diminished GFR, increased BUN and creatinine levels (due to dehydration and catabolic state), and renal calculi	Hypochloremic metabolic alkalosis
Electrolyte disturbances	Hypophosphatemia, hypokalemia, and hypomagnesemia	Hypokalemia, hyponatremia, and hypomagnesemia
Metabolic/endocrine	Hypercholesterolemia, hypoglycemia, hypercarotenemia, sick euthyroid (cold intolerance, bradycardia, constipation, and dry skin)	...
GYN	Amenorrhea, atrophy of vaginal mucosa, and dyspareunia	Amenorrhea or oligomenorrhea
Skeletal	Osteoporosis (compression fractures), (low serum estrogen level and low protein and calcium ingestion)	...

Hematologic	Bone marrow suppression, hypocellularity, anemia, leukopenia, and thrombocytopenia (rare)	...
Neurologic	Metabolic encephalopathies and delayed relaxation of DTRS	...
Neuroendocrine	See Section VI.	...

*HEENT = head, eyes, ears, nose, throat; ECG = electrocardiogram; + = positive; − = negative; NSSTT = nonspecific ST, T-wave changes; SVT = supraventricular tachycardia; AV = atrioventricular; PVCs = premature ventricular contractions; LV = left ventricular; GI = gastrointestinal; GFR = glomerular filtration rate; BUN = blood urea nitrogen; GYN = gynecologic; and DTRS = deep tendon reflexes.

TABLE 10-2.
Neuroendocrine Changes Associated With Eating Disorders*

Neuroendocrine System	Anorexia Nervosa	Bulimia Nervosa
A. Hypothalamic—pituitary—adrenal axis		
Cortisol: Morning plasma cortisol	—	N
Urinary-free cortisol	—	N
Metabolic clearance of cortisol	—	U
Urinary metabolites (17-hydroxycorticosteroids) (17-Ketosteroids)	R	U
Cortisol production rate	—	U
CSF corticotropin-releasing factor	—	U
Dexamethasone suppression test, failure to suppress cortisol adequately following 1 mg of dexamethasone	+	+/−
B. Hypothalamic—pituitary—gonadal axis		
Gonadotropins: serum LH and FSH	R or N	R or N
Loss of pulsatile secretion of LH	+	+/−
Serum estrogen	R	R or N
Serum testosterone	R	U
C. Hypothalamic—pituitary—thyroid axis		
T$_4$ and T$_3$	R or N	N
TSH	N	N

Eating Disorders

Reverse T₃	–	N
TRH stimulation test	R or N	R or N
D. GH		
Basal GH	I or N	N
E. PRL: serum PRL	R or N	–
Nocturnal rise in PRL	R	U
F. CSF vasopressin	I	U
G. Normal circadian rhythm of melatonin	+/–	+
H. Other neurophysiologic and endocrine systems		
Thermoregulation	R	N
Glucose and insulin metabolism		
Fasting glucose	+/–	N
Glucose tolerance test	R or N	N
Basal insulin	+/–	U
Insulin clearance	R	U
Insulin receptor sensitivity	–	U
Sleep patterns		
REM latency	R	N
Total sleep time	R	N
Stage 3 and 4 sleep	R	N

*I = increased; N = normal; U = unknown; R = reduced; CSF = cerebrospinal fluid; + = positive; – = negative; LH = luteinizing hormone; FSH = follicle-stimulating hormone; T_4 = thyroxine; T_3 = triiodothyronine; TSH = thyroid-stimulating hormone; TRH = thyrotropin-releasing hormone; GH = growth hormone; PRL = prolactin; and REM = rapid eye movement.

bulimia nervosa have lower plasma NE levels than normal controls. Long-term weight-recovered anorexics have diminished plasma MHPG, CSF MHPG, and CSF NE levels compared with controls. These findings may reflect a primary hypothalamic defect that contributes to the development of anorexia nervosa. This may also explain the persistent abnormal eating behavior and disturbed gonadotropin secretion in many weight-recovered anorexics. It has been suggested that binge eating may reflect a disruption in satiety mechanisms. Since 5-HT appears to decrease appetite (especially for carbohydrates) and play an important role in satiety mechanisms, bulimics may have diminished serotoninergic neurotransmission. The high frequency of affective illness in primary relatives of and in patients with bulimia nervosa and neuroendocrine disturbances similar to depressed patients, and the beneficial response to antidepressants, support theorizing a disturbance in 5-HT neurotransmission in bulimia nervosa.

B. **Endogenous opiate peptides (EOP).**

1. **Background.** The EOPs enhance food intake in a variety of animal models. Stress-induced hyperphagia in mice is opioid related. Starvation in rats increases the hypothalamic EOP dynorphin, a potent enhancer of feeding. Starvation also produces analgesia in rats. In humans, opioids enhance food intake, especially for highly palatable fatty foods. The EOPs modulate hypothalamic monoamine neurotransmitter systems that regulate mood, appetite, and many neuroendocrine functions.

2. **Relationship of EOPs to eating disorders.** Patients with anorexia nervosa have weight-dependent elevations in CSF EOP activity. Starvation, exercise, and elevated corticotropin-releasing factor are the proposed etiologies for increased CNS EOP activity. Opiates may contribute to the food craving in anorexia nervosa and to the binge eating in bulimia nervosa. Preliminary reports suggest opiate antagonists diminish binge-eating duration, frequency of binge-eating and

purging episodes, and the amount of food consumed in binges in subjects with bulimia nervosa. The EOPs are also believed to play a role in the abnormal gonadotropin secretion and menstrual disturbances in anorexia nervosa and bulimia nervosa. Theoretically, patients with eating disorders may become accustomed to high levels of CNS EOPs through patterns of dieting and weight loss. Starvation, bingeing, and purging may alter EOP levels that may perpetuate the pathologic eating behaviors.

VIII. Neurobiology of starvation.

A. Starvation in normal humans.

1. Starvation itself appears to play a major role in the pathogenesis of anorexia nervosa because prolonged starvation in normal volunteers causes the following physical signs and symptoms: amenorrhea, delayed gastric emptying that results in bloating, dyspepsia, and early satiety. These subjects develop hypotension, bradycardia, hypothermia, reduced sensitivity to pain, hair loss, and lanugo.

2. Behavioral and cognitive effects of long-term semistarvation.

a. Food-related behaviors: Increased preoccupation with food and increase in food-related dreams and thoughts. Subjects eat slower, have increased hunger, often remain hungry after eating, and may develop bulimic episodes. There are increased attempts to control appetite through the use of cigarettes and gum chewing and increased consumption of coffee and tea.

b. Affective symptoms: Irritability, anxiety, depression, apathy, mood lability, social withdrawal, and sleep disturbance.

c. Cognitive changes: Reduced attention and concentration abilities and indecisiveness.

3. Neuroendocrine changes associated with starvation.

a. HPA axis: Increased plasma cortisol level, nonsuppression of dexamethasone suppression test (DST), and decreased cortisol production rate.

b. HPO axis: Decreased serum LH level; loss of pulsatile LH secretion in >50% of subjects.

c. Catecholamines: Decreased plasma NE level; decreased urinary MHPG level.

d. Thyroid: Blunted thyrotropin-releasing hormone (TRH) stimulation test.

e. Growth hormone (GH): Increased GH secretion.

f. Prolactin (PRL): Loss of normal nocturnal rise in PRL level.

IX. **Relationship between eating disorders and affective disorders.**

A. **Background.** The high incidence of affective symptoms, FH of affective disorders, and neuroendocrine disturbances similar to those associated with depressive disorders have led many investigators to consider eating disorders as variants of affective disorders.

B. **Affective symptoms and family history.**

1. Anorexia nervosa: 35% to 55% have an affective illness (usually dysthymic or major depressive disorder); 30% have (+) FH of affective illness.

2. Bulimia nervosa: 30% to 80% have an affective illness; 60% have (+) FH of affective illness.

C. **Shared neuroendocrine disturbances.**

1. High incidence of abnormal DST in depression, anorexia nervosa, and bulimia nervosa.

2. Diminished GH response to insulin-induced hypoglycemia in both anorexia nervosa and depression.

3. Urinary MHPG level is reduced in both anorexia nervosa and depression. Urinary MHPG level increases

with weight gain and correlates with reduced depressive symptoms.

4. The TRH stimulation test is blunted in major depression and bulimia nervosa. In anorexia nervosa, TSH response to TRH is delayed.

5. The rapid eye movement latency is decreased in major depression and anorexia nervosa.

6. Response to antidepressants is favorable in depression, in a small percentage of patients with anorexia nervosa, and in a significant number of bulimics.

X. **Psychodynamic factors in the development of eating disorders.**

A. **Premorbid personality.**

1. Anorexia nervosa: Bright, polite, uptight, rigid, and high achievers strive for perfection; they are often precocious.

2. Bulimia nervosa: Egocentric, emotionally labile, impulsive, and dysthymic individuals; projective testing reveals narcissism, negativity, anger, feelings of being overwhelmed, and introversive-coping style.

B. **Psychodynamic theories.**

1. Anorexia nervosa.

a. Classic psychoanalytic perspective. Starvation serves as a defense against evolving female sexual development and the assumption of adult roles. Dieting and binge eating represent a phobic response to the anxiety created by the development of secondary sexual characteristics and menarche. The anorexic patient has fantasies of oral impregnation. Starvation serves as a means of rejecting the fantasy of becoming pregnant.

b. Self-psychologic perspective. Early empathic failures by mother and inadequate mirroring, result in development of false self and superficial precocious child. Overstimulating, eroticized father-daughter relationship develops as a compensatory response to inadequate mirroring by the mother. Oedipal conflict becomes intensified; father and daughter begin to separate. The daughter then uses starvation, exercise, and drive for perfection to maintain a sense of integrity and prevent fragmentation.

2. Bulimia nervosa. Early empathic disruptions and inadequate mirroring result in inadequate development of sense of self. Chronic empathic failures by parents and anxiety from life stressors reinforce feelings of emptiness and threaten sense of stability. Affects are experienced as threatening and are defended against through impulsive behavior. Food serves as an archaic self-object. Bulimic behavior serves to self-regulate affective states and feelings of emptiness in response to empathic failures and external stress.

C. **Family theories.**

1. Anorectic family: Restricted affect, with child as a narcissistic extension of parents.

2. Bulimic family: Labile affects; parents foster a dependent loyalty to family, creating powerful parents and helpless child.

3. Theory of Crisp: Anorexic child has a central role; carries family psychopathology. Adolescence is perceived as a threat to the family system.

4. Theory of Minuchin: Concept of psychosomatic families, i.e., "pathologically enmeshed transactional patterns." Four family characteristics that encourage somatization:

a. Enmeshment.

b. Overprotectiveness.

c. Rigidity.

d. Lack of conflict resolution. Symptomatic child becomes involved in parental conflicts through "triangulation" and protective "detouring." Sick child regulates family stability and reinforces the lack of conflict resolution.

5. Theory of Bruch: Conflict arises out of early feeding disruptions in mother-daughter dyad. Inappropriate maternal-feeding responses disrupt development of trust and create confusion and lack of confidence in self. False self develops as a superficial adaptation and need to please mother. Narcissistic injuries result in narcissistic rage toward a mother who is unable to tolerate this; therefore, child fails to express self and withdraws to perfectionism in attempt to gain control.

D. Proposed biopsychosocial model for anorexia nervosa (Figure 10–1).

XI. **Inpatient treatment of anorexia nervosa.**

A. **Criteria for hospitalization of patients with anorexia nervosa or bulimia nervosa.**

1. Suicidal behavior, severe depression, or psychosis.

2. Serious cardiac arrhythmias.

3. Electrolyte disturbances refractory to oral supplementation.

4. Progressive weight loss below 70% ideal weight.

5. Severe hypothermia or dehydration.

6. Bingeing/purging out of control.

7. Unremitting laxative abuse.

8. Family crisis.

B. **Assessment and medical stabilization.**

1. Physical examination and careful monitoring of vital signs and electrocardiographic (ECG) abnormalities.

2. Ensure adequate hydration.

3. Correct electrolyte disturbances (if hypokalemic, use potassium chloride).

4. If medically unstable due to hypotension, cardiac arrhythmias, and/or hypothermia, restrict to bed rest.

190 *Psychiatric Disorders*

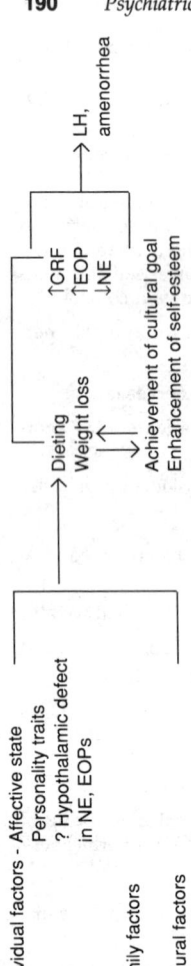
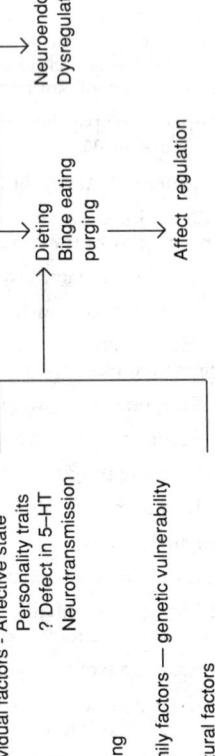

FIG 10–1.
Proposed biopsychosocial models for anorexia nervosa and bulimia nervosa. NE = norepinephrine; EOPs = endogenous opiate peptides; CRF = corticotropin-releasing factor; LH = luteinizing hormone; and 5-HT = 5-hydroxytryptamine (serotonin).

5. Psychiatric evaluation and psychologic testing.

6. Nutrition assessment and counseling.

7. Family assessment.

C. **Refeeding.**

1. Contract for an acceptable weight; aim for weight gain 1 to 2 lb during first week and 3 to 5 lb/wk subsequently.

2. Begin with 800 to 1,200 kcal/day in frequent small meals to avoid sensation of bloating.

3. Gradually increase intake to 1,800 to 3,000 kcal/day, depending on height and age.

4. Adjust composition of meals to provide nutritional balance while accommodating for patient's food preferences.

5. Liquid supplements to help achieve caloric goals.

6. Vitamin and mineral supplements, especially calcium (1,000 to 1,200 mg/day).

7. Soluble fibers from grain sources reduces constipation and promotes elimination.

8. Dairy products as tolerated (may be lactose intolerant due to starvation).

9. In severe cases, when adequate oral feeding is intolerable, begin total parenteral nutrition (TPN) at 800 to 1,200 kcal/day; gradually increase TPN to 1,800 to 3,000 kcal/day.

10. Limit caffeine intake.

D. **Refeeding complications and their treatment.**

1. Edema: Treat patient with leg elevation, support stockings, and salt restriction.

2. Abdominal distention and bloating: Reassure patient that this is expected and will resolve. If severe, give metoclopramide, 5 mg twice daily.

3. Congestive heart failure: Transfer patient to medical ward if necessary; treat with salt restriction and diuretics (inpatient use only due to abuse potential).

E. **Development of a behavioral treatment program.**

1. Set goals: Specific weight gain per week (reduction of food restriction, reduction of food preoccupations and food rituals, and limit ritualistic exercising).

2. Develop reward system to reinforce compliance with program.

3. Privileges contingent on meeting goals.

F. **Psychotherapy.**

1. **Individual psychodynamic.** In the early stages of treatment, development of a therapeutic alliance through empathic responses is essential. Resistance to the development of a therapeutic alliance is likely since the therapist is perceived as a threat to the anorexic's goal of thinness. As the relationship builds, an idealizing transference frequently develops. The patient is likely to display excessive compliance and extreme sensitivity to empathic failures by the therapist. This excessive compliance often can be understood in terms of the patient's submissive style as a means of pleasing parents through which she achieves a sense of wholeness. Empathic failures that stimulate the patient's narcissistic rage should not be interpreted early in treatment. Instead, empathic responses are appropriate and foster a self-object transference necessary for subsequent development of the self. Gradually, the therapist should help the patient become aware of her frustration and anger toward her unempathic parents. Slowly, there is internalization of the empathic self-object, allowing the therapist to interpret the patient's eating behavior, distortions, and narcissistic rage. Eventually, a more cohesive self develops, assertiveness is reinforced by the therapist, and the patient relies less on her abnormal eating behavior to deal with her world.

2. **Group therapy.** This therapy may be useful in

the treatment of anorexia nervosa by providing patients with an atmosphere where they can interrupt their experience of isolation through the group's shared symptoms. Group members develop relationships within the group, gradually allowing for the opportunity to deal with issues of trust, anger, and competition. Eventually, there is further exploration of feelings related to their symptom production. The risk of an unstructured group is the exchange of information on how to avoid weight gain and deceive their treatment team.

3. **Family therapy.** Various family therapies (structural, strategic, psychodynamic experiential, and family systems therapy) have been employed in the treatment of anorexia nervosa. There has been little formal study of the effectiveness of these treatments. Patients with onset of illness before the age of 18 years and duration less than 3 years appear most responsive to family therapy. In general, treatments that promote family differentiation and patient autonomy may be beneficial in anorexia nervosa.

G. **Adjunctive therapies.**

1. Impulse control program, i.e., relaxation training.

2. Assertiveness training.

3. Art therapy.

H. **Psychotropic medications.** The medications discussed below may have adjunctive uses in patients with anorexia nervosa.

1. **Antidepressants.** In patients with anorexia, most controlled studies have failed to show significant differences between tricyclic antidepressants (TCAs) and placebo. Some patients have shown a significant response to desipramine, imipramine, or amitriptyline with respect to improvement in weight gain and depressive symptoms. Monoamine oxidase inhibitors (MAOIs) and lithium have also been reported beneficial in the treatment of patients with anorexia nervosa. Antidepressants should be administered cautiously after

correction of hypotension and electrolyte and ECG abnormalities. Begin with a low dosage, i.e., desipramine (25 mg), and gradually increase dosage to 150 to 250 mg/day, monitoring closely for adverse effects. Many patients with anorexia nervosa reach therapeutic or toxic TCA levels at low dosages; therefore, monitoring TCA blood levels is indicated.

2. **Cyproheptadine.** This serotonin and histamine antagonist mildly enhances weight gain and reduces depressive symptoms in patients with anorexia nervosa when administered in high doses, i.e., 32 mg/day.

3. **Opiate antagonists.** Although double-blind placebo-controlled studies have not been reported, several recent case reports document improvement in weight gain with administration of naltrexone in dosages of 50 to 150 mg/day. Naltrexone is an attractive agent due to its minimal side effects.

4. **Phenothiazines.** Reduction in agitation and the delusional components of anorexia nervosa may be achieved through the use of phenothiazines. One should obviously consider the potentially serious risks of these agents vs. their potential benefits.

XII. **Inpatient treatment of bulimia nervosa.**

A. Criteria for hospitalization (see Section XI./A.).

B. Assessment and medical stabilization (see Section XI./B.).

C. Construct behavioral treatment program to interrupt bulimic behaviors; introduce normal-eating behaviors and cognitive restructuring (Table 10–3).

D. **Psychotherapy.**

1. **Individual.** Several studies have demonstrated cognitive behavior therapy superior to brief psychodynamic therapy or no therapy.

a. Cognitive behavior therapy.

Stage 1: Interruption of binge eating, vomiting, and

laxative abuse; introduce normal eating habits; develop awareness of affects leading to bulimic behavior; education regarding consequences of bingeing, vomiting, and laxative abuse; detailed self-monitoring, i.e., recording of diet, purging behaviors, and affective states leading to bulimic behavior.

Stage 2: Identification and examination of dysfunctional thought and responses to internal and external stimuli that result in bulimic behavior.

Stage 3: Maintain changes; preparation for future stressors.

b. Psychodynamic therapies.

2. **Group therapy.** As in the treatment of anorexia nervosa, several approaches to group therapy in the treatment of bulimia nervosa may be beneficial. These approaches include cognitive behavior, insight oriented, psychodynamic, experiential-behavioral, supportive, and self-help.

3. Family therapy (see Section XI./F./3.).

E. **Adjunctive therapies** (see Section XI./G.).

F. **Psychotropic medications.**

1. **Antidepressants.** The rationale for the treatment of bulimia nervosa with antidepressants stems from the high frequency of coexisting depressive symptoms, major depressive disorder, and other evidence, suggesting a relationship between bulimia nervosa and affective illness (see Section IX.). In addition, bulimics have a high frequency of coexisting generalized anxiety disorder (+/− panic attacks), which is often responsive to treatment with TCAs. In controlled trials, the TCAs imipramine and desipramine are more effective in reducing bulimic behavior and depressive symptoms than placebo. Desipramine appears to be particularly effective in reducing bingeing and purging even in patients without coexisting major affective illness. As in the treatment of anorexia nervosa, TCAs should be admin-

TABLE 10–3.
Inpatient Treatment Program for Bulimia (4 to 6 Weeks)*

	Goals	Strategies
Initial phase: abstinence (1-2 wk)	Response prevention, meal regularization, and staff monitoring of caloric intake	Close observation, active social support, unit restrictions, and food restriction except at mealtimes
Intermediate phase: inoculation (1-2 wk)	Stress inoculation (exposure in vivo) and weight maintenance	Relaxation of bathroom restriction, short passes and low stress, group and individual psychotherapy and family therapy
	Cognitive restructuring	Eating disorders milieu, monitoring of surreptitious binge eating or vomiting (active surveillance and amylase and electrolytes), and aerobics program

Termination phase: Outpatient transition (1-2 wk)	Transition to outpatient setting, weight maintenance off hospital diet, and maintenance of abstinence	Complete relaxation of bathroom restrictions, food preparation on the unit, longer passes (overnight), surveillance and physiologic monitoring, and continuation and intensification of psychotherapy (encouragement to express feelings, allow patients to share difficulties concerning adherence, and problem solving around life skills)

*From Kaye WH, Gwirstman HE: The Treatment of Normal Weight Bulimia. Washington, DC, American Psychiatric Press, 1985. Used with permission.

istered after correction of any electrolyte and ECG abnormalities, and with careful attention to side effects. The MAOIs also appear to be promising in the treatment of bulimia nervosa; phenelzine (60 to 90 mg/day) in one double-blind study was superior to placebo in reducing bulimic symptoms. Hypotension may preclude adequate dosing. Hypertensive reactions secondary to consumption of tyramine-containing foods may be serious in an impulsive bulimic patient on an MAOI. The new antidepressant fluoxetine hydrochloride, a specific 5-HT uptake inhibitor, may also reduce bulimic symptoms although no placebo-controlled studies have been published to date. Preliminary reports suggest that lithium may also benefit some bulimic patients.

2. **Anticonvulsants.** Both phenytoin and carbamazepine appear to reduce bulimic symptoms.

3. **Opiate antagonists.** Although long-term placebo-controlled studies are pending, preliminary reports suggest the opiate antagonist naltrexone reduces bingeing and purging in bulimic subjects.

XIII. **Prognosis and outcome.**

A. **Prognosis.**

1. Favorable prognostic indicators in anorexia nervosa.

a. Earlier age at onset, especially <17 years.

b. Return to normal menses.

c. Good premorbid school and work history.

d. Professional occupation.

2. Negative prognostic indicators in anorexia nervosa.

a. Late onset or chronic stage of illness at first presentation.

b. Large number of hospitalizations and treatment failures.

c. Male prognosis is often worse than female; more serious underlying psychopathology common in males.

d. Lower socioeconomic status.

e. Presence of bulimia in addition to anorexia nervosa.

f. History of premorbid obesity.

g. Presence of serious psychopathology in parents.

h. High-negative expressed emotion in family.

B. **Outcome.**

1. Problems that assess outcome of inpatients with anorexia nervosa and bulimia nervosa: High variability of outcome between studies.

a. The majority of studies are retrospective, depend on accuracy of medical records, and have significant problems with locating all patients for follow-up.

b. Diagnostic criteria have varied (especially for bulimia); criteria for determining improvement and recovery have been inconsistent.

c. Duration and method of follow-up have varied.

2. Outcome data: anorexia nervosa.

a. Status at follow-up.

(i) Recovered: 40% to 50%.

(ii) Improved: 20% to 30%.

(iii) Unimproved: 20% to 30%.

(iv) Mortality: 5% to 18%.

b. Serious morbidity due to chronic anorexia nervosa, depression, phobias, and medical complications: 30% to 40%.

c. Maintenance of dietary restrictions and/or anxiety associated with eating and body image distortions: 40% to 50%.

d. Bulimic symptoms: 20% to 40%.

e. Normal eating behavior: 35%.

f. Menstrual irregularity or amenorrhea: 25% to 50%.

g. Persisting depressive symptoms: 25% to 45%.

h. Social phobias: 10% to 40%.

i. Obsessive-compulsive symptoms: 10% to 20%.

j. Relationships: 70% recovered anorectics marry; 30% unimproved anorectics marry; 20% to 25% avoid heterosexual relationships, especially those with low body weight; and 40% to 50% maintain persistent hostile dependency on family.

3. Outcome in bulimia nervosa.

a. Outcome in bulimia nervosa is difficult to assess due to changes in diagnostic criteria for bulimia during the past several years, few studies in the literature, and the heterogeneity of treatments that patients have received.

b. Status at follow-up (2 to 5 years).

(i) Recovered: 30% to 40%.

(ii) Improved: 15% to 30%.

(iii) Unimproved: 20% to 40%.

c. Lifetime prevalence of associated Axis I disorders.

(i) Affective disorders: 70%.

(ii) Obsessive-compulsive disorder: 35%.

(iii) Panic disorder with or without agoraphobia: 15% to 25%.

(iv) Substance use disorders: 30% to 40%.

XIV. **Pica.**

A. *DSM III-R* **classification: diagnostic criteria for 307.52 pica.**

1. Repeated eating of a non-nutritive substance for at least 1 month.

2. Does not meet the criteria for either autistic disorder, schizophrenia, or Kleine-Levin syndrome.

B. **Epidemiology.** Prevalence, 27% to 55% pregnant women; 10% to 32% children under the age of 6 years. Age at onset, usually 1 to 2 years. Approximate equal frequency of male and female children. In children, the prevalence decreases with increasing age.

C. **Clinical features.** Ingested substances, e.g., dirt, clay, paint chips, plaster, paper, starch, hair, and/or stones. In children, pica most often resolves spontaneously with early adolescence and rarely persists. In pregnant women, pica usually resolves following termination of pregnancy.

D. **Evaluation.** Psychologic evaluation of child and family; evaluation of home environment. Careful medical evaluation, including metabolic screening.

E. **Medical complications.** Lead poisoning from ingestion of paint and plaster; intestinal parasites from ingestion of contaminated soil; and intestinal obstruction related to ingestion of hair, stones, etc.

F. **Etiologic theories.**

1. Through ingestion of non-nutritive substances, child attempts to correct for specific metabolic or mineral deficiencies.

2. Ingestion of these substances is an attempt to fulfill unmet oral needs related to maternal deprivation.

3. Child reacts to environmental deprivation or child abuse.

G. **Treatment.** Family counseling and behavioral therapies are most useful.

XV. **Rumination disorder of infancy.**

A. **DSM III-R classification: Diagnostic criteria for 307.53 rumination disorder of infancy.**

1. Repeated regurgitation, without nausea or associated gastrointestinal illness, for at least 1 month following a period of normal functioning.

2. Weight loss or failure to make expected weight gain.

B. **Epidemiology.** Prevalence, rare. Age at onset, 3 to 12 months of age. Approximate equal frequency of males and females.

C. **Clinical features.** Child appears to strain and take a characteristic position with arched back. Food is then brought into mouth, ejected, or chewed and reswallowed. There may be associated head banging, head rocking, or hair pulling. Infants are usually brought to medical attention due to failure to thrive or parents' concern about failing to feed the child properly.

D. **Differential diagnosis.** Pyloric stenosis and congenital anomalies of the gastrointestinal (GI) tract.

E. **Etiologic theories.**

1. Defect in autonomic nerves of GI tract.

2. Gastroesophageal reflux secondary to incompetent sphincter or hiatal hernia.

3. Disturbance in early maternal-infant relationship results in inadequate oral gratification. Rumination allows oral needs to be gratified.

F. **Complications.** Malnutrition, dehydration, and death in up to 25% cases. Interruption of early parent-child relationship due to parents' sense of failure at feeding.

G. **Management.** Careful medical evaluation; behavior therapy techniques.

REFERENCES

1. Kaye WH, Gwirtsman HE: *The Treatment of Normal Weight Bulimia*. Washington, DC, American Psychiatric Press, Inc, 1985.

11 Factitious and Somatoform Disorders

I. **Introduction.** Somatization, as opposed to somatization disorder, is best conceptualized as a symptom by which a patient communicates distress. The use of this mode of expression is multifaceted, however, and in addition to being a signal flare for help, this symptom can serve as a vehicle for having dependency needs met, for asserting one's autonomy, for avoiding psychologic or social pain or obligations, or for communicating feelings of fear, anger, or sadness.

Understandably, somatization is neither unique to certain psychiatric disorders nor to psychiatric illness in general. The transient hypochondriasis that follows an acute myocardial infarction, for example, is considered normal behavior. Thus, somatization as a symptom represents a continuum of illness behavior from normal to pathologic.

Pathologic illness behavior or disorders of somatization occur when that behavior interferes with normal occupational or social function. A number of such disorders have been described and are distinguished below.

II. **Somatization disorder.**

A. **Diagnostic criteria.**

1. Thirteen of 35 multisystemic physical symptoms

of sufficient severity to have required a physician visit, alteration of life pattern, or the need for prescription medication (see *DSM III-R* for details).

a. Two or more of the following seven screening symptoms suggest a high likelihood of occurrence (Table 11–1).

TABLE 11–1.

Mnemonic for Seven Screening Symptoms of Somatization Disorder

<u>S</u>omatization	<u>D</u>isorder	<u>B</u>esets	<u>L</u>adies	<u>A</u>nd	<u>V</u>exes	<u>P</u>hysicians
H	Y	U	U	M	O	A
O	S	R	M	N	M	I
R	M	N	P	E	I	N
T	E	I		S	T	F
N	N	N	I	I	I	U
E	O	G	N	A	N	L
S	R				G	
S	R	S	T			E
	H	E	H			X
O	E	X	R			T
F	A		O			R
		O	A			E
B		R	T			M
R		G				I
E		A				T
A		N				I
T		S				E
H						S

(i) Vomiting (other than during pregnancy).

(ii) Pain in extremities.

(iii) Shortness of breath at rest.

(iv) Amnesia.

(v) Difficulty in swallowing.

(vi) Burning sensation in sexual organs.

(vii) Painful menstruation.

2. Onset before third decade.

B. **Age/gender distribution/incidence/prevalence.**

1. Typical onset during adolescence.

2. Much greater incidence in females, with 1% to 2% of entire female population afflicted by some estimates.

3. More common in lower socioeconomic strata.

C. **Clinical features.**

1. Chronic/relapsing course.

2. Increased number of surgical procedures.

3. Anxiety/depression reported.

4. Suicide threats and occupational and marital instability.

5. Antisocial and histrionic personality disorders.

6. Hysterical cognitive style.

7. Alcohol or substance abuse.

8. Family history of antisocial personality disorder and/or alcohol or substance abuse.

D. **Theoretical features.**

1. Symptoms are not under voluntary control.

2. Somatization is a female correlate of antisocial personality disorder in males.

3. Symptoms communicate emotion or need for care.

E. **Differential diagnosis.**

1. Panic disorder.

2. Hypochondriasis.

3. Major depressive episode.

4. Other somatoform disorder.

F. **Treatment considerations.**

1. Long-term, stable relationship with physician-manager.

2. Minimization of medications.

3. Regular office visits and preferential reliance on physical examination rather than diagnostic tests.

III. **Conversion disorder.**

A. **Diagnostic criteria.**

1. Presentation with a physical symptom that does not derive from any known or identifiable organic disease.

B. **Age/gender/incidence/prevalence.**

1. Onset in early childhood to ninth decade.

2. Greater representation in females than males, with lifetime incidence of up to one third of normal women. Prevalence of 15 to 22/100,000 females and of 5% to 14% of all psychiatric consultations.

3. Youngest person in sibship more likely to be affected.

4. Higher prevalence among lower socioeconomic strata and in rural populations.

C. **Clinical features.**

1. Presence of precipitating stressor and sudden symptom onset.

2. Hysterical, passive-dependent personalities.

3. Increased suggestibility and field dependency.

4. Impairment of recent memory, vigilance, and attention on psychologic testing.

5. Drug and alcohol abuse.

6. La belle indifférence (minimization of symptom gravity).

7. Family history of conversion or somatization.

8. History of cerebral organic disease.

9. History of prior conversion symptoms.

10. Sexual disturbance.

11. Model for the symptom.

D. **Theoretical features.**

1. Symptoms are not under voluntary control.

2. Symptom choice serves primary gain.

3. Secondary gain serves to reinforce need for symptom.

4. Symptoms result from repression of anxiety.

5. Symptoms are the distillation of unconscious conflict.

6. "Conversion" as a diagnosis is questioned by many who view this as symptomatic of other psychopathology.

E. **Differential diagnosis.**

1. Central nervous system disorder.

2. Depression.

3. Anxiety disorder.

4. Somatization disorder.

5. Schizophrenia.

F. **Treatment considerations.**

1. Favorable prognosis is associated with:

a. Acute onset.

b. Identifiable stressor.

c. Good premorbid function.

d. Absence of organic disease or major psychiatric syndrome.

2. Multiplicity of treatment approaches include:

a. Catharsis.

b. Brief insight-oriented psychotherapy.

c. Suggestion (hypnosis/amobarbital [Amytal]).

d. Behavior therapy.

3. Confrontation with the psychologic nature of symptoms is rarely helpful and may make the establishment of rapport difficult.

IV. **Hypochondriasis.**

A. **Diagnostic criteria.**

1. Unrealistic or exaggerated interpretation of physical symptoms as abnormal in the absence of evident disease, of at least 6 months' duration.

2. This unrealistic fear persists despite repeated medical reassurance, but it is not of delusional intensity.

3. Primary hypochondriasis is distinguished from secondary hypochondriasis wherein anxiety or depression is present to a significant degree and believed to be causal, e.g., somatized depression or somatized anxiety.

B. **Age/gender/incidence/prevalence.**

1. Average age at onset in fourth or fifth decade.

2. Equal representation in males and females.

Factitious and Somatoform Disorders

3. Three percent to 13% of patients in general medical practice are affected.

C. **Clinical features.**

1. Obsessional worry/obsessional cognitive style.

2. Narcissistic/masochistic traits.

3. Depression often present.

D. **Theoretical features.**

1. Symptoms are not under voluntary control.

2. Symptoms derivate from aggressive or oral drives.

3. Symptoms serve as a defense against guilt or diminished self-esteem.

4. Symptoms represent the cognitive misinterpretation of amplified somatic sensations.

5. Patients seek interpersonal rewards for illness behavior (secondary gain).

6. Countertransference anger common.

E. **Differential diagnosis.**

1. Major depressive episode.

2. Physical illness.

3. Schizophrenia (somatic delusions are often vivid/bizarre).

4. Delusional disorder, somatic type.

F. **Treatment considerations.**

1. Ongoing relationship with physician-manager.

2. Regular office visits regardless of symptoms.

3. Encourage affective expression.

4. Group therapy.

V. **Psychogenic pain.**

A. **Diagnostic criteria.**

1. Presentation with severe and prolonged pain that is inconsistent with identifiable disease.

2. Psychologic factors seem to be responsible for the onset or perpetuation of pain.

B. **Age/gender/incidence/prevalence.**

1. Onset in adolescence or early adulthood.

2. Female preponderance.

C. **Clinical features.**

1. Addiction to analgesics and/or sedatives.

2. Alexithymia.

3. Obsessive focus on pain.

4. Pain related to chronic stress, loss, or other environmental stimulus.

D. **Theoretical features.**

1. Ego deficit in experience or expression of feelings.

E. **Differential diagnosis.**

1. Anxiety disorder.

2. Major depressive episode.

3. Schizophrenia.

F. **Treatment considerations.**

1. Depressed subgroup responsive to antidepressant medication.

2. Systems approach valuable (inclusive of family and significant of others).

3. Ongoing stable, trusting relationship with physician.

VI. **Factitious disorders.**

A. **Diagnostic criteria.**

1. Production of psychologic or physical symptoms under patient's control that is not explicable by the presence of another mental disorder.

2. Pseudologia fantastica (pathologic lies of self-aggrandizement) and peregrination (wandering) are necessary, in addition to simulation of illness, for the diagnosis of Munchausen syndrome.

B. **Clinical features.**

1. Character disorders, including histrionic, borderline, masochistic, and antisocial.

2. History of employment in health care is common.

3. Peregrination.

4. Pseudologia fantastica.

5. Approximate answers in patients simulating psychologic illness (Ganser syndrome).

6. Early contact with disease, death, and physicians/institutionalization.

7. Chaotic home environment.

8. Against-medical-advice discharges common.

9. Symptoms increase with observation.

10. History of organic disease common.

D. **Theoretical features.**

1. Symptoms are voluntarily produced to assume the patient role irrespective of secondary gain.

2. Patients are unaware of the underlying motive for their deception.

3. Patients have an inability to express affect; pregenital anger is acted out in the deception of physicians.

4. Noncompliance and self-mutilation may be considered variants of factitious illness.

E. **Differential diagnosis.**

1. Somatization disorder.

2. Malingering.

3. Character disorder.

4. Schizophrenia.

5. Organic disease.

F. **Treatment considerations.**

1. Noncondemning confrontation with clinical data coupled with expressed wish to help.

2. Patients rarely stay for treatment following the discovery of the factitious nature of their symptoms.

3. Therapeutic alliance.

4. Supportive, regular physician visits.

VII. **Malingering.**

A. **Diagnostic criteria.**

1. Voluntary production of physical or psychologic symptoms with an obvious and recognizable goal or purpose.

B. **Age/gender/incidence/prevalence.**

1. No information.

C. **Clinical features.**

1. Litigation pending.

2. Alcohol/drug abuse.

3. Antisocial, borderline, and/or histrionic personality disorders.

4. Self-mutilation by compliance, with extensive diagnostic workup, is unlikely.

D. **Theoretical features.**

1. Symptoms are an adaptive means of coping.

2. The diagnosis, which is an accusation, increases the likelihood of negative countertransference.

E. **Differential diagnosis.**

1. Factitious disorder.

2. Character disorder.

3. Physical illness.

F. **Treatment considerations.**

1. Symptoms resolve with resolution of external situation; little information exists regarding successful treatment.

VIII. **Somatized depression/anxiety.**

A. **Diagnostic criteria.**

1. Presenting complaints are somatic; however, evidence of vegetative symptoms of depression are present (e.g., insomnia, fatigue, anorexia, diurnal mood variation, and diminished libido). For somatized anxiety, symptoms consistent with autonomic excitement are predominant (tachycardia, flushing, dizziness, shortness of breath, etc.).

B. **Age/gender/incidence/prevalence.**

1. Probably similar to depression/anxiety disorders.

C. **Clinical features.**

1. Family history of affective disorder/anxiety disorder.

2. Prior episodes of depression/anxiety disorder.

3. Periodicity.

4. Symptoms are attributable to depression/anxiety (above).

D. **Theoretical features.**

1. Alexithymia results in preferential use of somatization to express symptoms.

2. Social/cultural factors influence presentation of depression or anxiety.

E. **Differential diagnosis.**

1. Somatization.

2. Organic disease.

F. **Treatment considerations.**
   1. Pharmacotherapy for depression/anxiety.
   2. Psychotherapy (encourage affective expression).

12 | Dissociative Disorders (or Hysterical Neuroses, Dissociative Type)

Early psychoanalytic investigators focused extensively on the study of hysteria, out of which grew the concept of dissociation. Pierre Janet is credited with introducing the concept of dissociation of consciousness in the late 1800s and building on the observations of Jean Charcot. Janet's conceptualization was further extended by the contributions of Morton Prince in his classic study of a case with multiple personalities. Although psychiatric interest in these disorders waned for a number of years, there has been a rejuvenation of interest recently with a number of publications that focus on dissociative disorders, particularly multiple personality disorder (MPD). Areas of contemporary investigation include the relationship between hypnotic phenomena and these disorders, and the role of trauma as an etiologic component in their development. The inter-relationship among the symptoms manifest in post-traumatic stress disorders, and that present in dissociative disorders is another area of promising inquiry. As current researchers "rediscover" the phenomena extensively described by early psychoanalytic investigators, important links may develop in our understanding of the relationships between the biologic foundations of psychiatry and psychodynamic theory.

In *DSM III-R*, the following five separate diagnoses are subsumed under the category of dissociative disorders[1]:

1. MPD

2. Psychogenic fugue

3. Psychogenic amnesia

4. Depersonalization disorder

5. Dissociative disorder not otherwise specified.

As described in *DSM III-R*, the essential feature of these disorders is a disturbance or alteration in the normally integrative functions of identity, memory, or consciousness. This leads to the presence of behaviors that are disconnected from the patient's usual actions and identity and may be outside of his/her awareness as well. The onset of the disturbance or alteration can be sudden or gradual, and its duration can be transient or chronic. *DSM III-R* deviates somewhat from previous classification systems in which fugue states, amnesia, somnambulism, and multiple personality were considered to be the four classic dissociative reactions. Somnambulism, now called sleepwalking disorder, is classified among the sleep disorders, and depersonalization disorder, in which the feeling of one's own reality is lost, is now included within the dissociative disorders.

Since the majority of the recent literature on dissociative disorders has focused on MPD and comparatively little is known about the other dissociative disorders, this chapter will concentrate primarily on MPD and will limit discussion of the other dissociative disorders to a brief description of their salient features. Psychogenic fugue and psychogenic amnesia share many elements with MPD, and their treatment is similar. The relationship between depersonalization disorders is not well elucidated.

PSYCHOGENIC FUGUE

This disorder is characterized by a sudden, unexpected flight from home or work and the assumption of a new identity, with an inability to recall one's previous identity, as well as no awareness that there was a previous identity. After the fugue ends, there is no recollection of the events that took place during the fugue. During the fugue state, the patient's behavior typically does not appear in any way abnormal, although it may be uncharacteristic for him/her. In rarer instances, outbursts of violent behavior have been known to occur during episodes of fugue.

There is relatively little information available about this disorder; sex ratio and familial distribution are not known. It is rarely diagnosed, although it is more frequently seen in times of war and natural disaster. Severe psychologic stress frequently precedes its development. Heavy alcohol use may be a predisposing factor in some instances. The age at onset is variable, and the course is usually of a brief duration although it may continue for many months in rare instances.

The differential diagnoses include MPD, psychogenic amnesia, and temporal lobe epilepsy. In MPD, the shifts in identity are recurrent, whereas fugue episodes are classically limited to a single occurrence. In psychogenic amnesia, there is an inability to recall elements of one's history, including one's identity; however, unexpected travel and the assumption of a new identity do not occur. In temporal lobe epilepsy, there is no assumption of a new identity, and psychologic stress is not a precipitating factor.

DSM III-R diagnostic criteria are as follows: (1) The predominant disturbance is sudden, unexpected travel away from one's home or customary place of work, with inability to recall one's past. (2) Assumption of a new identity is partial or complete. (3) The disturbance is not due to MPD or to an organic mental disorder (e.g., partial complex seizures in temporal lobe epilepsy).

PSYCHOGENIC AMNESIA

In psychogenic amnesia, the patient experiences a sudden inability to recall important personal information. In this disorder, there are four types of disturbance in memory that can occur. In localized (or circumscribed) amnesia, the most frequent type, there is amnesia for a circumscribed period of time, often the hours following an extremely stressful life event. In selective amnesia, there is a failure of recall for some but not all of the events that occurred during a circumscribed period of time. The least common types of amnesia are the generalized type in which the patient's entire past life is forgotten and continuous amnesia in which events cannot be recalled subsequent to a specific time up to and including the present.

Associated features include a puzzling indifference to the memory disturbance and the coexistence of posttraumatic stress disorder. It is most common in young females, but it also frequently occurs in young men during war. The onset of the amnesia is sudden and usually follows severe psychologic stress, often involving the threat of physical injury or death. The prevalence of psychogenic amnesia also increases during periods of natural disaster and war.

The differential diagnoses include MPD and organic mental disorder. In MPD, the amnestic periods correspond to periods when another personality has taken control of the person's behavior. The amnestic period is circumscribed and tends to be recurrent. The memory loss in psychogenic amnesia differs from that seen in blackouts secondary to psychoactive substance-induced intoxication, in that following a "blackout," there is a failure to regain full memory for the event. In alcohol amnestic disorder, there is a loss of short-term rather than immediate memory. Postconcussive amnesia most frequently involves retrograde amnesia, involving events preceding the trauma, whereas psychogenic amnesia is usually anterograde. Prompt recovery of the memories through hypnosis or amobarbital (Amytal) interview suggests a dissociative rather than an organic basis for the amnesia.

DSM III-R diagnostic criteria are as follows: (1) The predominant disturbance is an episode of sudden inability to recall important personal information that is too extensive to be explained by ordinary forgetfulness. (2) The disturbance is not due to MPD or to an organic mental disorder.

DEPERSONALIZATION DISORDER

In this disorder, the patient experiences a recurrent or persistent alteration in his/her experience of self, such that his/her sense of his/her own reality is temporarily lost. He/she may experience a sense of estrangement from his/her self, body, or surroundings. Patients may report that they feel like automatons or as if they were in a dream. Experiences of sensory anesthesia or not being in control of one's own speech or actions commonly occur. The patient is distressed by this alteration in perception and maintains intact reality testing. This diagnosis is not made if the symptom of depersonalization is secondary to another mental disorder, such as agoraphobia or panic disorder.

Associated features include derealization in which one's sense of the reality of the external world is altered. Symptoms of dizziness, depression, obsessive rumination, somatic concerns, anxiety, fear of going insane, and a disturbance in the subjective sense of time commonly occur. The onset of this disorder is usually in adolescence or young adulthood. Symptoms appear rapidly and diminish gradually. The course is chronic, with remissions and exacerbations often precipitated by mild anxiety or depression. Severe psychologic stress may predispose an individual to depersonalization disorder. Single brief episodes of depersonalization may occur in many people and should be differentiated from depersonalization disorder in which persistent and recurrent episodes cause significant distress.

The differential diagnoses include symptoms of depersonalization without significant social or occupational impairment. Depersonalization can occur in MPD, schizophrenia, mood disorders, especially intoxication, withdrawal, and epilepsy.

DSM III-R diagnostic criteria are as follows: (1) Persistent or recurrent experiences of depersonalization are indicated by (a) an experience of feeling detached from, and as if one is an outside observer of, one's mental processes or body, or (b) an experience of feeling like an automaton or as if in a dream. (2) During the depersonalization experience, reality testing remains intact. (3) The depersonalization is sufficiently severe and persistent to cause marked distress. (4) The depersonalization experience is the predominant disturbance and is not a symptom of another disorder, such as schizophrenia, panic disorder, or agoraphobia without a symptom of panic disorder but with limited symptom attacks of depersonalization, or temporal lobe epilepsy.

MPD

Multiple personality disorder is a chronic, complex, dissociative disorder in which the essential features are characterized in *DSM III-R* as the existence within a person of two or more distinct personalities or personality states, at least two of which recurrently take full control of that person's behavior. The different personalities, or alternate personalities, may each have their own complex social patterns and distinguishing behavioral characteristics.[1] Putnam et al.[2] observed, "The existence of multiple amnestic episodes, together with the presence of alternating separate and distinct identities, distinguishes multiple personality disorder from all other psychiatric syndromes."

Clinical Presentation

The classic MPD case description in which there are at least two fully developed personalities, with each having separate and distinct memories, behavior patterns, and social relationships, is one possible presentation of this disorder. As our knowledge and understanding of this disorder have grown in recent years, variations on this classic presentation have been recognized as occurring with some frequency. There may be only one distinct personality and one or more personality states, and there are variations in the degree to which memories, behavior patterns, and social relationships are shared among the differing personalities and personality states in a given individual. The alternate personalities often have different names, or failing that, may distinguish themselves by descriptive adjectives or numbers that have been attached to their names. Thus, the individual personalities in a system of alternate personalities may each introduce herself as "Jane"; however, the alert clinician discovers on inquiry that there is a Jane no. 1, and a Jane no. 2, a "main Jane," and a "Jane the pain."

The alternate personalities often exist within an internal structural framework that varies from simple groupings according to age, sex, function, shared memories, etc., to elaborate dynastic labyrinths of amazing complexity. There can be differing degrees of shared memory, communication, cooperation, and feeling among, across, and between these internal groupings.

In a review of 100 cases of MPD by Putnam et al.[3] in 1986, the numbers of alternate personalities ranged from 1 to 60, the mean number of personalities for each patient was 13.3, the median was 9, and the mode was 3. Cases of extreme complexity in which there are 100 or more alternate personalities have been reported.

In Putnam and colleagues'[3] case review, the most common alternate personalities were children (85% of the cases), and alternate personalities who reported themselves to be of a gender opposite to that of the biologic sex of the patient were found in 53% of the cases. In 68% of the cases, the personality that presented for treatment was unaware of the existence of other personalities. In 86% of the cases, there were alternate personalities that claimed to be aware of all of the other alternate personalities.

Episodes of amnesia often described as periods of "time loss" are an integral part of this disorder. Patients may not report this symptom, however, for fear of being perceived as "crazy." In Putnam and associates'[3] case review, episodes of amnesia were reported in 98% of the patients.

Associated Features

Several studies describe the typical presentation of MPD as polysymptomatic, in which the symptoms of MPD are hidden, and another more commonplace diagnosis is suggested. Symptoms of depression and anxiety, somatoform symptoms, self-destructive behaviors, phobias, hallucinations, and schneiderian first-rank symptoms are commonly found.[3-9] Putnam et al.[2] suggested that with such a plethora of manifestations suggesting other conditions, it is practical to consider MPD as a superordinate diagnosis.

The frequent experience that patients with MPD have, of hearing the alternate personalities in the form of voices talking to them or conducting conversations inside their head, has often misled clinicians into assuming the presence of a psychotic process in these patients.

Often, patients with MPD also meet diagnostic criteria for post-traumatic stress disorder.[1, 10-12]

Diagnostic Assessment

Given the complex presentation of this disorder and the frequency of symptom constellations suggestive of other conditions, the period from the initial mental health system contact to the diagnosis of MPD is frequently delayed, and patients with MPD have often received a number of prior diagnoses before the diagnosis of MPD is made.[3] In light of this, it is prudent to consider the possibility of this diagnosis in any patient who has been a diagnostic dilemma over time, receiving a number of different diagnoses and responding little to standard psychiatric treatment.

The typical patient with MPD exhibits symptoms that are hidden and subtle, unlike the multimedia depictions of patients with this condition. Patients often do not volunteer information about periods of amnesia and time loss, hallucinated voices, etc., unless these experiences are specifically inquired about.

Systematic inquiry should be carried out by finding oneself in a location with no recollection of going there, finding clothing or other objects in the home for which there is no recollection of buying, and finding material that is written in a different handwriting or has a content that is foreign to the individual. Passive influence experiences can occur in which some part of the body can appear to behavior autonomously, outside of the personal conscious control. A patient described this as follows: "I don't like that brand of cereal, yet, while I was shopping my hand seemed to reach up on its own and throw it in the cart. I knew I had better just go ahead and get it at that point."

A patient should be asked about accusations of lying or being told of behavior that he/she does not remember, as well as perplexing encounters in which a person seems to recognize the patient but calls him/her by a different name, and he/she has no recollection of meeting that person previously. There may also be reports of surprise at the presence, absence, or variability of knowledge, skills, etc., that have occurred at different times. A patient who is usually right-handed may find himself/herself playing a sport left-handed or may find himself/herself playing a musical piece with an unrecalled expertise.

Often taking a systematic and exhaustive life history from early childhood to the present, including events at home, school, etc., can reveal periods for which there is little or no memory or marked inconsistencies in memory.

Bernstein and Putnam[13] have developed a dissociation scale that can be useful as a screening tool in evaluating patients in whom dissociative symptoms are suspected.

Epidemiology

Multiple personality syndrome is considered to have

its onset in childhood although most cases do not come to medical attention until the patients are in their late 20s to early 30s.[3, 10, 14, 15] Several case reports do exist of MPD occurring in children.[10, 14, 16, 17] Multiple personality disorder is diagnosed 3 to 9 times more frequently in females than in males.[1] There are questions regarding whether this reflects a bias in diagnosis or presentation within the mental health system.

Several studies have shown that there is an increased prevalence of this disorder in first-degree relatives of patients with MPD.[18, 19] Children of parents with MPD should be evaluated for signs of a dissociative pathologic condition.

Etiologic Theories

Current etiologic theories of MPD point overwhelmingly to childhood trauma as a precipitating factor.[20-23] Putnam and colleagues'[3] case review reported a history of significant childhood trauma in 97% of the cases. The types of trauma reported in this series included sexual abuse (in 83%), incest (in 68%), and physical abuse (in 75%), and 45% of the subjects reported that they witnessed a violent death in childhood. Kluft[24] described etiologies other than those that involved child abuse, including the death of a loved one, accidents, war, severe pain, illness, near-death experiences, cultural dislocation, and family chaos.

The development of the dissociative defenses in MPD is thought to protect the child from the full psychologic impact of overwhelming trauma that is often severe and repetitive in nature. The forces of later development then pressure the child to act on the dissociated states of consciousness secondarily to structure and personify them into the various alternate personalities. Kluft[24] has proposed a four-factor theory of the MPD etiology. Briefly described, his factors are as follows: (1) a capacity to dissociate; (2) life experiences that traumatically overwhelm the adaptive capacities of the child's ego; (3) shaping influences and substrates that determine the form taken by the dissociative defense; and (4) inadequate provision of stimulus barriers and restorative experiences by significant others, e.g., insufficient "soothing."

Treatment

Recent reports in several clinical series have suggested a positive outcome in terms of symptom alleviation in many cases of MPD through the use of intensive, dynamically oriented psychotherapy, along with adjunctive hypnotherapy in some cases.[25-27]

Early therapy should focus on developing rapport with the alternate system and working to increase cooperation and communication between them, with the therapeutic goal of improving the patient's functional capacity. Therapy gradually moves toward a breakdown of the dissociative defenses as traumatic material is worked through and the alternate personalities increase their range of defensive capabilities. The eventual goal of integration of the alternate personalities into a single personality is a highly individualized matter. The idea of integration may be very frightening to a number of alternate personalities who fear their destruction in the process or who do not wish to be associated in any way with some of the other personalities. Therapists are wise to work toward improved cooperation, communication, and functioning, as well as a diminution of symptoms, not pushing the idea of integration until this is a goal that is desirable to the client and his/her alternate system.

There is no definitive pharmacotherapy for the "core" symptoms of MPD.[25] Psychopharmacologic agents have been tried with sporadic success in individual cases, mainly to diminish affective, anxiety, and post-traumatic symptoms. The agents tried have included antidepressants, lithium, carbamazepine, major tranquilizers, and benzodiazepines. No consistent pharmacologic response has been noted in patients with MPD by using any of these agents.[28]

At present, pharmacotherapy should be limited to symptoms that are clearly present and consistent across the alternate system. Medication dosages should be carefully titrated, with attention paid to reports that a medication is differentially effecting various alternate personalities since this is known to occur. Patients with MPD often have alternate personalities who are troubled by suicidal or otherwise self-destructive behaviors, so the risk of a potential overdose must be borne in mind, and medications should be prescribed with utmost caution, keeping their potential lethality in mind.

Differential Diagnosis

The differential diagnosis of a patient with symptoms suggestive of MPD includes the other dissociative disorders, temporal lobe epilepsy, and malingering. In temporal lobe epilepsy, there are no distinctly separate personalities. The other dissociative disorders have been previously described. The symptoms present in MPD may lead the clinician initially to suspect a mood disorder or a psychotic illness. A carefully elicited history, including detailed descriptions of symptoms, is helpful in distinguishing these disorders. All of the personality disorders can coexist with MPD; however, patients with MPD are commonly misdiagnosed as having borderline personality disorder when the instability in behavior and mood is not recognized as due to the alteration in the personalities.

DSM III-R diagnostic criteria are as follows: (1) The existence within the person of two or more distinct personalities or personality states (each with its own relatively enduring pattern of perceiving, relating to, and thinking about the environment and self). (2) At least two of these personalities or personality states recurrently take full control of the person's behavior.

REFERENCES

1. American Psychiatric Association: *Diagnostic and Statistical Manual of Mental Disorders*, ed 3 (revised). Washington, DC, American Psychiatric Association, 1980.
2. Putnam FW, Loewenstein RJ, Silberman EJ, et

al: Multiple personality disorder in a hospital setting. *J Clin Psychiatry* 1984; 45:172–175.
3. Putnam FW, Guroff JJ, Silberman EJ, et al: The clinical phenomenology of multiple personality disorder: Review of 100 cases. *J Clin Psychiatry* 1986; 47:285–293.
4. Coons PM: The differential diagnosis of multiple personality. *Psychiatr Clin North Am* 1984; 7:9–29.
5. Bliss EL: Multiple personalities. *Arch Gen Psychiatry* 1980; 37:1388–1397.
6. Horevitz RP, Braun BG: Are multiple personalities borderline? *Psychiatr Clin North Am* 1984; 7:69–88.
7. Bliss EL, Larson EM, Nakashima SR: Auditory hallucinations and schizophrenia. *J Nerv Ment Dis* 1983; 171:30–35.
8. Kluft RP: First-rank symptoms as a diagnostic clue to multiple personality disorder. *Am J Psychiatry* 1987; 144:293–298.
9. Coons PM, Milstein V: Psychosexual disturbances in multiple personality: Characteristics, etiology, and treatment. *J Clin Psychiatry* 1986; 47:106–110.
10. Kluft RP (ed): *Childhood Antecedents of Multiple Personality Disorder*. Washington, DC, American Psychiatric Press, Inc, 1985.
11. Spiegel D: Multiple personality as a post-traumatic stress disorder. *Psychiatr Clin North Am* 1984; 7:101–110.
12. Spiegel D, Rosenfeld A: Spontaneous age-regression. *J Clin Psychiatry* 1984; 45:522–524.
13. Bernstein E, Putnam F: Development, reliability, and validity of a dissociation scale. *J Nerv Ment Dis* 1986; 174:727–735.
14. Kluft RP: Multiple personality in childhood. *Psychiatr Clin North Am* 1984; 7:121–134.
15. Kluft RP: The natural history of multiple personality disorder, in Kluft RP (ed): *Childhood Antecedents of Multiple Personality*. Washington,

DC, American Psychiatric Press, Inc, 1985, pp .
16. Kluft RP: Treating children who have multiple personality disorder, in Braun BG (ed): *Treatment of Multiple Personality Disorder*. Washington, DC, American Psychiatric Press, Inc, 1986, pp 197–238.
17. Kluft RP: Hypnotherapy of childhood multiple personality disorder. *Am J Clin Hypn* 1985; 27:201–210.
18. Braun BG: The transgenerational incidence of dissociation and multiple personality disorder: A preliminary report, in Kluft RP (ed): *Childhood Antecedents of Multiple Personality*. Washington, DC, American Psychiatric Press, Inc, 1985, pp 127–150.
19. Coons PM: Children of parents with multiple personality disorder, in Kluft RP (ed): *Childhood Antecedents of Multiple Personality*. Washington, DC, American Psychiatric Press, Inc, 1985, pp 151–166.
20. Braun B, Sachs R: The development of multiple personality disorder: Predisposing, precipitating, and perpetuating factors, in Kluft RP (ed): *Childhood Antecedents of Multiple Personality*. Washington, DC, American Psychiatric Press, Inc, 1985, pp 37–64.
21. Wilbur C: Multiple personality and child abuse. *Psychiatr Clin North Am* 1984; 7:3–6.
22. Gelinas DJ: The persisting negative effects of incest. *Psychiatry* 1983; 46:12–32.
23. Bowman ES, Blix S, Coons PM: Multiple personality in adolescence: Relationship to incestual experiences. *J Am Acad Child Adolesc Psychiatry* 1985; 24:109–114.
24. Kluft RP: Treatment of multiple personality disorder: A study of 33 cases. *Psychiatr Clin North Am* 1984; 7:9–29.
25. Kluft RP: Aspects of the treatment of multiple personality disorder. *Psychiatric Ann* 1984; 14:51–57.

26. Braun BG (ed): *Treatment of Multiple Personality Disorder*. Washington, DC, American Psychiatric Press, Inc, 1986.
27. Coons PM: Treatment progress in 20 patients with multiple personality disorder. *J Nerv Ment Dis* 1986; 171:388–390.
28. Barkin R, Braun BG, Kluft RP: The dilemma of drug therapy for multiple personality disorder, in Braun BG (ed): *Treatment of Multiple Personality Disorder*. Washington, DC, American Psychiatric Press, Inc, 1986, pp 107–133.

13 | Axis I Disorders in Children and Adolescents

I. **General comments.** This chapter and Chapter 14 (Axis II Disorders in Children and Adolescents) are broad overviews of an entire subspecialty's diagnostic categories and treatment strategies. These chapters are intended to provide a context within which the reader can approach the child and adolescent patient seen for evaluation. The reader is strongly recommended to review the major texts by Rutter and Hersov[1] (or Shaffer et al.[2]) for a more in-depth review of a given syndrome.

A. **Assessment.** The assessment of children and adolescents requires data from interviews with the child and parents and often direct observations of family functioning. Questionnaires from and interviews with the schoolteacher are important in most cases. Formal psychologic and academic testing may be indicated. A careful prenatal and developmental history is crucial.

These data need to be interpreted within a developmental framework. Furthermore, the individual child's presenting symptoms should be placed in the family context. When did these complaints begin? What is the family functioning like now? What psychosocial developmental stages is the child evolving through? What is the degree and nature of the dysfunction?

A discussion of these issues can be found in Chapter

38, "Developmental, Diagnostic, and Psychotherapeutic Aspects of Childhood and Adolescence." The evaluation process leads to a tentative diagnosis and to treatment planning.

B. **Diagnostic categories: children and adolescents.**
DSM III-R[3] describes criteria that can be used to group individuals with specific behaviors. These categorizations, or syndromes, may group several "illnesses" together that may be etiologically distinct. The benefits of this classification system include provision of clear communication as a reference point for clinical and research endeavors.

More needs to be learned about the nature of these disorders in children and adolescents (herein abbreviated as "in children"). Because of the rapid developmental changes in children, the application of criteria originally established for adults may require modification. Some disorders primarily begin in childhood. If adults present with these disorders, they may be termed "residual type" (e.g., attention deficit hyperactivity disorder [ADHD] or autism). Some children present with disorders that are more commonly seen in adults. Thus, the "adult" categories in *DSM III-R* may be applied with age-specific considerations.

C. **Mood disorders in children and adolescents.**

1. **Clinical presentation.** *DSM III-R* indicates certain special features for diagnosing depression in children. These include irritable mood quality, failure to make expected weight gain rather than weight loss, and a shorter duration of illness. The onset of depression may be more insidious, with a younger age at onset associated with a more chronic course and often with more genetic loading. Mania may, more often, present in adolescence and be characterized with agitation, irritability, and confusion. Bipolar depressive episodes present more commonly with psychosis, psychomotor retardation, hypersomnia, and hyperphagia than do unipolar episodes.

Psychosocial withdrawal and academic difficulties can lead to significant impairment in normal functioning and development. The emerging sense of self during childhood and adolescence may be severely effected by the pervasive effects of a mood disturbance. Mood disorders in children are often recurrent and have long-term morbidity.

2. **Associated features.** Suicidal ideation may be present; completed suicide is far more common, with an alarmingly increasing rate, in adolescents. Somatic complaints are frequent in preadolescents in whom separation anxiety and overanxious disorder may also be present. Adolescents may have concomitant substance abuse. Impairment in social relations may be common in both age groups as is academic failure that is related to cognitive slowing and decreased motivation.

3. **Differential diagnosis.** Attention deficit hyperactivity disorder vs. agitated depression vs. mania may each present with restlessness and irritability. Conduct disorder and substance abuse may be secondary to the mood disorder or additional illnesses.

4. **Epidemiology.** Mania, hypomania, and cyclothymia are thought to have an onset more commonly in adolescence. Major depression and dysthymia may occur in both age groups. In 10-year-old children, 1.7% have been reported to meet the old *DSM III*[4] criteria for major depression or dysthymia.

5. **Etiology.** In mood disorders, adult-onset, genetic, biochemical, environmental, and psychologic factors have been proposed. Parental loss at certain ages has a higher association with depression. Of note is that prepubertal children do not have the same sleep architecture changes that are seen in adults and in adolescents.

6. **Assessment.** A thorough psychiatric examination is essential, especially regarding suicidal ideation, intent, plans, and history of attempts. Recent losses, including a suicidal death of a friend or public figure,

may be factors associated with an increased risk of suicide attempts. The degree of psychosocial impairment and withdrawal should be determined for both family and peer relations.

The developmental stage of the younger child may make reporting of certain aspects of the mood disorder different from that of adults. Quality of mood may not be described as "depressed" but rather as "feeling down in the dumps, sad, blue, or like crying." Younger children especially may have difficulty reporting duration or periodicity of episodes. These episodes and anhedonia may be better described by parental report.

Certain diagnostic tools that are helpful in evaluating children include the Child Behavior Checklist (CBC); Diagnostic Inventory for Children and Adolescents (DICA); Diagnostic Inventory Schedule for Children, Revised (DISC-R); Children's Depression Inventory (CDI); Kiddie Schedule for Affective Disorder Symptoms (K-SADS); and Modified Teacher's Connors' Rating Scale (see Chapter 3 [Psychological Testing] for full details).

7. **Treatment.** Few controlled studies have been carried out with children and adolescents. Cognitive techniques may be helpful. Behavioral interventions that focus on social skills training may be useful. Psychodynamic therapy and family involvement may be helpful in cases of loss. Pharmacotherapy has not been proved to be as effective in children as it has in adults. The use of tricyclic antidepressants and lithium in children and adolescents is under active investigation, and given the potential side effects and the risk of overdose (especially with adolescents with impulsivity), these should be used only with caution by experienced clinicians.

D. **Other adult classifications used in children and adolescents.** The following is a listing of other diagnoses usually of adult onset that are often used in children: schizophrenia (may have a distinct "childhood schizophrenia," not described in the *DSM III-R*, with neurodevelopmental lags and insidious onset); schizophreniform disorder; organic mental disorders; psychoactive substance disorders (especially in adolescents); somatiform disorder; obsessive-compulsive disorder (may be associated with Tourette disorder); sexual disorders; psychologic factors that affect physical condition; and adjustment disorder. See Chapter 14 (Axis II Disorders in Children and Adolescents) for a discussion of the use of personality disorder diagnoses. The V-codes, especially the parent-child problem, also are used.

Childhood trauma, including physical or sexual abuse and witnessing of violent events, may present in various forms in children. Post-traumatic stress disorder, dissociative disorders, mood disturbances, and disruptive behaviors may be sequalae. (See Chapter 42 [Abuse].)

The relationship between disorders in children and in adults needs further evaluation with longitudinal studies. Some authors argue that there are distinct entities, such as "childhood schizophrenia," which may be distinct from the "adult" counterpart. There may be no relationship between adult and pediatric disease (e.g., anxious adults generally were NOT anxious as children). There may also be "residual" disorders from childhood that persist into adulthood, as in attention deficit disorder, residual type (a *DSM III* diagnosis). Still, other disorders may evolve into more classic adult presentations from childhood through adolescence as may be true with bipolar mood disorder.

E. **Individualized treatment.** This is crucial no matter which diagnostic categories are chosen. A presentation of school dysfunction and inattention might yield diagnoses that range from schizophrenia, bipolar illness, ADHD, depression, or post-traumatic stress disorder. Treatment interventions might all include school programs, family therapy, individual therapy, and perhaps the use of appropriate medications. The age and developmental stage of the child will also shape which interventions are selected.

II. (*DSM III-R* Axis I) disorders usually first evident in infancy, childhood, or adolescence.

A. **Disruptive behavior disorders.** (1) three groups (ADHD, conduct, disorder, and oppositional disorder); (2) "externalizing" symptoms (socially disruptive); and (3) conduct and oppositional disorders may be degrees of severity along a spectrum, and ADHD appears to be relatively distinct from these two disorders.

1. ADHD.

a. **Definition and clinical presentation.** Inattention, impulsiveness, and hyperactivity are in excess of age-appropriate levels. Usually, it is present at 4 years of age, and dysfunction is evident from the beginning of school (vs. episodic or later onset, rule out other disorders). Symptoms may not be present in office setting.

Attention deficit hyperactivity disorder may lead to academic dysfunction, social ostracism, and low self-esteem. Impairment may be severe or mild. Children with ADHD may continue with symptoms into adulthood (residual type). Some children meet *DSM III* criteria for attention deficit disorder "without hyperactivity"; these are called "undifferentiated attention deficit disorder" in *DSM III-R*.

Diagnostic criteria include at least eight symptoms during 6 months of the following:

(i) Hyperkinesis (fidgety, restless, and excessive talking)

(ii) Impulsivity (blurts out answers, cannot wait turn, unable to finish projects, shifts in activities, interrupts others, and dangerous activities)

(iii) Inattention (distractible, difficulty in sustaining attention, frequent shifts in attention, does not listen, and loses things)

(iv) Severity designated as mild, moderate, and severe impairment

b. **Associated features.** Attention deficit disorder in *DSM III-R* may be associated with conduct disorder/oppositional disorder and specific developmental disorders. Child may have school dysfunction with poor academic performance secondary to inattention/disruptive behavior; child may become "scapegoat" in family or classroom setting; and neurologic soft signs may be present.

c. **Differential diagnosis.** Inattention due to mood disorder, PTSD, dissociative disorder, and overanxious disorder; impulsiveness due to other disruptive disorders, TLE, and chaotic environment; and hyperactivity due to age-appropriate "overactivity," anxiety, and mood disorder.

d. **Epidemiology.** Prevalence (depending on definition and assessment tools): From 0.1% to 5%, with most studies clustering at 2% to 3%. Sex ratio: 6 to 9 males to 1 female. Familial/genetic patterns: More studies are needed. Suggestion of higher incidence is in first-degree relatives. Attention is very sensitive to both central nervous system (CNS) dysfunction and environmental stress.

e. **Etiology.** Measures of attention are very sensitive to CNS dysfunction, environmental stress, and psychiatric disturbance. This disorder attempts to classify a syndrome of inattention, impulsivity, and hyperkinesis that is more than a transient inability to attend.

Various etiologies have been suggested, but none have been proved by research as yet. The association of learning disorders and ADHD suggest subtle brain damage. Research on the response to certain medications suggests a possible neurochemical dysfunction that involves the monoamine neurotransmitter systems. Findings from familial studies support a genetic predisposition to the disorder. Some authors suggest that the disorder represents a developmental delay in normal maturation. Another view holds that the psychologic response to the social milieu may increase the chance of initiation or enhancement of the disorder. The validity of different subgroups of children with ADHD needs further study.

f. **Assessment.** Office observation may be unrevealing. Reports from parents and teachers are essential in making a diagnosis. Connors' Scales are useful for evaluating hyperactivity and impulsivity, but less helpful for evaluating actual inattention. Aspects of attention changes, in response to treatment, can be measured with continuous performance tests and other computerized measures; a standardized format needs to be developed.

g. **Treatment.** Psychosocial approaches are used.

(i) Cognitive/behavioral approach, theoretically used to reduce disruptive behaviors, enhance response to limit setting, and improve availability to teaching efforts, has had minimal additive effect over medications alone as recently suggested by Gittleman-Klein[5] in 1987.

(ii) School placement: Patient may require special classroom setting.

(iii) Family involvement: To support family, reinforce parent effectiveness, and encourage compliance with multimodality treatment efforts.

(iv) Psychotherapy may be indicated in selected cases, especially in older children, to deal with low self-esteem, demoralization, and alienation. Psychotherapy is not effective alone for core deficits.

(v) Medications have been shown to be crucial for enhanced attention and reduced disruptive/inappropriate behaviors.[5]

(a) First-line medications are the *stimulants*:

(i) Methylphenidate (Ritalin): 1- to 2-week trial

(ii) Dextroamphetamine (Dexedrine): 1- to 2-week trial

(iii) Less often: pemoline (Cylert): 4-week trial

Clinical response is usually seen within hours for the first two medications; 2 to 3 weeks for pemoline. Seventy percent of patients are responders to stimulants. Each stimulant may be effective by different biochemical mechanisms; therefore, a nonresponder to one type may respond to another stimulant.

(b) Second-line medications are the *tricyclic antidepressants*: Improvement may be rapid or occur in several weeks with dosages less than those used for depression. Dose is given in the morning.

(c) Third-line medication is *clonidine*.

Note: These medications are used to improve attention and reduce activity. Unfortunately, excessive dosing (especially of stimulants) may lead to impaired cognitive functioning. Careful monitoring of target symptom changes with drug dosage is crucial.

2. Conduct disorder.

a. Definition and clinical presentation. Repetitive persistent pattern of behaviors that violate the rights of others and age-appropriate general societal norms. Physical aggression is usually present, but not essential. Behaviors include stealing, lying, damaging other's property, and inflicting injury on others. These behaviors may occur covertly or overtly in a socially underdeveloped individual (*DSM III* "undersocialized") or one who is social ("socialized"). This is distinct from the *DSM III-R* classification of the setting in which these behaviors occur ("solitary" vs. "group" type). Those with the solitary aggressive type tend to have an earlier (preteen) onset and a worse prognosis with greater probability of developing adult antisocial personality disorder.

Diagnostic criteria require the persistence for 6 months of three of thirteen characteristic symptoms (e.g., stealing, running away, lying, destroying property, sexual forcing of others, and physical cruelty to people or animals). Subtyping includes severity (mild, moderate, and severe) and type (group, solitary aggressive, and "undifferentiated").

b. **Associated features.** Large families, common with the middle ordinal position, are highly represented. School dysfunction is common. Family environments may have inconsistent parental figures, an absent father, or parental alcohol abuse. Substance abuse and legal problems also may be present.

c. **Differential diagnosis.** Persistence over 6 months distinguishes conduct disorder from single acts of antisocial behavior. Severity in symptoms distinguishes this disorder from a diagnosis of oppositional defiant disorder; ADHD may be present additionally, as can specific developmental disorders. Antisocial behavior secondary to episodes of psychosis or affective illness should be ruled out.

d. **Epidemiology.** Prevalence studies range around 6%. Sex ratio: male-female, 4:1. Familial patterns: High overlap with family history of substance abuse, ADHD, antisocial personality disorder.

e. **Etiology.** Adoption studies suggest (1) genetic predisposition and (2) additional environmental influence toward conduct disorder. Family dysfunction, inconsistency, and hostility are frequent findings.

Thus, etiology is thought to be multifactorial, including biologic, psychologic, and social factors. Biologic studies of low-norepinephrine metabolites suggest that hypoarousal may be a source for certain associated disruptive behaviors and psychoactive substance abuse.

f. **Assessment.** A thorough evaluation (Child Behavior Checklist, psychiatric evaluation, and family assessment) is crucial to rule out other complicating disorders (especially ADHD, affective disorders, and specific learning disorders).

Poor prognosis factors include early age at onset, pervasiveness across situations, and more types of antisocial behavior.

g. **Treatment.** The following six types are used.

(i) Behavioral treatment involves limit setting, time-outs, reinforcement for prosocial behavior, and negative reinforcement for aversive acts.

(ii) Cognitive treatment involves teaching new problem-solving skills.

(iii) Parent management involves parents in a consistent behavioral approach to child rearing.

(iv) Functional family therapy involves a systems and behavioral approach to reduce hostility, enhance consistency, and modify scapegoating behaviors.

(v) Time-limited community-based interventions: Follow-up studies have NOT shown good responses, suggesting that interventions probably need to be *chronic* and *individualized*.

(vi) Medications.

(a) NOT a first-line treatment and should NOT be used without concomitant multimodal therapy as described above. Rule out need for treatment of other disorders (e.g., ADHD and depression).

(b) Aggressive behavior in children and adolescents may be responsive to adjunctive medication treatment in addition to intensive, long-term behavioral approaches.

(c) Two medications described as effective in the literature are lithium, according to Campbell and Spencer,[6] and haloperidol. Use of medications in this disorder needs further controlled studies.

3. Oppositional defiant disorder.

a. **Definition and clinical presentation.** An age-inappropriate behavior pattern of hostility and defiance without the severity is seen in conduct disorder. This disorder often begins by latency age and rarely after adolescence. The characteristic behavior may be seen in only certain situations (with family, friends, and teachers) and may not be evident in the office initially. The course is unclear but may include resolution, increasing severity toward conduct disorder, or emergent mood or thought disorder. Six months of several diagnostic symptoms (e.g., temper, argues, refuses, annoys, and blames) are required.

b. **Associated features.** Dysfunction in specific environments (school and home) may be evident; low-frustration tolerance, temper tantrums, and irritability may be present. Externalization as an explanation for behavior is common. Substance abuse and smoking are common.

c. **Differential diagnosis.** Conduct disorder is superordinate. If criteria are met during episodes of mood or thought disorder, then these disorders pre-empt oppositional defiant diagnosis.

d. **Epidemiology.** Prevalence is unknown. Sex ratio: Males greater than females, prepubertal equal to postpuberty.

e. **Etiology.** Familial/genetic patterns are unknown. Theories involve family dysfunction and child's excessive developmental separation tasks. Reinforcing attention from parents may play a significant role in maintaining behavior pattern.

f. **Assessment.** Thorough assessment, including family evaluation, is critical. Life history and developmental stage of child important in understanding role of oppositional behavior.

g. **Treatment.** The following types are used.

(i) Family therapy: If family issues/dysfunction appear directly related to patient's symptoms, especially for younger children.

(ii) **Individual therapy (behavioral/cognitive):** Establish limit setting and point system for reinforcement of cooperative behaviors.

(iii) **Psychodynamic:** May be helpful for adjustment difficulties, low self-esteem, and frustration tolerance, especially in older children and adolescents.

(iv) **Substance abuse treatment** to eliminate psychoactive substance use is critical.

(v) **Medications:** None are indicated.

B. **Anxiety disorders of childhood or adolescence.**

1. **Separation anxiety disorder.**

a. **Definition and clinical presentation.** At least 2 weeks of developmentally excessive anxiety that is focused specifically on separation from people to whom the patient is psychologically attached. Anxiety or panic emerges when separation is imminent (older children) or actually occurs. This then may lead to a refusal to leave the parental figure, interfering with establishment of peer relationships, school attendance, or independent activities. Sleeping alone may evoke fears and lead to clinging behavior. Disorder usually begins before adolescence and as early as the preschool period.

It should be noted that a developmentally normal 6- to 8-month onset separation anxiety reaches a peak at 10 to 24 months with a subsequent decline. Clinically, patients present at 5 and 12 years of age with school initiation and changes.

Diagnostic criteria include at least 2 weeks with three of nine symptoms (e.g., worries about harm or event that leads to separation, reluctance to separate, nightmares about separation, physical symptoms, and separation distress).

b. **Associated features.** Physical complaints (in younger children: headaches, earaches, stomachaches, nausea, and vomiting; in older children and adolescents: these symptoms plus cardiovascular symptoms, e.g., tachycardia, palpitations, and faintness, may also occur) may lead to medical evaluation. Separation leads to fears of accidental loss of attachment figures or dangers that will permanently separate them from their parents. Social withdrawal and general discomfort may accompany separation. Children may also be attention seeking, demanding, and irritable when separated.

c. **Differential diagnosis.** May occur with concomitant other anxiety disorders or mood disorders. Do not confuse with syndrome of pervasive developmental disorder or thought disorder. Some degree of separation anxiety is a normal developmental phase, especially during preschool period. In avoidant disorder, behavior to avoid school may be present, and anxiety here is focused on avoidance of an uncomfortable situation rather than fear of separation.

d. **Epidemiology.** Prevalence is unknown. Sex ratio is probably equal. Familial/genetic patterns: Some suggestions of maternal history of anxiety disorder.

e. **Etiology.** Separation is essential to development. Theories of etiology in this disorder involve psychosocial views of disturbances in this normal developmental task due to the inability of the child to tolerate fear of loss of parental figures. Family stress may be important when parental ambivalence toward individuation inhibits normal separation. The child may also identify with parental fear of separation and learn to feel anxious at times that require separation. Familial studies suggest a possible genetic predisposition for this anxiety disorder.

f. **Assessment.** Evaluating the child with and without the presence of a major attachment figure is important. Teacher input is critical. Assess any degree of regressive behavior, and ritualization or somatization that might reflect underlying anxiety.

g. **Treatment.** The following types are used.

(i) Family therapy facilitates normal separation-individuation process.

(ii) Individual therapy can help the patient deal with separation anxiety in a progressively desensitizing manner.

(iii) Medications: No studies are available.

2. Avoidant disorder of childhood or adolescence.

a. **Definition and clinical presentation.** At least 6 months of withdrawal from contact with unfamiliar people, leading to impairment in social functioning with peers. Relationships with familiar people are maintained and close. Discomfort and shyness in unfamiliar situations may occur.

Several symptoms may meet criteria for avoidant personality disorder that pre-empt this diagnosis. Age at onset is usually in school years but may occur after $2^1/_2$ years of age when developmentally appropriate stranger anxiety should be significantly diminished.

b. **Associated features.** Often accompanied by another anxiety disorder of childhood or adolescence. Isolation and depression may be present. School avoidance may lead to academic failure.

c. **Differential diagnosis.** Other anxiety disorders may be present. Generalized social withdrawal may be present in mood and thought disorders. Shy temperament may appear similar but without significant peer impairment.

d. **Epidemiology.** Prevalence is unknown. Sex ratio is unclear. Familial/genetic patterns possibly may have a higher incidence of maternal anxiety disorder.

e. **Etiology.** More studies are needed. Inadequate development of social skills may lead to this social withdrawal. Origins for this inadequacy may include combinations of temperamental traits (e.g., shyness) and presence of language and speech disturbances or early traumatic experiences that lead to social isolation only with close family members.

f. **Assessment.** Focus on ruling out specific physical disorders and assessing nature of fears that lead to avoidant behavior. "Why now?" is an especially important question in this disorder.

g. **Treatment.** The following types are used.

(i) Behavior/cognitive: Systematic desensitization and guided imagery.

(ii) Psychotherapeutic: Insight work around source of fears that lead to anxiety.

(iii) Family therapy: Systemic, behavioral, or dynamic may be helpful to explore nature of anxiety in family and ability to deal with fears and tolerate unfamiliarity.

(iv) Medications: School-avoidant behavior has been shown by Gittleman-Klein and Klein[7] to be responsive to imipramine. This is the only specific subset of anxiety disorders in children with a clearly indicated medication. This should be carried out in conjunction with the above treatments.

3. Overanxious disorder.

a. **Definition and clinical presentation.** Generalized and persistent worries about the past and future and preoccupation with performance ability; these may lead to marked self-consciousness, somatic complaints, and an inability to relax. Children may require constant reassurance. The anxiety here is generalized and not a focus on one particular area (e.g., separation). Children often present in early teens and may have other anxiety disorders as well.

Diagnostic criteria include 6 months of excessive anxiety or worry revealed as four of seven symptoms (e.g., worries about the future, past, or competence, somatic complaints, and/or self-consciousness).

b. **Associated features.** Simple or social phobias may be present as well. Approval-seeking behavior and perfectionism may be evident.

c. **Differential diagnosis.** May be present with

other anxiety disorders; ADHD may appear anxious but without worries about past or future. Psychosis and mood disorders are associated with anxiety but are supraordinate diagnoses.

d. **Epidemiology.** Prevalence is unknown. Sex ratio is equal. Familial/genetic patterns may have more maternal anxiety disorders.

e. **Etiology.** Various theories have been evoked to explain anxiety in children and adults. Familial studies suggest that there may be a genetic predisposition to anxiety. Psychodynamic theories suggest internal psychic conflicts specific for developmental tasks. Family factors may play a role in intensifying a child's anticipatory fear and generalized anxiety.

f. **Assessment.** It is the same as with prior anxiety disorders.

g. **Treatment.** The following types are used.

(i) Individual psychotherapy focuses on fears underlying anxiety.

(ii) Behavioral/cognitive: Relaxation techniques.

(iii) Family: Help family to support child's ability to tolerate anxiety and reduce fears.

(iv) Medications: No studies have shown their efficacy in children.

C. **Gender identity disorders.** *DSM III-R* categorizes three types of disorders of gender identity. Generally, these disorders are characterized by a disturbance in the individual's sense of being female or male. Certain definitions are important in understanding these disorders. "Gender identity" refers to one's own sense of being "male or female." "Gender role" indicates a social expression to others of maleness or femaleness. "Assigned sex" is the gender that has been determined at birth based on physical appearance. "Sexual orientation or preference" refers to the gender of the source of erotic stimulation.

Green[8] has reviewed three basic phases in typical

psychosexual development. The first phase (roughly between 1 and 3 years of age) of sexual identity development is the awareness of belonging to one of the genders. Thus, early on, young children begin to recognize the world as composed of males and females and to establish their identification with one of these groups. The second phase, established between 3 and 4 years of age, is the development of gender role behaviors or "sex-typed behaviors." In a given culture, certain activities, play, dress, and interactive styles are found to be "masculine" or "feminine." The third component is that of the development of a direction of erotic or romantic preference. This latter component may become clearly evident during adolescence and have precursors earlier in life. The inter-relationships of these three components is fascinating and complex but too detailed to describe here. (The reader is referred to Green[8] and Stoller.[9])

In the gender identity disorders, there is an atypical psychosexual development characterized by distress in one's assigned sex and gender role expectations. Thus, one's gender identity is not syntonic with external sexual features or with societal expectations. The three disorders vary based on the age (prepubertal or postpubertal) and the degree to which the individual is preoccupied with changing their sexual characteristics (postpubertal: nonsexual or transsexual).

1. **Epidemiology.** These are rare disorders. Clinically, many more boys present than girls during childhood. Furthermore, individuals presenting for transsexual surgical procedures are more commonly men than women. *DSM III-R* states that for transsexualism, males are 1/30,000, and females are 1/100,000. Rates for the other disorders are unknown.

2. **Etiology.** Several theories that explore the origin of atypical gender development exist. Studies of sexual activity in animals suggests a predominant role for a hormonal influence on the fetus and neonate in the type of sexual behavior exhibited later in life. Chro-

mosomal abnormalities in humans influence both primary and secondary sexual characteristics. Gender identity appears to be more a function of psychosocial factors during early childhood than of a biologic abnormality. Although physical abnormalities of the sex organs are rarely associated with gender identity disorder of childhood, the *DSM III-R* categories do not exclude making the diagnosis if they are present.

The theory that gender identity forms from between 1 and 3 years of age evokes several interactive variables that may be involved in atypical development. Normally, gender identity, assigned sex, and gender role correspond. The discontinuity between gender identity and assigned sex could be a result of constitutional factors (i.e., the child's temperamental traits), parental expectations and behaviors (e.g., desires for a child of opposite sex and treating him as a her), and the resultant internalization of this child-parent interaction in the formation of gender identification. Older psychosocial theories include the psychoanalytic view of identification with the parent of the opposite sex as a maladaptive resolution to the oedipal conflict.

At this point, more research is required to determine the etiologies of these uncommon disorders. A description of the three categories of disorders follows.

a. **Gender Identity Disorder of Childhood.** In prepubertal children, this is the finding of (1) distress about one's assigned sex or insistence that one is of the other sex and (2) an aversion for normative behavior or preference for clothes of the opposite sex OR persistent repudiation of the same sex anatomic features.

Criteria are defined for boys and for girls.

Socially, these children may become alienated from peers or family. This social distress may be the presenting complaint.

This diagnosis should not be made in children whose behavior does not fit cultural expectations unless they meet the full criteria.

The course of this disorder is being studied. At present, our knowledge of outcome comes from studies of children with certain behavioral tendencies who may not have met the full criteria for this disorder. The results of these studies are included here, but their direct applicability to this disorder has not been determined.

Follow-up studies of boys with a high degree of "femininity" suggest that about one half of these children may be "preheterosexual," with a much higher than average probability that, in adulthood, they will emerge as transsexuals, transvestites, or homosexuals.

Girls studied with "tomboyish" behavior were found to come for psychiatric evaluation much less frequently than boys and expressed much less social or intrapsychic conflict. Green[8] noted that retrospective studies of lesbians suggest a higher rate of tomboyism, but prospective data are unavailable at this point.

(i) **Assessment.** Intervention with a child with gender identity disorder raises several ethical issues. The child may express present internal conflict and social distress, and the family may express concerns about future outcome. The child may feel alienated in the family, as well as with peers.

The approach to assessment should thus be at many levels: family evaluation (to determine the nature of parental concerns, feedback loops that enhance alienation between father and "not-so-masculine" son who is perhaps portrayed as a "sissy," family roles and expectations, attention to individual child's unique personality style, etc.) and individual assessment of the degree of alienation and demoralization, impairment in social functioning, and other concomitant disorders.

(ii) **Treatment.** The goals of intervention overall are to reduce social stress for the child and to enhance healthy family functioning and dyadic relationships that may be "too close" to the parent of opposite sex and "too distant" to that of the same sex.

Ethical issues are raised regarding interventions to alter the gender identity of the child. Even if it were clear whether this could, in fact, be accomplished, the debatable issue is in applying a cultural standard to a given therapeutic goal. Parents may request that the child be psychologically "changed," whereas the child desires to not "be" the assigned sex or act in the gender role. This division, itself, creates a conflict that may "pigeonhole" the child into feeling that his/her constitutional tendencies are unacceptable in a person of that sex. This lack of flexibility in gender role may thus heighten distress in the family and alienate the child further.

Psychoanalytic, behavioral, and "eclectic" approaches have been tried with boys to reduce "feminine" behavior. Although these behaviors can be modified, there is presently no evidence that this reduction alters later patterns of erotic arousal or sexual orientation. Further outcome studies are needed to determine what effects interventions may have on eventual outcome in adulthood.

b. **Transsexualism.** This disorder is defined for individuals who have reached puberty and have had at least 2 years of a persistent preoccupation with the inappropriateness of the assigned sex. There is a desire to get rid of primary and secondary sex characteristics and acquisition of those of the opposite sex.

Most individuals have had gender identity disorder of childhood (although only a small percentage of those with gender identity disorder emerge as transsexuals).

There may be a distaste for dressing in assigned sex clothes; therefore, cross-dressing may be present. (This should be distinguished from transvestite fetishism, wherein cross-dressing is associated with sexual arousal.)

Subtypes include sexual orientation, i.e., asexual, homosexual, heterosexual, or unspecified.

(i) **Assessment.** Thorough psychiatric history and

evaluation. Need to assess for concomitant character pathologic condition (especially borderline personality disorder) or depression that may be common. Thought disorder needs to be considered. "Belief that one is of the opposite sex" is considered as "I feel as if I was of the opposite sex" and is therefore not considered a delusion in *DSM III-R*.

(ii) **Treatment.** Psychosocial: Psychotherapy for transsexualism has not been shown to be effective. Therapy for concomitant character difficulties and depression may be helpful. Family intervention may be useful for support.

Sex reassignment surgery: Generally, an irreversible procedure to remove primary and secondary sex characteristics and reconstructively create new features with supplementation with exogenous hormone. This requires a thorough psychiatric presurgical evaluation and a several months to yearlong trial period of (reversible) hormone therapy and cross-gender living. About one half go on to complete the surgical intervention. Outcome measures and results vary. Suicide has been reported in over 1% of cases postoperatively.

c. **Gender identity disorder of adolescence and adulthood, nontranssexual type.** Postpubertal individuals who have persistent discomfort with their assigned sex and who have recurrent cross-dressing (fantasy or reality) that is NOT for sexual excitement. They do not have a preoccupation with getting rid of their genitals or acquiring those of the opposite sex. Diagnostic subtypes also include sexual orientation. This is a newly defined disorder without sufficient data to describe the course, assessment, or unique treatment approaches.

D. **Tic disorders.** *DSM III-R* outlines three disorders in this group: Tourette disorder, chronic motor or vocal tic disorder, and transient tic disorder. Some authors argue that these disorders are on a spectrum with decreasing severity. They each have symptoms of tics, defined as an "involuntary, sudden, rapid, recurrent, nonrhythmic, stereotyped motor movement or vocalization." (*DSM III-R,* p 78) These tics are generally enhanced by stress, can be temporarily suppressed, and are diminished by absorption in other activities or by sleep.

Motor and vocal tics are divided into simple or complex. A few examples of common tics are as follows:

Simple motor: eye blinking, neck jerking, and facial grimacing

Simple vocal: coughing, throat clearing, grunting, and snorting

Complex motor: facial gestures, grooming behaviors, hitting self, touching, and smelling an object

Complex vocal: repeating words or phrases out of context, coprolalia (use of socially unacceptable, often obscene words), palilalia (repeating one's own sounds or words), and echolalia (repeating the last heard word or phrase)

Tic disorders need to be distinguished from disorders that also are associated with abnormal movements. Thus, certain neurologic disorders with athetoid (cerebral palsy), choreiform (Sydenham chorea), myoclonic (Wilson disease), or dystonic (dystonia musculorum deformans) movements should be in the differential diagnosis. Other abnormal movements should also be distinguished, such as in stereotypy and habit disorder (see end of this chapter). Mentally retarded and autistic children may have overlapping tic movements.

Use of psychostimulants has been associated with a new onset or worsening of tics. This may be due to uncovering of a latent tic disorder, especially in individuals with a family history of tics.

Two important distinguishing features of tics are

that they are *involuntary* and usually *dystonic* (i.e., distressing). These features help differentiate tics from compulsions that are intentional.

For all the tic disorders, age at onset is around 7 years, with a wide range from 2 to 14 years. The course and impairment differ for each category.

1. **Transient tic disorder.** This disorder involves time-limited episode of single or multiple motor and/or vocal tics for less than 12 months. Impairment is also limited unless it develops into a chronic tic disorder that, by definition, presents initially as this disorder.

a. **Differential diagnosis.** Distinguished from other tic disorders by duration: 2 weeks to 12 months and not exclusively during drug use or illness.

b. **Epidemiology.** Theories include neurotransmitter dysfunction as primary and/or with psychogenic (stress)-related factors.

c. **Assessment.** Evaluate features of tics, including precipitants and degree of distress and impairment, and follow over time.

d. **Treatment.** As course is initially unclear, intervention should be conservative. Reassurance and support of family in lowering their reaction to tics may be helpful and possible if symptoms are not severe. Behavioral techniques for relaxation and habit reversal may be effective. Pharmacotherapy should be initiated only in very severe initial cases.

2. **Chronic motor or vocal tic disorder.**

a. **Definition and clinical presentation.** Duration of at least 1 year of frequent motor OR vocal tics (BOTH = Tourette disorder). As in transient tics, involvement of the face and head initially is most common, followed by the arm and hand, then the body, and lower extremities in the evolution of motor tics. Respiratory and gastrointestinal involvement constitute the "vocal" tics and are more rare than the motor tics. Vocal tics in this disorder are less intense than those in Tourette disorder. Course varies but, in some cases, may be limited to about 5 years, ending during adolescence. Impairment depends on severity and its effect on social functioning.

b. **Epidemiology.** Data are insufficient.

c. **Etiology.** Theories involve neurochemical dysfunction (especially of dopaminergic or noradrenergic pathways) secondary to genetic or traumatic factors. Psychologic factors, including stress, anxiety, and conditioning, have also been discussed.

d. **Assessment.** This is the same as in transient tic disorder.

e. **Treatment.** The degree of distress and impairment from tics will help guide the decision to treat and the nature of intervention. Psychotherapy aimed at reducing emotional distress and social alienation may be indicated. Pharmacotherapy may be initiated after weighing the risks of side effects (with the use of haloperidol) with the nature of impairment.

3. **Tourette disorder.**

a. **Definition and clinical presentation.** This disorder requires multiple motor and one or more vocal tics at some time (not necessarily concurrently). The tics occur many times a day or intermittently for at least a year. With time, the characteristics of the tics change in location, frequency, complexity, and severity. First symptoms vary but often are single motor tics that involve the face (especially the eye). Motor tics may become very complex (including hopping, skipping, and squatting) and may be in various combinations with the vocal tics. Vocal tics involve a diaphragmatic component and include various sounds (clicks, grunts, sniffs, coughs, or words). Coprolalia is a frequently cited finding that only occurs in roughly one third of cases, often beginning in adolescence.

b. **Associated features.** Patients have findings of

obsessions, compulsions, mental coprolalia (sudden intrusive thoughts of socially unacceptable or obscene words or phrases without an attempt to ignore or suppress the thoughts). Attentional difficulties and impulsivity may also be present.

c. **Epidemiology.** Lifetime prevalence ranges from 0.5 to 1000. Male-female ratio is 3:1. There is a high familial incidence, with an overlap with obsessive-compulsive disorder and ADHD.

d. **Differential diagnosis.** This requires both motor and vocal tics at some point in the absence of other neurologic disease or drug use.

e. **Etiology.** Various neurochemical hypotheses are supported by drug effects: Dopaminergic (antagonists, e.g., haloperidol, lead to improvement, and agonists, e.g., amphetamine, worsen or precipitate tics); noradrenergic (α-receptor agonists, e.g., clonidine, lead to improvement). Family studies suggest genetic factors important.

f. **Assessment.** Careful evaluation of the evolution of the syndrome over time and the degree of severity of distress and social impairment (in family and with peers) and family history.

g. **Treatment.** The following types are used.

(i) Psychosocial: Secondary to pharmacotherapy in this disorder. Support for the child is needed in the face of potential concerns around alienation and demoralization from the family and peer group. Family and education are important. It is unclear if behavioral techniques that reduce the frequency in other tic disorders are as effective when applied to patients with Tourette disorder. Further studies are needed.

(ii) Pharmacotherapy.

(a) First-line medication: Haloperidol has a good (70% to 80%) response rate but high discontinuation rate. Low doses are needed (see Chapter 25 on pharmacotherapy in children).

(b) **Second-line medication:** (if no response to a trial of haloperidol or unacceptable side effects): Pimozide (a postsynaptic dopamine receptor inhibitor) has been recently approved for use in Tourette disorder. Watch for significant cardiac side effects. Do not administer with haloperidol.

(c) **Third-line medication:** Clonidine has been shown to be less effective for tic reduction but does seem to improve attention and maladaptive behaviors (see Campbell and Spencer[6]).

E. **Elimination disorders.**

1. **Functional encopresis.**

a. **Definition and clinical presentation.** For a 6-month minimum, the child has at least a monthly repeated passage of feces in inappropriate places. Primary: after the age of 4 years with no fecal continence for more than a year; secondary: continence for at least 1 year after the age of 4 years.

This category includes youngsters who may soil intentionally or more commonly involuntarily, including overflow secondary to functional fecal retention. This may persist for years but rarely past midadolescence. The degree of impairment is related to effects on the family, peer relationships, and self-esteem.

b. **Associated features.** Twenty-five percent have functional enuresis as well. Social alienation and humiliation may be present.

c. **Differential diagnosis.** Rule out physical disease (e.g., aganglionic megacolon).

d. **Epidemiology.** One percent of 5-year-old children; males greater than females; higher in lower socioeconomic class; and familial distribution unknown.

e. **Etiology.** Multifactorial theory: Physiologic predisposition to a certain pattern of bowel function, bowel-training history, parent-child relationship, and family function and structure combined with environmental stresses to produce functional encopresis.

f. **Assessment.** Physical examination to rule out other illness, including anal fissure (which might produce pain and a subsequent functional retention to avoid pain). Evaluation of the type of soiling (timing, toilet availability, stool consistency, and location of soiling). Psychologic factors, parent-child dyadic relationship, and family pathology need a thorough evaluation. Assess for other psychopathologic condition in the child. Establish any precipitating events, such as birth of a sibling, divorce, and/or start of school. The relationship of the child's developmental stage, history of toilet training, and the social milieu changes needs to be examined.

g. **Treatment.** Hersov[10] has described a comprehensive approach to treatment. Only the most severe cases require inpatient treatment. The type of intervention is dependent on the nature of the soiling and associated etiologic factors. Appropriate management may include the following types.

(i) **Primary.** Behavioral reinforcement for appropriate behaviors. Functional retention with secondary overflow: Physical intervention (e.g., initial enema and stool softener) to reduce pain with defecation. Fear of parental intervention may require parental therapy to alter their style of response to the child.

(ii) **Secondary.** Multimodal approach, i.e., constipation relief and behavioral methods to reward appropriate behavior. Family intervention and psychotherapy to focus on potential rigidity in family interactions and on guilt and shame in the child. Biofeedback has been described as effective for older children.

2. **Functional enuresis (FE).**

a. **Definition and clinical presentation.** *DSM III-R* defines FE for children of at least a chronologic age of 5 years and mental age of 4 years as a repetitive urinary voiding in clothes or bed, voluntarily or unintentionally. These events must occur twice per month between 5 and 6 years old and at least once per month for older children. Two groups are defined: primary, without a year's history of urinary continence (80%); secondary, has had a year's history of urinary continence (20%). Diurnal (daytime) and nocturnal timing is also used in the classification of FE.

Functional enuresis is usually self-limited, even without intervention. However, secondary sequalae and resultant embarrassment can be minimized with efforts that more rapidly produce dryness.

   b. **Associated features.** The vast majority of children do NOT have other psychiatric disorders, but FE (especially combined diurnal and nocturnal) is associated with a higher rate of concomitant disorders. These include functional encopresis, sleepwalking disorder, and sleep terror disorder. Also, FE is associated with twice the likelihood of nonenuretic children for developmental delays. Enuresis may also be associated with subsequent low self-esteem, social embarrassment, alienation, and familial conflict.

   c. **Differential diagnosis.** Organic causes of enuresis (e.g., diabetes, urinary tract infection, renal disease, and seizure disorder) should be ruled out.

   d. **Epidemiology.** Age, 5 years: 7% males and 3% females. Age, 10 years: 3% males and 2% females. Age, 18 years: 1% males and nearly nonexistent in females.

   e. **Etiology.** Developmental delay in bladder musculature with impaired ability of bladder to fill without increased pressure, reproducing a lower volume threshold before voiding occurs. This biologic predisposition may then combine with an acute psychosocial stressor, such as entering school or the birth of a sibling. Other predisposing factors include a history of hospitalization (especially between the ages of 2 and 4 years) and a history of delayed toilet training.

   f. **Assessment.** Organic causes should be ruled out. Evaluate the onset of the illness, associated psychiatric disorders, and family interactions (especially around toilet training). Assess factors that might reinforce enuretic behavior and what role it plays in the family at this time.

g. **Treatment.** Establish a baseline record of wetting before active intervention. Encourage parents to reinforce dry nights. Educate family as to sleep and toilet habits: nighttime fluid restriction, bringing the child to the toilet before bedtime, and reinforcement for appropriate behaviors.

Behavioral interventions: If the above steps are not sufficient, the most effective and long-lasting intervention is the classic conditioning paradigm of the "bell and pad." This involves placing a pad under the child that sets off an alarm when wetted. Ideally, the initial urination then awakens the child who can then get up and urinate. Parental and child understanding and compliance are essential.

Fifty percent of cases respond in several weeks' time with no relapse. Those with or without other psychiatric disturbance have similar response rates to this intervention.

Pharmacotherapy: Under certain conditions, imipramine may be used. It has several drawbacks that include its characteristic side effects, development of tolerance, and a high relapse rate for the enuresis after discontinuation.

Shaffer[11] has suggested certain situations that might call for the use of imipramine: when wetting is the focus of significant masked hostility and requires rapid reduction of stressors, when immediate short-term effect is needed (e.g., during travel), and when use of the bell and pad is temporarily impossible or the family is noncompliant after an attempted trial.

Psychotherapy: This has not been shown to be effective alone for enuresis. It may be helpful for concomitant psychiatric disturbance in the child or family.

F. Speech disorders not elsewhere classified.

1. Cluttering.

a. Definition and clinical presentation. Usually, cluttering occurs in a child after the age of 7 years who has the onset over a few weeks to months of this disorder of speech fluency (rate and rhythm). Speech is dysrhythmic with jerky bursts of speech with faulty phrasing patterns (unrelated grammatically to other parts of sentence structure). Patients may be unaware of the deficit.

b. Associated features. There are fewer associated features than stuttering. Fragmented and incomplete sentences can produce impaired intelligibility and subsequent poor peer relations, family stress, and emotional difficulties. Also, children may have articulation deficits, expressive language errors, academic skills disorder, ADHD, and visuomotor impairments.

c. Differential diagnosis. Stuttering and spastic dysphonia (but children have awareness of disorder). Normal childhood dysfluency (around 2 years of age, transient).

d. Epidemiology. New category, insufficient data.

e. Etiology. Unknown.

f. Assessment. Involves a thorough psychiatric examination, including a speech and language evaluation and assessment of academic or neuropsychologic deficits. Patient's awareness of disability should be explored, and degree of social impairment should be assessed.

g. Treatment. Outcome studies have not yet been established for this newly classified disorder. Theoretically, speech therapy may be helpful, as well as supportive individual therapy, if social alienation is significant and distressing to the patient.

2. Stuttering.

a. Definition and clinical presentation. Children

present usually between 2 and 7 years of age with an impairment in speech fluency that is characterized by frequent repetitions of prolongations of sounds or syllables. They may also have other dysfluencies that involve blocks of sounds or interjection of words. This disturbance is also called "stammering" in the United States. Onset is gradual and, in almost all cases, is before the age of 10 years. Eighty percent recover by midadolescence (60% spontaneously).

b. **Associated features.** Impairment in peer relationships is common. Avoidance of speaking may produce academic difficulties. They may have anticipatory fear of stuttering and avoid certain situations or words. Abnormal movements may also be present, including eye blinks, tics, and mouth tremors. Emotional sequalae include fear, frustration, depression, and anxiety. Other developmental disorders (articulation and expressive language) may be present.

c. **Differential diagnosis.** Cluttering (patient with stuttering may be initially unaware but then becomes cognizant of the disturbance). Spastic dysphonia (has concomitant breathing pattern abnormality). Normal childhood dysfluency, at the age of 2 years, may be indistinguishable from stuttering.

d. **Epidemiology.** Male-female ratio, 3:1; 5% of children in population; higher (10%) in younger children; 1% in adults; high monozygotic twin concordance; and high familial incidence.

e. **Etiology.** Multiple theories, including: biologic predisposition (hypothesis about cerebral dominance deficiency); psychogenic models (stuttering as a neurotic symptom or as a learned behavioral response); and feedback (cybernetic) models. Recent twin and family data support a genetic predisposition.

f. **Assessment.** This is the same as with cluttering. Also, careful assessment of patient's awareness of and emotional reactions to the disturbance, including mechanisms employed to avoid the dysfluency. These latter avoidance efforts may enhance anxiety and worsen the underlying stuttering. Family response to the disorder should also be assessed.

g. **Treatment.** Several approaches have been attempted. One view of intervention is focused on target symptoms and behaviors.

(i) **Anxiety.** Education around the cycle of avoidance that enhances stuttering. Provision of support and anxiety-reducing cognitive/behavioral techniques. Also, highlight the view of stuttering as a modifiable behavior itself, not the sign of a hidden illness.

(ii) **Stuttering.** Some behavioral alterations in articulation have been tried with limited success. More effective seems to be the reduction of elements that may be secondary to the stuttering (e.g., fear, anxiety, and avoidance techniques) but maintain and intensify the dysfluency. Thus, supportive encouragement to speak and not avoid may provide a reduction in the impairment associated with stuttering.

(iii) **Emotional sequelae.** If demoralization and low self-esteem have become significant effects of the stuttering, then individual psychotherapy may be warranted to focus on these sequalae.

(iv) **Family issues.** Family intervention and education may be indicated if the family's response to the disorder has become a significant source of distress for the child and family.

G. **Other disorders of infancy, childhood, or adolescence.**

1. **Elective mutism.**

a. **Definition and clinical presentation.** This is an uncommon disorder characterized by a persistent refusal to talk in one or more significant social situations (e.g., school). Onset follows a period of normal development. Language comprehension and expression are generally intact, although some children may have delays and disarticulation. Onset is usually before the age of 5 years; duration is weeks to months, occasionally years. School and social impairment may be severe.

b. **Associated features.** Occasionally, speech disorders (developmental articulation disorder) or physical abnormalities that lead to disarticulation may be present. Social withdrawal, school refusal, temper tantrums, and other oppositional behavior may be present. Enuresis and encopresis have a higher incidence in elective mutism.

c. **Differential diagnosis.** Children with an inability to speak due to mental retardation or pervasive developmental disorder or due to developmental expressive language disorder. Children from countries with another primary language who have not yet mastered the new country's language. Transient mutism due to anxiety.

d. **Epidemiology.** Less than 1%, with females slightly more represented than males.

e. **Etiology.** Most theories indicate psychologic mechanisms that lead to the withholding of verbal output, usually only away from the family. Temperamental features (shyness), family dynamics (enmeshment with parent), and anxiety away from the home have been observed. This category also includes the finding of mutism as a sequela of a stressful event, or "traumatic mutism."

f. **Assessment.** Determine history of speaking in certain situations and ability to comprehend. Precipitant to onset should be assessed (e.g., changes in home and traumatic experiences). Family assessment of aggression, depression, and parental discord should be obtained. Determination of temperament and personality styles in child and family members should be made.

g. **Treatment.** Intervention will vary, depending on the etiologic factors in each case. Thus, treatment may include individual psychotherapy, family therapy, and behavioral interventions (including reciprocal inhibition, social skills training, and reinforcement schedules).

2. **Identity disorder.**

a. **Definition and clinical presentation.** Identity disorder usually occurs in late adolescence and is defined by a severe subjective distress regarding issues that relate to one's identity (including goals, career choice, friendships, sexual orientation and behavior, religion, morals, and group loyalties). This distress must last greater than 3 months, is independent of other psychiatric disorders at some point, and there is subsequent impairment in social academic or occupational functioning.

b. **Associated features.** The degree of inner turmoil is severe compared with the apparent external stressors. Ambivalence and oppositionality may be present. If persistent, these features may severely impair the individual's ability to reach certain goals, including separation from family or establishing a career direction.

c. **Differential diagnosis.** Identity problems secondary to other psychiatric illness (schizophrenia and mood disorders). Borderline personality disorder may also initially appear as identity disorder, but the concomitant disturbance in other areas distinguishes this disorder. Normal adolescence is not associated with the severity of distress or impairment as in identity disorder.

d. **Epidemiology.** Insufficient data.

e. **Etiology.** Theories suggest that the possible increase in the prevalence of this disorder in modern society might be due to an inability to achieve normal developmental integration of the self during adolescence in the face of an overwhelming number of choices that the individual must make regarding life-style, occupation, religious beliefs, and moral values. Thus, a cultural effect on the psychologic process of development of the self is suggested as a possible cause for this disorder.

f. **Assessment.** Evaluate the presence of other Axis I or II disorders. Determine the severity of distress and impairment. Assess the relationship of patient to family and nature of family function with respect to patient's developmental tasks of establishing independence and self-integration.

g. **Treatment.** Individual psychotherapy may be helpful to enhance the developmental task of identity consolidation and coherent integration of different aspects of the self. In certain cases, family issues may be intensifying the difficulties with this normal developmental task, and family intervention may be required.

3. **Reactive attachment disorder of infancy and early childhood.**

a. **Definition and clinical presentation.** This category defines a broad spectrum of disorders with an onset before the age of 5 years that are characterized by markedly disturbed social relatedness in the setting of pathogenic care.

This disturbed relatedness includes a failure to initiate or respond to most social interactions (e.g., lack of interest or visual tracking) or indiscriminant sociability (e.g., excessive friendliness with strangers). These are not due to mental retardation or a pervasive developmental disorder.

Pathogenic care needs to be present and persistent and includes (1) disregard for child's basic emotional needs (neglect and punishment); (2) disregard for child's physical needs (safety, nutrition, and housing); and (3) repeated change of caregiver (e.g., many foster homes).

This category presumes causality if the onset of the disordered relatedness is subsequent to the pathogenic care.

It may be helpful to view this category as relating

to a caregiver-child dysfunction. This dysfunction, if persistent, can result in significant impairment in the overall functioning of the child, leading to physical problems and possible death.

b. **Associated features.** Physical problems may be present (starvation and dehydration). Feeding and sleeping disturbances and hypersensitivity to touch and sound may be observed. Infection and death are potential complications.

c. **Differential diagnosis.** Mental retardation and pervasive developmental disorder can be associated with deficits in social relatedness. Severe neurologic abnormalities (including sensory deficits) or chronic medical illness should be distinguished from this disorder. According to *DSM-III-R*, psychosocial dwarfism has most of the features of this disorder, except for grossly pathogenic care.

d. **Epidemiology.** Insufficient data.

e. **Etiology.** The disorder assumes a pathogenic caregiver as the cause for the abnormalities in the social interactions of the child. Intervention by placement in a nurturing environment with subsequent improvement supports this view.

f. **Assessment.** Observation of the child-caregiver interaction and direct interaction between the child and examiner; look for eye contact, affective responsiveness, flexibility and complexity of interchanges, reciprocal interactions (games and responsivity), and age-appropriate child behaviors. Attempt to determine potential "mismatch" between the child's constitutional traits ("temperament") and the caregiver's ability to respond to these individual characteristics.

Home environment should be assessed: What is the living situation like, how many other children are provided for, and what are the stresses on the caregiver? Ask the caregiver about the "pleasure-distress" ratio in caring for this child. What support systems are available and being utilized?

g. Treatment. The child's safety is an over-riding concern. Thus, the acuteness of the situation needs to be assessed, and in some cases, placement is a necessary intervention.

In cases of the caregiver being motivated to improve the deficits in care, several combined approaches may be helpful: educational (child's needs and proper care), supportive (providing practical help, support groups, and financial counseling), and psychotherapeutic (individual or family therapy).

Because of the potential lethality of this disorder, close supervision of progress and involvement of child protective services may be necessary.

4. Stereotypy and habit disorder.

a. Definition and clinical presentation. This disorder includes children of any age with intentional, repetitive behaviors that cause physical injury to themselves or interfere with their normal activities. Examples of these nonfunctional behaviors include handshaking or handwaving, body rocking, head banging, nail biting, or picking at nose or skin. Course varies with etiology and ranges from brief to chronic with severe impairment.

b. Associated features. More severe forms are associated with mental retardation. Congenitally blind individuals may have this disorder. Occasionally, there are self-restraint behaviors, such as keeping hands in pockets, to prevent injuries.

c. Differential diagnosis. *DSM III-R* diagnosis cannot be made in pervasive developmental disorder or tic disorder, although these disorders frequently are associated with these behaviors. With tics, the movements are involuntary (although suppressible) and distress producing. Normal behaviors include rocking and thumb sucking in infants are normal and not associated with impairment or injury.

d. Epidemiology. New classification: insufficient

data. However, in mental retardation, it is estimated that 10% to 23% of children may have this disorder.

e. **Etiology.** There are various etiologic theories in different groups.

(i) **Abnormal development.** Exacerbation of normal patterns of self-stimulation seen in young children as in mental retardation.

(ii) **Psychosocial.** This may be secondary to a lack of stimulation, leading to self-stimulation or to attention-seeking behavior (that may be reinforced by the caregiver's response).

(iii) **Biochemical.** Psychoactive substances may produce these behaviors (e.g., amphetamines).

(iv) **Neurologic abnormalities.** This disorder is seen in several diseases (temporal lobe epilepsy, Lesch-Nyhan syndrome, and postencephalitic syndrome).

(v) **Psychiatric disorder feature.** This may be a component of other severe disorders (e.g., schizophrenia and obsessive-compulsive disorder).

f. **Assessment.** Evaluate the nature of the movements, i.e., their timing frequency and degree of severity. Assess the environment for lack of stimulation, possible reinforcers for behaviors, and exogenous medications. Determine the coexistence of other psychiatric or neurologic disorders.

g. **Treatment.** Interventions will depend on etiology. Provision of a safe environment is important. Increase external stimulation, if indicated. Reduce sources of reinforcing patterns of interaction for self-injurious behaviors and provide positive reinforcement for new adaptive behaviors. Eliminate psychoactive substance use. Provide treatment for other psychiatric disorders that may include psychotropic medications.

REFERENCES

1. Rutter M, Hersov L (eds): *Child and Adolescent Psychiatry: Modern Approaches*. London, Blackwell Scientific Publications, Inc, 1985.
2. Shaffer D, Ehrardt AE, Greenhill L (eds): *The Clinical Guide to Child Psychiatry*. New York, The Free Press, 1985.
3. American Psychiatric Association: *Diagnostic and Statistical Manual of Mental Disorders*, ed 3 (revised). Washington, DC, American Psychiatric Association, 1987.
4. Kaplan HI, Sadock BJ: *Synopsis of Psychiatry: Behavioral sciences and clinical psychiatry*, ed 5. Baltimore, Williams & Wilkins, 1988.
5. Cantwell DP, Carlson GA (eds): *Affective Disorders in Childhood and Adolescence: An Update*. New York, Spectrum Publications, 1983.
6. Strober M, Hanna G, McCracken J: Bipolar illness, in Last C, Hersen M (eds): *Handbook of Child Psychiatric Diagnosis*. New York, John Wiley & Sons, Inc, in press.
7. American Psychiatric Association: *Diagnostic and Statistical Manual of Mental Disorders*, ed 3. Washington, DC, American Psychiatric Association, .
8. Gittleman-Klein R: Pharmacology of childhood hyperactivity: An update, in Meltzer HY (ed): *Psychopharmacology: The Third Generation of Progress*. New York, Raven Press, 1987, pp 1215–1224.
9. Campbell M, Spencer EK: Psychopharmacology in child and adolescent psychiatry: A review of the past five years. *J Am Acad Child Adolesc Psychiatry* 1988; 27–3:269–279.
10. Gittleman-Klein R, Klein DF: Controlled imipramine treatment of school phobia. *Arch Gen Psychiatry* 1971; 25:204–207.

11. Green : , in Rutter M, Hersov L (eds): *Child and Adolescent Psychiatry: Modern Approaches*. London, Blackwell Scientific Publications, Inc, 1985, pp 638–649.
12. Stoller RJ: *Presentations of Gender*. New Haven, Conn, Yale University Press, 1986.
13. Hersov L: Faecal soiling, in Rutter M, Hersov L (eds): *Child and Adolescent Psychiatry: Modern Approaches*. London, Blackwell Scientific Publications, Inc, 1985, pp 482–489.
14. Shaffer D: Enuresis, in Rutter M, Hersov L (eds): *Child and Adolescent Psychiatry: Modern Approaches*. London, Blackwell Scientific Publications, Inc, 1985, pp 465–481.

14 | Axis II Disorders in Children and Adolescents

Axis II diagnoses in children include the rare use of personality disorder diagnoses and the developmental disorders. These latter disorders cover a wide range of syndromes, including mental retardation, pervasive developmental disorders, and specific developmental disorders.

I. **Developmental disorders.**

A. **Mental retardation.**

1. **Definition.** Most current definitions of mental retardation include consideration of both intellectual and adaptive functioning. Intellectual functioning is assessed by formal intelligence testing. Adaptive functioning is assessed clinically and includes the ability or trainability in personal health habits, motor skills, speech, nonverbal communication, social awareness, independence, and self-sufficiency.

2. **Diagnosis.** This is based on the American Association of Mental Deficiency (AAMD) standard of 1983. There must be concurrent impairment in adaptive functioning and a measured IQ below 70, with ranking of severity as follows:

55–70	Mild
40–55	Moderate
25–40	Severe
0–25	Profound

Borderline mental functioning, defined as an IQ between 70 and 85, was deleted as a diagnosis by the AAMD in 1973. It is included as a condition not attributable to a mental disorder in *DSM III-R*.[1]

3. **Associated features.** Other mental disorders (especially pervasive developmental disorders, attention-deficit hyperactivity disorder, and stereotypy/habit disorder) have a higher prevalence. Certain behavioral patterns may be present, including passivity, dependency, low-frustration tolerance, and aggressiveness with poor impulse control. Specific neurologic disorders have characteristic findings.

4. **Epidemiology.** The overall prevalence of mental retardation in the United States and Great Britain is around 1% when current *DSM III-R* criteria are applied. Studies that have reported prevalence rates of 2.5% to 3% are based on less restrictive diagnostic criteria; in these studies, almost 90% would fall in the mildly retarded category.

Mildly retarded individuals often develop skills that are sufficient to allow independent living, including full occupational independence; frequently children with IQs between 55 and 70 are not singled out from the general population. More severely retarded individuals generally require considerable adult support throughout their lives.

5. **Etiology.** In about 50% of cases, the etiology is unknown. Approximately one fourth of cases are at-

tributable to a genetic factor, and one fourth to an environmental factor, such as infant meningitis, fetal malnutrition, or maternal rubella. Down syndrome causes the highest proportion of the genetic cases.

6. **Assessment.** A thorough medical and neurologic evaluation is essential. A specific assessment of cognitive, motor, emotional, and social development is important. An evaluation of a patient's ability to perform or learn activities of daily living is helpful for caregivers.

7. **Treatment.** This includes family support, appropriate school or living placement, and behavioral intervention. Aggressive behavior, if not diminished by behavioral interventions, may require pharmacotherapy.

B. **Pervasive developmental disorders.**

1. **Autistic disorder.** Infantile autism or autistic disorder is a syndrome of behavior and perceptual deficits of unknown etiology, probably present at birth, that presents symptomatically in infancy or very early childhood.

a. **Clinical presentation.** Gaining familiarity with the clinical picture of autism is most easily acquired by seeing an autistic child. Characteristics include the following.

(i) **Social indifference.** There is a lack of facial responsiveness or eye contact with new people in the child's field of vision, an absence of social smiling and the anticipatory response to being picked up, and an absence of stranger anxiety. There is a tendency to avoid physical contact and cooperative play.

(ii) **Abnormal response to sensory input.** There may be no response to loud, frightening noises, a heightened response to other (e.g., distant) sounds, and an apparent fascination with certain textures, odors, or lights. There is often intense scrutiny of fine surface details of objects and of self-induced stimuli, such as with rubbing fabrics, sifting soil through hands, or flicking the ears.

(iii) **Communication disturbance.** There may be echolalia, both immediate and delayed (delayed even to the following day), aprosodic speech (speech without the emotional tone conveyed by rhythm, inflection, and tone), and pronoun reversals (e.g., "you for 'I'").

(iv) **Peculiarities of activity.** There are motor stereotypies or mannerisms, such as moving the hands rhythmically in the near visual field, hand flapping, walking on the toes, preoccupation with spinning (both objects and self), and posturing.

(v) **Uneven developmental progress.** There is often an associated diagnosis of mental retardation. However, there are often rapid developmental spurts and lengthy plateaus, and quite frequently, there are circumscribed areas of considerable developmental advance.

b. **Diagnosis.** *DSM III-R* defines the syndrome as consisting of disturbances in social interaction, communication, and imaginative activity, and a repertoire of activity and interest. It includes certain disturbances in cognition, motor behavior, and response to sensory input, as well as certain other common symptoms, as associated features, not essential to the diagnosis.

c. **Epidemiology.** Incidence ranges from 2 to 20/100,000, depending on the breadth of definition.

d. **Course.** Onset is early during infancy or before 36 months of age, rarely after 5 or 6 years of age. Good prognostic factors include a higher IQ and less severe language and social disturbances. Most autistic adults are severely handicapped. Of the fewer than one of six adults who attain some degree of independent occupational and social function, most retain a shallow affect, poor interpersonal skills, constricted and unusual interests, and a remarkable lack of awareness of others' feelings and social responses. Some may develop seizures before reaching adulthood, most often in early adolescence.

e. **Etiology.** Early theories of a family dysfunction that causes autism have been unsupported by all studies. Autism is a syndrome that may have a collection of causations. Data support several abnormalities, including genetic (siblings have 50 times the increased chance of having autism), biochemical (serotonin abnormalities), and cognitive (higher prenatal and perinatal complications).

f. **Treatment.** This includes family support, appropriate educational placement, and behavioral management. Studies support the clinical practice of pharmacotherapy for certain target behaviors (especially haloperidol, but less support for fenfluramine).

2. **Pervasive developmental disorders—not otherwise specified.** A grouping for children with qualitative impairment in reciprocal social interaction and of verbal and nonverbal communication skills.

C. **Specific developmental disorders.** These do not meet criteria for autism, schizophrenia, or schizotypal or schizoid personality disorder.

1. **General.** These disorders are determined by academic and neuropsychologic testing and are diagnosed when the child reveals inadequate development of specific skills (academic, language, and/or motor). Mental retardation and pervasive developmental disorder are supraordinate diagnoses. While the deficits may be remediable, they may not develop to normal function despite interventions.

2. **Assessment.** Autism may present with varying degrees of severity. Determination of functioning in the realms defined under "clinical presentation" is important. A detailed developmental history is essential. Family reaction to an "unusual child" should be determined. Theories vary for each disorder. The academic skills disorders may be due to maturational lags, cognitive dysfunction, and interacting effects of emotional and educational factors. There also may be a genetic predisposition. The language and speech disorders

may be due to similar influences that involve developmental delays (especially in articulation) and genetic predisposition to cerebral dysfunction. The high association of psychiatric morbidity with the language disorders may be secondary to or a primary feature of the language deficit. Developmental delays and cerebral trauma may be causal in the motor skills disorder. A further reason is needed to elaborate these theories of etiology.

3. **Evaluation.** Formal academic/motor testing should be compared with intellectual capacity.

4. **Differential diagnosis.** Other psychiatric diagnoses should be ruled out, including social deprivation, anxiety, depression, or specific physical or neurologic disorders.

5. **Diagnosis.** Each category of specific developmental disorder has functionally defined diagnostic criteria in *DSM III-R*. The essential clinical features are summarized briefly here.

a. **Academic skills disorder.**

(i) **Developmental arithmetic disorder.** Impairment in the development of arithmetic skills that interferes with academic functioning is less common than reading disability.

(ii) **Developmental expressive writing disorder.** This is a marked impairment in the ability to compose expressive writing tests; it may have a familial pattern and be associated with developmental language and reading disorders.

(iii) **Developmental reading disorder.** This marked impairment in the development of reading comprehension and work recognition skills may be associated with a personal history or family history of language and expressive writing disorders.

b. **Language and speech disorders.**

(i) **Developmental articulation disorder.** There is a wide range in the severity of impairment in the development of correct articulation of spoken sounds. Misarticulation, omissions, and substitutes that are characteristic of speech may be very responsive to therapy. Association with language disorders is common, and a familial pattern has been described. Often, early speech milestones are within normal limits.

(ii) **Developmental expressive language disorder.** This is an impairment in linguistic functioning in the ability to organize and express language (oral or written). It may be mild to severe with long-term impairment higher if associated with a receptive language component. Many patients recover without therapy if mild; it may be very responsive to speech therapy with attainment of normal speech by adolescence. Mild cases may first be recognized in late childhood/early adolescence.

(iii) **Developmental receptive language disorder.** This impairment in the comprehension of language varies from an inability to understand phrases to more severe forms with marked deficits in auditory processing. If this diagnosis is present, it usually has an earlier onset from other specific developmental disorders with which it is often associated. More severe forms are associated with disruptive behavioral disorders and generally higher psychiatric morbidity even with intervention (see Cantwell and Baker,[2] 1988).

c. **Motor skills disorder.** Motor coordination deficits present as developmental delays in motor milestones or as clumsiness in motor activities; it may be associated with other nonmotor developmental disorders and developmental delays.

6. **Treatment.** This should include intervention, i.e., school involvement designed to focus on the specific disability is crucial. Psychotherapy may be important for an associated disruptive behavior disorder

(behavioral/cognitive approaches) or depression, demoralization, and anxiety (supportive/dynamic therapy). Family involvement for education and exploration of the meaning of a disabled child in the family system can be important in many families. Guilt over genetic etiology in one spouse may be present.

II. **Personality disorder diagnoses.** Personality characteristics are shaped by inherited, temperamental, and environmental factors. Personality disorder traits may be present in childhood or adolescence. As childhood developmental stages may significantly affect personality traits, characteristics that will persist into adulthood are difficult to predict. For this reason, personality disorder diagnoses are usually not given to children or young adolescents. In unusual cases with clearly persistent and pervasive manifestations that meet the full criteria, a personality disorder diagnosis can be made.

The *DSM III-R* outlines a diagnostic correspondence between certain Axis I disorders in childhood and adolescence and Axis II diagnoses (in adults). Preliminary studies have suggested that many children with these Axis I diagnoses do NOT go on to have the corresponding Axis II diagnosis in adulthood. Thus, the nosologic relationship in these pairs is yet to be determined. The described diagnostic correlates are as follows:

Axis I	Axis II
Conduct disorder	Antisocial personality disorder
Avoidant disorder of childhood or adolescence	Avoidant personality disorder
Identity disorder	Borderline personality disorder

Personality traits that lead to social alienation from family and peers may contribute to demoralization and dysphoria. The role of therapeutic intervention needs further elaboration.

REFERENCES

1. American Psychiatric Association: *Diagnostic and Statistical Manual of Mental Disorders*, ed 3 (revised). Washington, DC, American Psychiatric Association, 1987.
2. Cantwell DP, Baker L: *Developmental Language and Speech Disorders*. New York, Guilford Press, 1988.
3. Graham P: *Child Psychiatry: A Developmental Approach*. Cambridge, England, Oxford University Press, Inc, 1986.
4. Grossman HJ: *Classification in Mental Retardation*. Washington, DC, American Association on Mental Deficiency, 1983.
5. Rutter M, Hersov L: *Child and Adolescent Psychiatry: Modern Approaches*. London, Blackwell Scientific Publications, Inc, 1985.
6. Shaffer D, Ehrhardt AE, Greenhill L (eds): *The Clinical Guide to Child Psychiatry*. New York, The Free Press, 1985.
7. Weiner J (ed): *Diagnosis and Psychopharmacology of Childhood and Adolescent Disorders*. New York, John Wiley & Sons, Inc, 1985.

15

Personality Disorders

Personality disorders are one of the most frequently encountered clinical entities in psychiatric practice. They are also one of the most difficult to define, to understand in terms of etiology, and to treat.

I. **Personality disorders—general issues.**

A. **Definition.**

1. *Personality* is the sum total of the characteristic patterns of feeling, thinking, and behaving that constitute the unique way a person interacts with his/her environment and with himself/herself.

2. *Personality traits* are subaspects of personality that are identifiable and consistent and are found in various combinations or patterns to form characteristic *personality types* (i.e., the submissive trait is frequently a part of dependent, histrionic, and avoidant personalities, and exploitiveness is frequently a part of narcissistic, borderline, and antisocial personalities, but each is grouped with different, other distinguishing traits in each case). Personality traits do not imply a pathologic condition as they are equally identifiable in normal personality types.

B. **Characteristics of personality.**

1. Personality (and thus a personality disorder) is

pervasive—it includes all aspects of the self, including both conscious and unconscious factors.

2. It is *stable*—the patterns and traits endure over time.

3. It is *consistent*—it replicates its characteristic responses across various situations and social contexts.

C. **Origin of personality.** The pervasive, stable, and consistent nature of personality is explained by its origin—rooted in a biologic and long-formed, environmentally shaped development.

1. *Temperament* refers to the unique constitutional subsets of personality—the energies, rhythms, sensitivities, and dispositions that are biologically endowed and are at least partially identifiable from birth. Heredity and prenatal factors contribute to temperament.

2. *Character* refers to the aspects of personality determined by environmental forces and are reflected in a person's adherences to and departures from the values and customs of his/her society and societal subgroups. Social learning theories are helpful explanations of this process.

3. *Personality* comprises both temperament and character and is a larger, more encompassing term than either.

4. Early developmental factors are more significant than later life experiences in the formation of personality; thus, both normal and unhealthy (abnormal) personalities emerge in childhood/adolescence and remain relatively stable throughout life. Continued social learning/adaptation throughout life may result in the diminishment of personality dysfunction in middle and later life in many cases.

D. **Normal vs. abnormal personality.**

1. An ideally healthy (normal) personality is characterized by the capacity to function autonomously and competently, a tendency to adjust to one's social en-

vironment effectively and efficiently, a subjective sense of contentment and satisfaction, and the ability to self-actualize and fulfill one's potentials. While most normal people may not achieve this ideal, they will approximate it through good social and occupational function and a sense of general well-being.

2. An abnormal or unhealthy personality is characterized by maladaptive, inflexible patterns of thinking, feeling, and relating. Emotional stability is either tenuous or maintained by a stultifying rigidity. There is a tendency to repeat vicious, self-defeating cycles of behavior. High levels of stress produce serious, interpersonal disturbances and/or physically or emotionally disabling symptoms.

3. Normality and abnormality are relative concepts that refer to broadly defined points on a behavioral continuum. Thus, abnormal personalities (personality disorders) are maladaptive extensions or extremes of normal personality patterns.

4. An example of how personality traits that may be adaptive and highly functional in their more flexible and moderate forms become maladaptive disorders in more extreme, inflexible cases is found in Table 15–1.

5. Personality is recognizable as pathologic when its maladaptivity is of sufficient severity to cause consistent impairment in social and/or occupational functioning or produces marked subjective distress.

II. **Personality disorders—classification.**

A. *DSM III-R* **personality disorders—accepted.**
DSM III-R provides diagnostic criteria for 11 widely accepted personality disorders. These have been further grouped into three clusters. Table 15–2 depicts these three clusters with associated terminology and features.

B. *DSM III-R* **personality disorders—provisional.**
DSM III-R includes an appendix that lists criteria for

TABLE 15-1.
Multidimensional Criterion List for Normal and Abnormal Personality*

Normal Personality Type	Abnormal Personality Type	Behavioral Appearance	Interpersonal Conduct	Cognitive Style	Affective Expression	Self-perception
Forceful	Antisocial	**Adventurous** Reckless	**Intimidating** Antagonistic	**Subjective** Personalitistic	**Angry** Malevolent	**Assertive** Competitive
Confident	Narcissistic	**Poised** Arrogant	**Unempathic** Exploitive	**Imaginative** Expansive	**Serene** Optimistic	**Confident** Admirable
Sociable	Histrionic	**Animated** Affected	**Demonstrative** Seductive	**Superficial** Flighty	**Dramatic** Fickle	**Charming** Sociable
Cooperative	Dependent	**Docile** Incompetent	**Compliant** Submissive	**Open** Naive	**Tender** Timid	**Weak** Inept
Sensitive	Passive-aggressive	**Erratic** Stubborn	**Unpredictable** Uncooperative	**Divergent** Inconsistent	**Pessimistic** Irritable	**Unappreciated** Mistreated
Respectful	Compulsive	**Organized** Perfectionistic	**Polite** Respectful	**Circumspect** Constricted	**Restrained** Solemn	**Reliable** Conscientious
Inhibited	Avoidant	**Watchful** Guarded	**Shy** Aversive	**Preoccupied** Distracted	**Uneasy** Anguished	**Lonely** Rejected
Introversive	Schizoid	**Passive** Lethargic	**Unobtrusive** Aloof	**Vague** Impoverished	**Bland** Flat	**Placid** Complacent

*From Millon T, Everly GS: Personality and Its Disorders. New York, John Wiley & Sons, Inc, 1985.

TABLE 15–2.
Diagnostic Criteria for Three Clusters of Personality Disorders

DSM III Clusters	DSM III-R Personality Disorder Diagnoses	Psychodynamic Descriptive Terminology	Genetic, Temperament, or Constitutional Terms (Spectrum of Illness)	Postulated Defense Mechanisms
Odd, eccentric, erratic, fantasy	Schizoid, paranoid, schizotypal	Autistic, narcissistic, prepsychotic	Schizophrenic spectrum (psychoticism)	Projection, schizoid distortion
Dramatic, emotional, erratic	Histrionic, antisocial, narcissistic, borderline	Extroverted, hysterical, character disorder	Psychopathic spectrum	Acting out, splitting, externalization, sexualization, somatization
Anxious, fearful, introverted	Avoidant, dependent, obsessive-compulsive, passive-aggressive	Introverted, sadomasochistic, pathologic neuroticism	Neurotic spectrum (neuroticism)	Isolation, regression, passive-aggression, reaction formation, hypochondriasis

Personality Disorders   285

two additional personality disorders that need further study before widespread acceptance is established.

1. **Self-defeating personality disorder.** A particular personality pattern in which a person is drawn to situations or relationships in which he/she will suffer, undermines pleasurable experiences, and prevents others from helping him/her.

2. **Sadistic personality disorder.** A particular personality in which a person demonstrates a pervasive pattern of cruel, demeaning, and aggressive behavior, not directed only toward one person, and not only for the purpose of sexual excitement (as in sexual sadism).

III. **Personality disorders—relationship to other psychiatric diagnoses.**

A. **Personality disorders—relationship to neurotic and psychotic disorders.** Spectrum of dysfunction: On a continuum of mental health, personality disorders generally fall between neurosis and psychosis.

1. **Psychosis.** Psychosis implies a gross impairment in reality testing and the creation of a new, alternative reality. When a person is psychotic, he/she incorrectly evaluates the accuracy of his/her perceptions and thoughts and makes incorrect inferences about external reality even in the face of contrary evidence. Direct evidence of psychotic behavior includes the presence of delusions, hallucinations, or grossly disorganized thinking.

a. **Psychotic disorders.** Most psychotic disorders are attributable to schizophrenia, bipolar disorder, depression, substance abuse, or organic mental disorders.

b. **Psychosis and personality disorders.** Persons with personality disorders generally do not experience psychosis. The eccentricities of schizotypal disorders and the suspiciousness of paranoid personality disorders reveal traits that approximate the more serious psychotic disorders, but these traits are comparatively minor distortions of reality that involve matters of relative judgment.

Borderline personality disorder may include brief (micro) psychotic episodes. These are generally the result of extreme stress and are of insufficient severity and duration to warrant an additional diagnosis. While they do not generally experience the gross disruptions of a fundamental function characteristic of psychosis, people with personality disorder uniformly have trouble in maintaining stable work and love relationships.

2. **Neurosis.** Neurosis is a term that is difficult to define due to its changing use in psychiatric practice. For this reason, and because of its psychoanalytic theoretical and somewhat hypothetical nature, its use is notably minimized in the *DSM III-R*. It originally referred to all emotional disturbances other than psychosis, although its use currently is generally limited to disorders (primarily anxiety disorders) in which neurotic processes are seen as the underlying cause.

a. **Neurotic disorder.** A neurotic disorder is a mental disorder in which the predominant disturbance is a distressing *symptom* or *group of symptoms* that one considers unacceptable and alien to one's personality (ego-dystonic). These symptoms are seen as the result of a neurotic process (see below).

(i) There is no marked loss of reality testing or gross disturbance of behavioral pattern in terms of social appropriateness.

(ii) The symptoms frequently are mild, but in severe cases, they can be disabling.

(iii) The disturbance is relatively enduring or recurrent without treatment and is not limited to a mild transitory reaction to stress.

(iv) There is no demonstrable organic etiology.

b. **Neurotic process.** A neurotic process is a specific etiologic process that involves the following sequence: unconscious conflicts between opposing wishes or between wishes and prohibitions lead to unconscious perceptions of dysphoria or anticipated danger. This leads to the use of a psychologic defense mechanism that results in symptoms and/or personality disturbance. In specific psychoanalytic terms, there is frequently a conflict between the intrapsychic demands of the id and the superego, and an inadequate ego is unable to resolve the conflict in a functional way. The purpose of therapeutic intervention, then, is to strengthen the ego through the development of more mature defense mechanisms (see below), thus enabling the person to resolve the intrapsychic conflict in a satisfactory way.

c. **Neurotic disorders and *DSM III-R*.** In *DSM III-R*, the neurotic disorders are included in the classifications for affective, anxiety, dissociation, somatoform, and sleep disorders. In the *DSM III-R* phenomenologically based classification, the term neurosis is not generally used, and the theoretical explanation of symptom etiology is not assumed. Some of the commonly identified neuroses and their *DSM III-R* equivalents are listed below.

(i) **Anxiety neurosis.** An unresolved internal conflict that results in chronic and persistent apprehension manifested by autonomic hyperactivity (sweating, palpitations, dizziness, etc.), musculoskeletal tension, and irritability. Somatic symptoms may be prominent. This is referred to in *DSM III* as either generalized anxiety disorder or panic disorder.

(ii) **Depersonalization neurosis.** An unconcious internal conflict that results in feelings of unreality and estrangements from one's body, one's self, or one's surroundings. Reality testing remains intact. This is referred to as depersonalization disorder in *DSM III-R*.

(iii) **Depressive neurosis.** Excessive reaction of depression due to a long-standing internal conflict (often involving a loss of a loved person or possession). This is labeled dysthymic disorder in *DSM III-R*.

(iv) **Hysterical neurosis (conversion type).** A psychiatric syndrome in which the predominant disturbance is a loss or alteration in physical function that suggests a physical disorder, but which is instead an expression and/or resolution of an extrapsychic conflict. Classic conversion symptoms include those that suggest neurologic disease, such as blindness, deafness, paralysis, coma, seizures, or somatosensory changes (i.e., anesthesias, pain, or paresthesias). This is referred to in *DSM III-R* as conversion disorder or somatoform pain disorder.

(v) **Hysterical neurosis (dissociative type).** An intrapsychic conflict that results in alterations in the state of consciousness or identity, producing such symptoms as amnesia, fugue, somnambulism, or multiple personality. In *DSM III-R*, classification is based on the most prominent symptom, i.e., psychogenic amnesia, psychogenic fugue, sleepwalking disorder, or multiple personality disorder.

(vi) **Obsessive-compulsive neurosis.** An unconscious internal conflict produces the persistent intrusion of unwanted and uncontrollable egodystonic thoughts and/or urges (obsessions) and actions (compulsions). The thoughts may consist of single words or phrases or whole trains of thought, all of which seem irrational. Actions may vary from single movements to complex rituals (repeated hand washings and checking behaviors). The *DSM III-R* classifies this as obsessive-compulsive disorder.

(vii) **Phobic neurosis.** An unconscious internal conflict that results in intense fear of an object or situation that the person consciously recognizes as harmless. Symptoms may include faintness, fatigue, palpitations, nausea, tremor, and even panic. The *DSM III-R* further classifies phobias as organic phobia, social phobia, or simple phobia.

d. **Neurosis and personality disorders.**

(i) **Similarities.**

(a) Neurotics and persons with personality disorders generally have intact reality testing.

(b) Depression and anxiety are common affect states in both a neurosis and a pathologic personality.

(ii) **Differences.**

(a) Neurotic disturbances are largely experienced as an intrapsychic dysfunction, and symptoms are ego-dystonic, whereas a personality pathology is largely experienced as an interpersonal dysfunction, and maladaptive behavior patterns are frequently experienced as ego-syntonic ("the problem is somebody else's fault"). For example, a person with an obsessive-compulsive disorder will be distressed at his/her own inability to control thoughts or behavior, while obsessive-compulsive personalities are frequently irritated at and intolerant of the imperfections or disorganization of other people.

(b) Generally, a neurosis is less pervasively disabling than personality disorders. Most neurotics have conflicts in more discreet, limited areas of their lives, resulting in manageable levels of anxiety or depression. In severe cases or under more severe stress, acute neurotic disorders with more severe symptoms may emerge. Most neurotics, however, are able to maintain reasonably stable relationships and occupations. In contrast, a personality dysfunction is pervasive and generally disrupts social and occupational function in a pervasive, repetitive way.

(c) Neurotics are generally more amenable to treatment than persons with personality disorders. Neurotic symptoms are ego-dystonic, so neurotic patients are motivated. Their disturbance is less pervasive, so they have greater personal and social resources to draw on. The abandonment of maladaptive neurotic defenses leads to the subjective relief of anxiety and depression, so that treatment is self-reinforcing. In contrast, persons with personality disorders tend to be less motivated and have less robust resources, and treatment is not self-reinforcing. The abandonment of maladaptive defenses tends to increase anxiety and depression previously abolished by these defenses.

(iii) **Overview of spectrum of illness.** The relationship of psychotic personality and neurotic disorders can be visualized on a continuum. This can be done in two ways: (1) a psychodynamic one (through an analysis of ego-defense mechanisms) and (2) a more genetic/descriptive one.

(a) **Defense mechanisms and the spectrum of illness.** Defense mechanisms are patterns of feelings, thoughts, or behaviors that are relatively involuntary (unconscious) and arise in response to perceptions of psychic danger. Their purpose is to keep psychic conflict and/or pain (along with any associated anxiety or distress) out of conscious awareness. Some of these defense mechanisms, such as projection, splitting, and acting out, are almost invariably maladaptive. Others, such as suppression and denial, may be either adaptive or maladaptive, depending on their severity, their inflexibility, and the context in which they occur. Others, such as altruism, sublimation, and humor, are usually adaptive.

Table 15–3 shows the spectrum of mental health. While there is some overlap, narcissistic defenses are largely found in psychotic disorders, immature defenses in personality disorders, neurotic defenses in neurotic disorders, and mature defenses in healthy, high-functioning adults. More primitive defenses are normal in young children, and all people tend to resort to more primitive defenses during periods of severe stress.

(b) **Genetic descriptive relationships and the spectrum of illness.** A broad, descriptive review of the relationship among neurotic, personality, and psychotic disorders is illustrated in Table 15–4.

B. **Personality disorders—relationship to affective disorders.** Research has shown that a subpopulation

TABLE 15–3.

Spectrum of Defenses*

Narcissistic (or Psychotic) Defenses	Immature Defenses	Neurotic Defenses	Mature Defenses
Denial (psychotic)	Acting out	Controlling	Altruism
Distortion	Blocking	Displacement	Anticipation
Projection (psychotic)	Hypochondriasis	Dissociation	Asceticism
	Introjection	Externalization	Humor
	Passive-aggressive behavior	Inhibition	Sublimation
	Projection (nonpsychotic)	Intellectualization	Suppression
	Regression	Isolation	
	Schizoid fantasy	Rationalization	
	Somatization	Reaction formation	
		Repression	
		Sexualization	
		Somatization	

*Developed from glossary of defenses in Kaplan H, Sadock B (eds): Comprehensive Textbook of Psychiatry, ed 4. Baltimore, Williams & Wilkins, 1985.

of patients present with interpersonal problems that suggest a personality disorder with an underlying affective or subaffective disorder. They may or may not have neurovegetative symptoms, but they do tend to have some fluctuation or cycling of their symptoms. Furthermore, significant objective improvement in social/occupational function and in reported subjective mood has been obtained through the use of antidepressant medication. The borderline personality disorder has been most thoroughly studied in this regard, although some evidence also exists for a subaffective component to some narcissistic, histrionic antisocial, and obsessive-compulsive personality disorders. Furthermore, patients with an underlying cyclothymic disorder may present a clinical picture that suggests a chaotic borderline disorder that is substantially improved with lithium therapy.

C. **Personality disorders—relationship to organic disorders.** The *DSM III-R* personality disorders are, by definition, etiologically unrelated to any identifiable organic disturbance and, as such, are coded on Axis II. There are, however, personality disturbances that are or appear to be causally related to organic factors. These are categorized as organic personality syndrome in *DSM III-R* and, as such, are coded on Axis I. This is a nonspecific term that applies to a wide range of clinical presentations and a variety of organic etiologies, all of which reveal a persistent personality disturbance. The most common etiologies include neoplasms (e.g., meningiomas), head trauma, cerebrovascular disease, dementing illnesses, and post-central nervous system infection. The most common clinical presentations are as follows:

1. **Frontal lobe syndromes**—Two primary types.

a. Convexity syndrome—characterized by pervasive apathy, lack of motivation, passivity, and blunted affect.

b. Orbital-medial syndrome—characterized by dis-

TABLE 15–4.
Relationship Among Neurotic, Personality, and Psychotic Disorders

	Neurotic Disorders	Personality Disorders	Psychotic Disorders
Ego function	Mild to moderate impairment but reality testing is intact	Mild to moderate impairment, but reality testing is intact	Severe impairment, reality testing always is impaired
Nature of disorder	Intrapsychic distress, symptoms of anxiety and depression	Interpersonal conflict or dysfunction, may have symptoms of anxiety or depression	Intrapsychic and interpersonal disruption with perceptual and cognitive disturbance
Developmental stage	Conflicts generally related to later (oedipal) stages	Conflicts generally related to earlier (pre-oedipal) stages	Regression to very earliest stages of fragmentation and disintegration, strong biologic/genetic loading makes

Basic ontologic fear	"Loss of the love of the object"	"Loss of the object"	developmental explanation less compelling "Loss of the self"
Onset	Chronic or acute	Chronic	Usually acute
Attitude of patient toward disorder	Symptoms viewed as ego-alien/ego-dystonic	Maladaptive behavior seen as ego-syntonic	Variable
Attitude of others toward patient	Moderate concern	Annoyance, anger	Great concern, fear
Genetic and underlying biologic factors	Undetermined, possibly present in some subgroups	Undetermined, probably present in some subgroups	Present in some subgroups

inhibition, social inappropriateness, poor impulse control, and affective lability.

2. **Temporal lobe epilepsy.** A highly idiosyncratic disturbance that often includes a deepening of affect, a humorless verbosity, hypergraphia, a vicious social style, a preoccupation with religion or supernatural ideas, and an altered sexual interest and behavior.

3. **Early-stage dementia.** One of the earliest indications of dementia may be an abnormal change in personality. This is particularly notable in Pick disease and multiple sclerosis, but may also be true for other dementing illnesses (i.e., Alzheimer disease, Huntington chorea, etc.).

D. **Personality disorders.** There is a relationship to childhood disorders. The *DSM III-R* classification indicates the following correspondence between disorders of childhood and adolescence and adult personality disorders.

Disorders of Childhood Adolescence	Personality Disorders
Conduct disorder	Antisocial personality disorder
Avoidant disorder of childhood or adolescence identity disorder	Avoidant personality disorder
	Borderline personality disorder

Disorders of childhood may or may not emerge in adulthood as the corresponding personality disorder. Since personality disturbances in childhood may reflect unusual social stresses and/or incomplete or delayed development, a diagnosis of personality disorders in childhood should be made with caution and only (if at all) when the disturbance is pervasive, persistent, and unlikely to be limited to a developmental stage. Indiscriminate labeling may confirm and contribute to the pathologic condition that it seeks to describe.

IV. Personality disorders—diagnosis and treatment.

The most broadly accepted criteria for diagnosing personalities are the phenomenologic/descriptive ones provided in the *DSM III-R*. Data from a thorough history and mental status examination, supplemented by psychologic testing, can be compared with those criteria in formulating a working diagnosis. A distillate of the major features of each personality disorder with corresponding differential diagnoses and distinguishing features is provided in Table 15–5.

The treatment of personality disorders is built around a central core of psychotherapy. Since a personality pathology is largely exercised in an interpersonal arena, the interpersonal nature and focus of psychotherapy are particularly well suited to addressing these disorders. Cognitive and behavioral approaches are generally used adjunctively for skill development and symptom control. Medication is also largely adjunctive and should be prescribed and monitored with regard to identified target symptoms and clearly formulated treatment goals that are determined and developed with the patient. For the patient, the meaning of taking psychotropic medication needs to be explored, clarified, and, if necessary, interpreted; otherwise, medication can complicate treatment rather than enhance it. A summary of basic treatment approaches for each of the personality disorders is included in Table 15–5.

TABLE 15–5.
Major Personality Disorder Features and Corresponding Differential Diagnoses and Distinguishing Features[*]

Diagnosis	Major Features	Diagnostic Factors		Distinguishing Features	Treatment Factors		
		Personality Disorders With Overlapping Criteria	Other Major Differential Diagnoses		Psychotherapy	Behavior Therapy	Pharmacotherapy
Cluster A (odd, eccentric)							
Paranoid personality disorder	Pervasive unwarranted suspiciousness, hypersensitivity to criticism, or restricted affectivity	Schizoid, schizotypal, avoidant, compulsive	Paranoid disorder schizophrenic, paranoid type antisocial personality disorder	Hypervigilance, suspiciousness, nonpsychotic presentation	Utilize direct, consistent, professional style; humor or intimate style easily misinterpreted; tendency to oversimplify; identify activating stressors	Reduce hypersensitivity to criticism, improve social skills	Consider low-dose neuroleptics
Schizoid personality disorder	General social indifference, isolative, restricted range of affect and expression	Schizotypal, paranoid, avoidant, compulsive	Schizophrenia	Social isolation without psychotic symptoms or excessive sensitivity to rejection	Major concern is developing working therapeutic relationship; gradually encourage other social activities and relationships	Possible social skills development in later stages of therapy	Minimal
Schizotypal personality disorder	Idiosyncratic pattern of thought, appearance, and behavior; social nonconformity;	Schizoid, paranoid, avoidant, compulsive	Schizophrenia, depersonalization disorder, paranoid disorder, borderline personality disorder	Cognitive/perceptual distortions without formal psychotic symptoms	Understand and clarify patient's feelings; therapist to convey acceptance and consistency	Social skills training, strengthen cognitive processing skills, anxiety control for social anxiety	Consider low-dose neuroleptics

Personality Disorders

Disorder	Features	Differential Diagnosis	Associated Types	Psychotherapy	Behavioral/Social Treatment	Pharmacotherapy
Cluster B (dramatic, emotional, erratic)	discomfort of isolation					
Antisocial personality disorder	Consistent pattern of irresponsible and antisocial behavior identifiable before age of 15 yr and continuing into adult life	Attention deficit disorder, substance abuse, mania, depressive disorder	Borderline, histrionic	Consistent violation of rights of others, lack of loyalty in interpersonal relationships	Group therapy, institutional setting; individual therapy of limited value	Treat with respect, firmness and consistency of program, rechannel into more prosocial activities	Consider antidepressants, manage drug/alcohol associated conditions
Borderline personality disorder	Pervasive pattern of instability of mood, interpersonal relationships, and self-image	Bipolar disorder, cyclothymic disorder, depressive disorders, attention deficit disorder, brief reactive psychosis, substance abuse disorders	Antisocial, histrionic, narcissistic	Intense, unstable relationships; impulsive, often self-destructive behavior; unstable mood, often shifting rapidly in parallel with shifts in interpersonal relationships	Empathic, consistent, and insightful management of therapeutic relationship; careful atten to boundaries and interpersonal distance (engulfment-abandonment dilemmas); focus on fragile sense of self-identity, contradictory impressions of self and others, and nature of conflicts in close relationships	Impulse-control training, problem-solving skill training, social skills training, vocational skills training	Consider antidepressants, lithium, low-dose neuroleptics, carbamazepine

(Continued.)

TABLE 15-5 (cont.)
Major Personality Disorder Features and Corresponding Differential Diagnoses and Distinguishing Features*

Diagnosis	Major Features	Personality Disorders With Overlapping Criteria	Other Major Differential Diagnoses	Distinguishing Features	Psychotherapy	Behavior Therapy	Pharmacotherapy
Histrionic personality disorder	Pervasive pattern of excessive emotionality and attention and attention-seeking behavior	Borderline, antisocial	Dysthymic disorder, depressive disorder, somatization disorder, brief reactive psychosis	Hyperemotional responses, superficial claim but shallow relationships, seductive behavior, highly dependent relationships	Careful attention to professional boundaries, emphasize calm reasonable approaches to dealing with crisis, identify maladaptive patterns for obtaining gratification of dependency needs	Moderate emotional expression and decrease of manipulative behaviors, reinforce genuineness and empathy	Consider antidepressants, particularly MAOIs for hysteroid dysphoria
Narcissistic personality disorder	Inability to satisfactorily maintain and regulate self-esteem, resulting in maladaptive patterns of thinking and behavior: self-aggrandizing fantasy, behavior entitlement, and interpersonal exploitiveness, lack of empathy,	Antisocial, borderline, histrionic, obsessive-compulsive	Depressive disorder, dysthymic disorder	Fragile self-esteem, exaggerated self-importance, constant seeking of admiration	Maintain empathic consistent therapeutic relationship, careful attention to boundaries and shifting transference (idealized vs. devaluing), focus empathically on patient's vulnerability and ways of defending against awareness of	Moderate extremes—patient's tendency to overvalue and devalue, reinforce expressions of empathy	Consider antidepressants, lithium

300 *Psychiatric Disorders*

Personality Disorders

Disorder	Description	Differential	Axis I	Key features	Psychodynamic approach	Behavioral approach	Pharmacology
Avoidant personality disorder	Pervasive pattern of social discomfort, fear of negative evaluation; timidity and social isolation; these are in the presence of deep desire for affection, acceptance, and attachment hypersensitivity to criticism	Schizoid, schizotypal, dependent	Social phobias	Sensitivity to rejection combined with avoidance of relationships	Gentle, careful building of trust in therapeutic relationship; facilitation of opportunities to enhance self-esteem	Systematic desensitization, social skills training, cognitive	Consider MAOIs, beta blockers
Dependent personality disorder	Pervasive pattern of dependent passive and submissive behavior	Avoidant, borderline, narcissistic	Agoraphobia	Subordinates own needs, avoids self-reliance	Interpretation dynamics that sustain dependency, assessment of capacity for independent function	Anxiety management program, assertiveness training, social/occupational skills training if applicable	Consider antidepressants, MAOIs
Obsessive-compulsive personality	Pervasive attempts to manage inner anxieties through inflexible attempts to perfectly master and control one's environment (including other people).	Schizoid, schizotypal, paranoid	Obsessive-compulsive disorder	Perfectionism and scrupulosity, stubbornness and rigidity	Dream analysis and use of unconscious material, interpretation of wishes and fears underlying "controlling" behavior, avoid overintellectualizing	Social skills training, reinforce affective responsivity while decreasing intellectualized processes	Consider clomipramine

(Continued.)

TABLE 15-5 (cont.)
Major Personality Disorder Features and Corresponding Differential Diagnoses and Distinguishing Features*

Diagnosis	Diagnostic Factors			Treatment Factors		
	Major Features	Personality Disorders With Overlapping Criteria	Other Major Differential Diagnoses	Distinguishing Features	Psychotherapy	Behavior Therapy	Pharmacotherapy
	insistence on perfection is reflected in indecisiveness, difficulty in task completion, and devotion to work, order, and productivity						
Passive-aggressive personality disorder	Pervasive pattern of passive resistance to demands for adequate social and occupational performance	Obsessive-compulsive narcissistic	Oppositional disorder	Passive resistance to demands of others	Avoid advice giving, rescuing, or struggles for control; interpret anger/hostility behind passive behavior; confront expressions of passive resistance (i.e., late payments, arrivals, or missed sessions, etc.)		

*PDO = personality disorder; ETOH = alcohol; MAOIs = monoamine oxidase inhibitors.

REFERENCES

1. American Psychiatric Association: *Diagnostic and Statistical Manual of Mental Disorders*, ed 3 (revised). Washington, DC, American Psychiatric Association, 1987.
2. Liebowitz, MR, Stone MH, Turkat ID: Treatment of personality disorders, in Frances AJ, Hales RE (eds): *Psychiatry Update*, vol 5. Washington, DC, American Psychiatric Press, Inc, 1986, pp 356–450.
3. Millon T, Everly GS: *Personality and Its Disorders*. New York, John Wiley & Sons, Inc, 1985.
4. Meissner WW: Theories of personality and psychopathology: Classical psychoanalysis, in Kaplan H, Sadock B (eds): *Comprehensive Textbook of Psychiatry*, ed 4. pp 337–418.
5. Vaillant GE, Perry JC: Personality disorders, in Kaplan H, Sadock B (eds): *Comprehensive Textbook of Psychiatry*, ed 4. pp 958–986.
6. Waldinger RJ: *Fundamentals of Psychiatry*. Washington, DC, American Psychiatric Press, Inc, 1986.

16
Sleep: Its Order and Disorder

I. **Definition.** Sleep can be defined as a regular, recurrent, easily reversible state characterized by relative quiescence and an increase in the threshold of response to external stimuli relative to the waking state. It is both a behavioral and a biologic state.

II. **Normal sleep cycle.**

A. Major theories.

1. Sleep is a passive process. This theory postulates that sleep (nonwakefulness) is the normal state and that wakefulness is produced by the ascending reticular activating system. This theory is currently falling out of favor.

2. Sleep is an active process. This theory postulates that sleep is produced by certain structures, specifically the hypothalamus (preoptic area), the nucleus solitarius, and the raphe nuclei, overcoming the activating influences that are associated with wakefulness.

B. Physiology.

1. The neurotransmitters involved in sleep have not been clearly delineated, but serotonin, acetylcholine, norepinephrine, gamma-aminobutyric acid (GABA), and perhaps dopamine all appear to be involved. Recent

evidence suggests that serotonin may allow for the induction of sleep by another factor, possibly a peptide, and acetylcholine levels appear to be increased in cerebrospinal fluid during rapid eye movement (REM) sleep. Gamma-aminobutyric acid has also been implicated in the sleep process, particularly because of its role as a major inhibitory transmitter in the central nervous system (CNS), because the benzodiazepines appear to work as potentiators of GABA. A recent discovery is DSIP (delta sleep-inducing peptide), a "hypnotoxin" that induces sleep in animal studies. It is found in greatest concentration in the thalamus and has effects similar to the benzodiazepines.

2. Sleep-wakefulness is cyclic, showing a circadian rhythm related to similar rhythms for body temperature, hormone release (i.e., growth hormone, melatonin, and cortisol), urinary excretion, and even hepatic enzyme activity. These cycles are modulated by light-dark cycles that affect the human internal clock, which, it seems, runs on a 25-hour cycle when not influenced by external clues.

C. Stages.

1. There are three discrete levels of activity of the human CNS identified: (1) waking or arousal, (2) the synchronized or non-REM stages of sleep, and (3) desynchronized or REM sleep. Normal people have relatively similar sleep patterns. During a night's sleep, they will have four to five REM-non-REM cycles characterized by increasing lengths of the REM stage in successive cycles. The first REM sleep period generally occurs around 90 minutes after the initiation of sleep. Non-REM sleep constitutes from 75% to 80% of normal sleep time and is divided into four stages characterized by increasing depth of unconsciousness and specific electroencephalographic (EEG) patterns (Fig 16–1).

2. Non-REM sleep is divided into four stages. Stage 1 is a normally brief state that lasts from 1 to 7 minutes during which, if the subject is awakened, he/she will

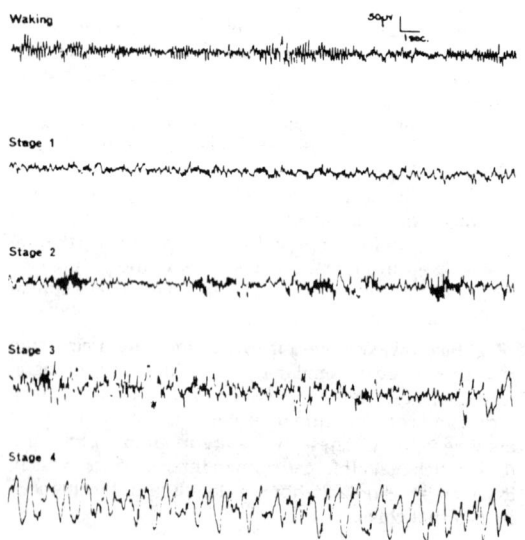

FIG 16–1.
Human sleep stages: the EEG of sleep in a human adult. A single channel of recording—a monopolar recording from the left parietal area, referred to the ears as a neutral reference point—is shown for each stage. (From Hartmann EL, Sleep, in Kaplan HI, Sadock, BJ (eds): *Comprehensive Textbook of Psychiatry*, ed 4. Baltimore, Williams & Wilkins, 1985, pp 55–67. Used with permission.)

report no dreams and feel as if he/she was only half asleep. In stage 2, the patient is truly asleep, and muscle tone, heart rate, and blood pressure all tend to decrease. Stage 3 is behaviorally similar to stage 2 but is characterized by delta activity on an EEG recording, which represents more than 20% of the background activity. Stage 4 is similar to stages 2 and 3 but is characterized by delta activity that represents more than 50% of the background activity. Most mental and physical recovery obtained from sleep occurs during stages 3 and 4 of non-REM sleep.

3. Rapid eye movement or desynchronized sleep is characterized by rapid and jerky, but symmetric, eye movements that give this state its name, by an EEG pattern very similar to the waking state, and by skeletal muscle atonia. It is also associated with an increase in pulse rate, blood pressure, cerebral blood flow, muscle metabolism, and penile erection in males. There is so much mental, EEG, and physiologic activity during this stage, that it is often referred to as paradoxical sleep.

III. Variations in the sleep cycle.

A. Significant changes in the sleep cycle occur with the various sleep and arousal disorders listed in Section IV, but variations occur in other situations also.

B. Infants may spend 16 to 20 hours each day sleeping, 50% of this time in REM sleep. Children may spend 10 to 13 hours asleep, 30% of this in REM sleep. After puberty, REM constitutes from 20% to 25% of the time asleep, which varies from 6 to 8 hours for most people, with the lower numbers being more common in the elderly for both total sleep time and for REM percentage. However, a wide variability of sleep needs exist in the general population, with some requiring less than 6 hours of sleep and others requiring more than 8 hours. With advancing age, stage I increases, while stages III and IV tend to decrease, until by the age of 60 years, very little stage III or IV sleep remain. Also in the elderly, sleep becomes more fragmented with frequent awakenings and increasing difficulty in returning to sleep.

C. Following sleep deprivation, REM sleep may occur almost immediately after the initiation of sleep, and it constitutes a greater proportion of sleep time (REM rebound); sleep time itself is generally increased. An REM rebound may also occur after suppression of REM sleep by selective awakening and after suppression by the use of alcohol or other hypnotic agents. Deprivation of the delta stages of non-REM sleep will cause a rebound of delta sleep.

D. Drugs frequently affect sleep architecture. The commonly used antidepressant medications, the heterocyclics, the monoamine oxidase inhibitors (MAOIs), and lithium, all cause a decrease in REM sleep. Studies with the heterocyclic agents indicate that tolerance to this REM suppression does not develop, and rebound occurs following discontinuation of these drugs. An REM rebound does not appear to occur with lithium. Interestingly, electroconvulsive therapy and cocaine also cause a decrease in REM sleep. The neuroleptic agents may increase drowsiness and REM sleep; however, high doses of chlorpromazine suppress REM. L-Tryptophan has variable and uncertain effects on sleep. The benzodiazepines cause a decrease in stages I, III, and IV, an increase in stage II, and an increase in REM latency, as well as a decrease in REM sleep. Tolerance develops rapidly to the sedative-hypnotics, and their long-term use results in irregular sleep latency, REM suppression, and frequent awakenings.

IV. **Sleep disorders by DSM III-R classification.** *DSM III-R* restricts its sleep disorders to those disturbances of sleep that are chronic (more than one month's duration), not including the transient disturbances that are part of everyday life due to psychosocial stressors. Other classifications of sleep disorders, such as the Association of Sleep Disorders Centers (ASDC) classification, have included transient and situational sleep problems.

A. **Dyssomnias.** The dyssomnias refer to disturbances in the amount, quality, and timing of sleep.

1. **Insomnia disorders.** These are disorders of initiating or maintaining sleep (DIMS), or of not feeling rested after sleep. They must occur at least three times per week for at least 1 month and result in significant

daytime fatigue. Approximately 15% of the general population complains of insomnia, but the social and occupational impairment is relatively mild in most cases. It may manifest as initial, middle, or terminal insomnia and can be treated, if severe, with a brief (2-week) course of a short-acting benzodiazepines (Table 16–1). Tolerance to the sedative effects of the hypnotic agents develops rapidly, and long-term treatment is useless. Biofeedback and relaxation techniques may be helpful.

a. **Insomnia related to another mental disorder (nonorganic) (*DSM III-R* 307.42).** This is an insomnia disorder due to an Axis I or II nonorganic mental disorder. Depression and anxiety are probably the most common associated disorders. With major depression, terminal insomnia is typical as is a shortened REM latency, a lengthened first REM period, and reduced stages 3 and 4 sleep. Manic and hypomanic patients generally do not complain of a sleep problem and appear to have a true reduction in the need for sleep. Of importance is that a sleep disturbance may herald the onset of a psychotic decompensation.

b. **Insomnia related to a known organic factor (*DSM III-R* 780.50).** This is an insomnia disorder related to a known organic factor or physical disorder, such as sleep apnea, Parkinson disease, myoclonus, pain syndromes, or psychoactive substances. Under the ASDC classification, this category has been divided up further, including (1) sleep apnea DIMS syndrome due to a central breathing cessation or upper airway obstruction, (2) the alveolar hypoventilation DIMS syndrome, and (3) the DIMS associated with nocturnal myoclonus or restless legs.

A wide variety of agents may cause sleep disorders, both with long-term use and with withdrawal. These include cancer chemotherapeutic agents, steroids, stimulants, depressants, antihypertensives, thyroid preparations, MAOIs, oral contraceptives, anticonvulsants, opiates, and hallucinogens. Long-term alcohol use may

TABLE 16–1.
Treatment of Transient Insomnia*

Hypnotic Agents	$T_{1/2}$, hr	Dose, mg (Given at Bedtime)
Lorazepam (Ativan)	9–12	1–2
Oxazepam (Serax)	3–21	15–30
Flurazepam (Dalmane)	3–8	15–30
Temazepam (Restoril)	5–15	15–30
Triazolam (Halcion)	2–3	0.125–0.5

*$T_{1/2}$ = half-life.

also result in a severe disintegration of sleep architecture with reduced sleep time, as well as fragmented and reduced REM sleep. During alcohol withdrawal, insomnia may last for weeks.

c. **Primary insomnia (*DSM III-R* 307.42).** This is an insomnia disorder that is not associated with another mental disorder or known organic factor. The person may be preoccupied and worry excessively about his/her sleep difficulties. This tension may exacerbate nighttime sleep difficulty; yet, the person may inadvertently fall asleep easily during the day.

2. **Hypersomnia disorder.** This category was formerly called the disorders of excessive somnolence (DOES) and has the essential feature of excessive daytime sleepiness or prolonged transition to the fully awake state (sleep drunkenness). The prevalence of these disorders is 1% to 2%, with social and occupational impairment highly variable.

One of these disorders, the Kleine-Levin syndrome, is an interesting but relatively rare condition characterized by recurrent periods of hypersomnia. It is often associated with hyperphagia, apathy, irritability, confusion, loss of sexual inhibitions, and withdrawal from social interactions. Onset is between the ages of 10 and 21 years, favoring males. It is often self-limited, ending by the age of 40 years.

In women, a menstrual-associated syndrome marked by hypersomnolence and voracious eating, occurring shortly before or at the onset of menses, has been described.

Sleep drunkenness is a form of confusional state and clouded sensorium that occurs when the transition from sleep to full wakefulness is prolonged and exaggerated. This rare condition may be familial.

a. **Hypersomnia related to another mental disorder (nonorganic) (*DSM III-R* 307.44).** This is a hypersomnia disorder due to an Axis I or II nonorganic mental disorder. This may be associated with bipolar disorder, unipolar depression, and/or cyclothymic and dysthymic syndromes. It is, however, unusual for bipolar depressed persons to show the degree of excessive somnolence seen in the other hypersomnias.

b. **Hypersomnia related to a known organic factor (*DSM III-R* 780.50).** This is associated with a known organic factor, such as a physical disorder, psychoactive substance, or medication. The physical disorder may not be readily apparent, and a patient presenting with complaints of daytime somnolence often warrants referral to a sleep disorders specialist.

Under the ASDC classification, this category has been divided up further, including (1) sleep apnea DOES syndrome and (2) alveolar hypoventilation DOES syndrome.

These are relatively common disorders that are marked by central or obstructive apnea. Predisposing factors include advanced age, male sex, and extreme obesity (pickwickian syndrome), but these may not be present. Patients may show irritability, emotional lability, depression, loud snoring, or gasping. Serious medical complications of the persisting syndrome include pulmonary and systemic hypertension, congestive heart failure, cardiac arrhythmias, sinus arrest, impotence, morning headache, impairment of memory, attention, and cognition. Polysomnography and oximetry are helpful in determining the diagnosis and severity of the disorder. Treatment includes weight reduction for obese patients, sleeping in an upright position, and surgical correction in the obstructive syndromes. Low-flow oxygen and occasional mechanical assistance devices, pharmacologic agents, such as imipramine, clomipramine, protriptyline, and theophylline, as well as the avoidance of depressant agents, including alcohol, hypnotics, and beta blockers, may also be helpful.

Also under this subgroup, in the ASDC classification, would be the sleep-related myoclonus and restless legs syndromes and narcolepsy.

Narcolepsy is a syndrome of excessive daytime sleepiness with sleep-onset REM periods that may be associated with hypnagogic hallucinations, cataplexy, or sleep attacks, and sleep paralysis. The onset is generally between the ages of 10 and 30 years, favoring males. Diagnosis is frequently made clinically when patients present with one or more of the classic tetrad of symptoms mentioned above. Diagnosis may be confirmed by polysomnographic detection of REM immediately on sleep onset. Forced daytime naps are helpful although stimulant medication is often needed, with methylphenidate being the drug of choice. Antidepressants have been used when cataplexy is a problem. Non-REM narcolepsy is a disorder of recurrent daytime sleepiness but without the sleep attacks and other accompanying symptoms. The sleep-onset REM is not present, and there is little response to stimulant medication. The serotonin blocker, methysergide, may be useful.

c. **Primary hypersomnia (*DSM III-R* 780.54).** This is a hypersomnia that is not related to another mental disorder or known organic factor.

d. **Sleep-wake schedule disorder (*DSM III-R* 307.45).** This disorder results from a mismatch between the normal circadian rhythms and the normal sleep-wake cycle demanded by the environment. These occur transiently when one changes time zones rapidly (jet lag) or changes a job schedule, such as when a work period is scheduled during one's habitual sleep period. There are three types of sleep-wake schedule disorder: (1) the advanced or delayed type, (2) the disorganized type, and (3) the frequently changing type.

In the advanced or delayed type, the onset and offset of sleep are considerably advanced or delayed from what the person wishes. The delayed type is more frequently observed in those persons who previously had few scheduled work or social commitments. This is often too aggressively treated with medication. The advanced type is more frequently observed in the elderly. It may result in early-morning awakening and may be difficult to differentiate from depression. The disorganized type shows a random and unpredictable pattern of sleep and wake times. It may occur in people who sleep haphazardly or nap frequently, especially elderly or bedridden persons. The frequently changing type is associated with airplane flights or with changing work schedules.

The only effective treatment approach is chronotherapy that involves a systematic daily change of environmental stimuli until the sleep-wake cycle is adjusted to meet personal and environmental needs. Sedative-hypnotics are frequently prescribed in these disorders but are of little, if any, help.

e. **Dyssomnia not otherwise specified (*DSM III-R* 307.40).** This includes insomnias, hypersomnias, or sleep-wake schedule disturbances that cannot be classified in any of the specific categories noted above.

B. **Parasomnias.** These disorders constitute about 15% of sleep disorder diagnoses. They do not cause complaints of insomnia, hypersomnia, or sleep-wake schedule problems but rather are disorders that involve an abnormal event that occurs during sleep or at the threshold between wakefulness and sleep. Sleep-related seizures compose approximately 11% of this group and should be looked for with a sleep EEG recording, as no abnormality may be seen with a waking EEG recording.

1. **Dream anxiety disorder (nightmare disorder) (*DSM III-R* 307.47).** This disorder consists of repeated awakenings from sleep with a detailed recall of vivid frightening dreams. They may increase during periods of mental stress and decrease with fatigue. They occur during periods of REM sleep, often at the end of the night when REM sleep is more abundant. An increased frequency of nightmares can be associated with depres-

sion and anxiety, as well as with withdrawal from drugs, such as reserpine, beta blockers, alcohol, and thiothixene. However, if drugs or alcohol are clearly precipitating factors, then the disorder is classified as parasomnia NOS (*DSM III-R* 307.40) (see below). Psychotherapy and behavioral treatment have been described as effective treatment methods. As contrasted with sleep terror disorder, large-body movements are not a feature, due to the REM-related loss of muscle tone, and the patient rapidly becomes oriented on awakening.

2. **Sleep terror disorder (pavor nocturnus) (*DSM III-R* 307.46).** This disorder involves repeated episodes of abrupt awakening that are often incomplete and usually begin with a panicky scream. The person may report having had a sense of terror and fragmentary dream images before arousal. It occurs more commonly during the first third of the major sleep period during stages 3 and 4 of non-REM sleep and lasts from 1 to 10 minutes. The person may show signs of acute anxiety with dilated pupils, profuse perspiration, tachypnea, tachycardia, and piloerection. The person is unresponsive to the comforting efforts of others until the agitation and confusion subside, and has morning amnesia for the episode. It usually begins between the ages of 4 and 12 years but may appear in early adulthood, and it favors males. Benzodiazepines and imipramine are the agents of choice for treatment.

3. **Sleepwalking disorder (somnambulism) (*DSM III-R* 307.46).** This disorder involves repeated episodes of a sequence of complex behaviors, including leaving the bed and ambulating without cognizance or later memory. Like sleep terror disorder, it occurs during the first third of the major sleep period (during stage III or IV non-REM sleep) during the delta activity on the EEG recording. It generally lasts up to 30 minutes. The episode generally starts with perseverative motor movements and progresses to complex motor acts, such as walking, dressing, eating, and going to the bathroom. During sleepwalking, the person is relatively un-

responsive and is difficult to awaken. Coordination is poor, and sleepwalkers may injure themselves. The person may return to bed without ever awakening or may awaken in a strange place. Sometimes, the person awakens during the event and is disoriented for several minutes. Frequency of occurrence is increased by fatigue and stress. The disorder begins between the ages of 6 and 12 years, and most persons outgrow it by their 20s. It is important to rule out a seizure disorder. Although many cases are not treatable by medication, diazepam and imipramine are sometimes effective.

4. **Parasomnia NOS (*DSM III-R* 307.40).** This disorder involves a disturbance during sleep that cannot be classified in the above categories.

5. **Sleep-related enuresis.** This was previously categorized by ASDC criteria as a parasomnia. It has been reclassified by the *DSM III-R* as a functional enuresis under elimination disorders. This disorder is characterized by involuntary or intential voiding of urine during day or night, after the age of 5 years and the mental age of 4 years. It is considered secondary if it has been preceded by a period of urinary continence that lasts 1 year and primary if it is not.

Generally, the child awakens with no memory of a dream or having urinated. It occurs most frequently during the first third of the sleep cycle. However, sometimes, it may occur during REM sleep, and the child may recall a dream that involved the act of urinating. It is slightly more common in males, and 75% of children with the disorder have a first-degree biologic relative with a history of the disorder. Most cases resolve by adolescence, but 1% persist into adulthood.

Imipramine and behavioral treatments are the mainstay of therapy.

17
Pain

I. **Introduction.** Pain is frequently the predominant or only clinical manifestation of a wide variety of disease processes. Because pain is subjective, the history is of utmost importance. The average patient may not consider himself/herself ill if not in pain. Pain may be analyzed in psychologic terms (attention to it, feelings about it, and behavior due to it). Pain also includes an affective component of suffering, discomfort, distress, and misery. One must discern if the pain is acute or chronic and whether it has a physical cause.

Pain may be methodically analyzed by localization, character, exacerbating and ameliorating factors, associated phenomena, and time relationships. A report of pain may reflect any one, or a combination, of the following:

A. The presence of a local tissue injury.

B. A local afferent input that has become associated in the mind with the threat of injury or disease.

C. Peripheral or central nervous system damage that interferes with the normal modulation of small-fiber afferent input, i.e., neuralgias.

D. A psychologic need to suffer or to be punished.

E. A conscious and deliberate attempt to deceive others for personal gain, i.e., malingering.

F. A report of no pain may indicate:

1. No injury or neuronal stimulation sufficient to stimulate the threshold, indicating tissue damage.

2. Receptors or pathways are damaged and, therefore, do not transmit pain.

3. The tissue or structure has no afferent pain fibers, i.e., lung parenchyma.

4. The pathologic process does not activate pain fibers, i.e., lymphoma.

5. The patient's level of consciousness or attention is insufficient to interpret the quality of the sensory input as pain, i.e., stupor/coma, phencyclidine use.

6. Psychologic factors are influencing the patient to reject or not attend to the injury or suffering, and body sensations are not experienced as pain.

II. **Assessment.** In the initial evaluation, consider what motivated the patient to seek help. For example:

A. Interpersonal crisis.

B. The perceived interference of the symptom with the interpersonal or social relationships.

C. "Sanctioning," i.e., seeking medical attention because a family member or friend insists.

D. The idea that the symptom will interfere with a vocational or physical activity.

E. Expiration of an externally imposed time limit to the abatement of the symptom.

If in the assessment process, physical illness has been ruled out, then somatic symptoms may be the principal symptoms of an acute or chronic psychiatric disorder. Acute disorders are often precipitated by environmental stressors and present with symptoms that, for the most part, are somatic expressions of anxiety and mood disturbance. The onset of chronic disorders may be traced to adolescence or early adulthood, and by later life, there may be a global disturbance in functioning. These patients are more likely to use symptoms and the sick role to establish some unsatisfactory level of functioning.

Acute pain usually responds well to an analgesic and is less often attributable to psychologic factors. In chronic pain, the localization, character, and timing of the pain may be more vague, and because the autonomic nervous system adapts, signs of autonomic hyperactivity disappear. Chronic pain also responds less well to analgesics, and psychologic factors may be more prominent.

Chronic pain often falls into one of three categories.

1. Category 1—Chronic structural disease, e.g., rheumatoid arthritis, metastatic cancer, and sickle cell anemia, characterized by prolonged episodes of pain alternating with pain-free intervals or by unremitting pain waxing and waning in severity. Psychologic factors may plan an important role in exacerbating or relieving pain, but treatment of the pain by analgesics or therapy directed to the underlying disease is usually more helpful.

2. Category 2—Psychophysiologic disorders, - e.g., a history of disk disease or torn ligaments where the present problem is psychologically induced muscle spasms that produce pain long after the underlying deficit has healed. These patients respond poorly to analgesics but respond well to other therapies.

3. Category 3—Somatic delusions (neither structural or physiologic disorders) that include affective disorders, schizophrenia, somatization disorder, conversion disorder, and personality disorders.

A careful history should include signs and symptoms of depression, the degree to which the pain has interfered with the patient's activities, sleeping difficulties, anxiety, chronic anger, interpersonal withdrawal, somatic preoccupation, a change in appetite or bowel habits, and a change in sleep patterns.

A careful general physical examination should be performed, with special attention to the site of the presumed pathologic changes. This should include skin, joints, and neurologic examinations. A complete laboratory examination should also be done, including, as appropriate, x-ray films, and blood studies. Pain behavior should be measured with pain intensity scales, the Minnesota Multiphasic Personality Inventory (MMPI), and charting of activities of daily living and visual analogue scales.

III. **Psychogenic pain disorder.**

A. Occurrence is in women (two thirds more common than men).

B. It primarily occurs in people aged about 45 years, almost always older than 18 years, with at least a high school education.

C. Patients are usually from large families, without a significant psychiatric history but with a history for chronic pain syndromes.

D. There is a history of iatrogenic drug addiction (meperidine [Demerol], Dilaudid, Percodan, codeine, morphine, methadone, Darvon, Talwin, minor tranquilizers or benzodiazepines, and possibly other substance abuse); there is a family history of substance abuse.

E. Medical and surgical evaluation and treatment are unrevealing and unsuccessful; no cause is found.

F. There is a chronic duration, but this often exacerbates suddenly and usually after stress; it is similar to conversion disorder, except that the predominating symptom is pain rather than a neurologic deficit.

G. It serves, possibly, one of two psychologic purposes:

1. Primary gain: Symptom "buries" an unconscious mental conflict, i.e., unacceptable, painful thought that is repressed, and the emotional energy is converted to a physical pain, with the part of the body representing the symbolic conflict.

2. Secondary gain: Patient gets something that he/she wants (dependency, drugs, and/or vacation) or avoids something. Usually, the patient is unaware of the relationship (unconscious) or does not appreciate the significance (lack of insight).

IV. Emory model: classes of psychogenic pain disorder.

A. Class I, e.g., chronic back pain (high behavior; low pathologic condition; patients exhibit pain behaviors in excess of medical findings, low activities of daily living (ADL), high social/psychologic malfunctions, and drug misuse, and they do not improve with medical or psychiatric intervention but improve with rehabilitation programs).

B. Class II, e.g., chronic headache (low behavior, low pathologic condition, highly dramatic complaints without anatomic patterns, normal ADL, no drug abuse, no neuroticism, and successful treatment with relaxation training).

C. Class III (high pathologic condition and patient behavior; poor coping with significant illness, but when pathologic condition resolves, behavior continues as in the morbid state, and there is a poor response to all forms of treatment).

D. Class IV (high pathologic condition, low behavior, and successful treatment with self-management and relaxation training).

V. Chronic pain-associated features.

A. Many (25%) psychologic pain syndromes have associated organic disorders. The pain crisis is marked by symptoms and incapacity rather than a precise knowledge of its origins.

B. There is a recurrent, sudden appearance of the symptom. Often, there is a concurrent personality disorder (dependent, histrionic, antisocial, passive-aggressive, borderline, or narcissistic).

C. There is an association with at least moderate anxiety and depression.

D. Patients are often immature, shallow, demanding, of limited insight, and lower socioeconomic stature.

E. Hypochondriasis/hysteria.

F. Disease conviction (somatic vs. psychologic).

G. Irritability.

H. Denial of psychologic component.

I. Affective inhibition.

J. Universal helplessness.

K. Marked dependency.

L. There is a poor prognosis in those people with social passivity, history of substance abuse, long duration of pain, increased pain-related behavior, or an injury state associated with financial compensation.

VI. **Common pain syndromes.**

A. Post-traumatic (causalgia).

B. Musculoskeletal (disk, lower back pain, and headaches).

C. Iatrogenic pain from previous surgery.

D. Central or phantom pain following amputation.

E. Neuralgias (trigeminal and postherpetic).

VII. **Psychiatric diagnosis associated with chronic pain.**

A. Primary affective disorder.

B. Psychosis.

C. Early organic brain syndrome.

D. Substance abuse.

E. Conversion disorder.

F. Somatization disorder.

G. Psychogenic pain disorder.

H. Hypochondriasis.

I. Histrionic personality disorder.

J. Malingering.

VIII. **Treatment.** Treatment is primarily done on an outpatient basis unless the patient meets the admission criteria listed below. Detoxification or dependency treatment often needs to be done in a hospital setting, especially in the case of benzodiazepine withdrawal or concomitant medical problems that would make the detoxification process dangerous. Those patients unable to care for themselves at home during dependency treatment may also need to be hospitalized. The geriatric population frequently requires hospitalization when debilitated. Patients with the potential for substance abuse may also be hospitalized to minimize the chance for development of covert substance abuse. Lastly, patients who require rigorous, daylong physical therapy may require hospitalization.

A. **Admission criteria.**

1. After a complete physical and psychiatric workup.

2. Chronicity greater than 6 months.

3. Absence of malignancy but pain is progressive.

4. No specific other approach applicable.

5. Patient's acceptance of hospitalization for psychogenic pain.

B. **Initial steps in treatment.**

1. Detoxify the patient if necessary.

2. Develop trust by taking their complaints seriously and by regular visits. Direct confrontation often causes withdrawal.

3. Develop reasonable goals and an expectation of continued functioning, thus avoiding hospitalization.

4. Discourage long-term administration of analgesics secondary to their limited efficacy and possible risks. If drugs are used, use nonaddicting drugs (i.e., antidepressants, antihistamines, and vitamins/amino acids). Codeine is the preferable narcotic if necessary. Medicine should be given in regular doses, not as needed (PRN) to avoid reinforcement of drug-seeking behaviors.

a. The most efficacious tricyclic antidepressant is serotonergic, primarily amitriptyline, although others have been used as well (i.e., doxepin and trazodone) Doses are usually 25 to 75 mg/day, although oftentimes, patients are given higher doses if a major depression is concomitantly being treated.

b. Tryptophan (2 to 6 gm/day) with vitamin B_6 (100 mg/day) and, occasionally, vitamin C (500 to 2000 mg/day) are good adjunctive pharmacologic therapies.

5. The patient should keep a pain diary to help determine what worsens and improves the pain.

6. Psychotherapy effects few changes although the support is helpful; family therapy is oftentimes more helpful.

7. Allow ventilation, stress identification, and environmental restructuring.

IX. **Treatment modalities.**

A. **Anesthetic.**

1. Trigger-point injection.

2. Temporary and permanent peripheral nerve blocks.

3. Autonomic nerve blocks.

4. Intrathecal blocks.

5. Continuous epidural and intrathecal infusion.

B. **Physical medicine.**

1. Physical therapy.

2. Splinting and bracing.

3. Transcutaneous electrical stimulation.

4. Acupuncture.

5. Dorsal column stimulation.

6. Rhizotomy.

C. **Behavior programs.**

1. Cognitive/behavioral, i.e., operant conditioning, implosion therapy, and systematic desensitization.

2. Hypnosis (actively initiated, structured, and intense concentration for the achievement of agreed-on reduction of chronic pain).

3. Guided imagery.

4. Group and family therapy.

5. Modeling.

6. Biofeedback information about biologic functioning in a patient in a moment-to-moment measurement. There are two types: direct (immediate feedback about a patient's biologic activity like muscle contraction control) and indirect (where the symptom is not directly measured on a moment-to-moment basis but the patient is taught a skill that seems to produce a desirable effect on the symptom). The indirect type is used most frequently in pain management, but this requires frequent practice to be successful.

7. Relaxation techniques, i.e., "The patient is in control of his/her own pain." This works most successfully with hypnotizable patients, and self-hypnosis used as an adjunct improves the success of this therapy.

D. **Pharmacologic therapy.**

1. Nonsteroidal anti-inflammatory agents.

2. Aspirin.

3. L-Tryptophan and pyridoxine.

4. Vitamin therapy (controversial).

5. Non-narcotic pain medicines (i.e., Flexen, etc.).

6. Antidepressants (primarily serotonergic-mediated antidepressants, i.e., amitriptyline, on the basis that pain pathways are centrally mediated at least in part by serotonin). This also successfully treats the affective component of the syndrome, if any as well as any associated insomnia (25 to 75 mg/day).

NOTE: There is no standard dose although some feel that serum levels of certain medicines are helpful, i.e., aspirin and antidepressants.

X. **Examples of a behavioral program for pain control.**

A. **Supportive psychotherapy.**

1. Use your understanding of the patient's illness to gain maximum benefit in alleviating the patient's anxiety and disorganization about his/her illness.

2. Give a simple factual explanation of the illness, the treatment that is intended, expectations of the outcome, and any unpleasant effects that the treatment may bring. Also prepare the patient for changes in body image if that is part of the treatment (i.e., hair loss from cancer therapy, colostomy, or amputation).

3. Be sure to involve and gain support of the family.

4. Group therapy can also be of assistance to alle-

viate the patient's sense of being alone, being alienated, and being different from others. This is primarily used in pain centers.

B. **Operant conditioning.**

1. This is based on the premise that chronic pain is a learned behavior and that this may be corrected without direct intervention with the patient's deeper mental life. This is also primarily utilized in pain centers.

a. Consequences (that govern behavior) that increase a behavior are positive reinforcers and that decrease a behavior are negative reinforcers.

b. Pain can be controlled by use of these reinforcers. Positive reinforcers include attention, sympathy, concern, rest, and analgesic drugs. Therefore, these are withdrawn to rid the patient of undesirable behaviors like lying in bed, etc., returning them when these behaviors extinguish. Desirable behaviors will be noticed, complimented, and reinforced.

c. Hypnotherapy and Guided Imagery. Hypnosis is a state of mind in which the patient has an increased susceptibility to suggestions made by the hypnotist. This has been shown to induce analgesia, both while under hypnosis and afterward, in about 20% of patients. This is most appropriate in patients where the pain is chronic and not severe, and anxiety and tension play a major role. The primary goal is to have the patient relax by assisting him/her in progressive muscle relaxation and deep breathing.

After the patient is relaxed, the physician may guide him/her through relief of his/her pain (hypnosis), including a posthypnotic suggestion that this pain will be relieved in the future.

In guided imagery, when the patient is fully relaxed, the physician "escorts" the patient to a very relaxed environment, i.e., a warm stream in a sunbathed forest, and allows the environment to soothe and relieve the patient's pain. With this technique, making a tape for the patient for future use and practice is often helpful in pain relief (often daily) when you, as his/her physician, are not available.

d. Biofeedback. This is used for the same group of patients as those who would benefit from hypnosis or guided imagery but who you are concerned would not be able to comply with those techniques.

(i) Patients for whom it would be detrimental to relinquish "control" to a therapist.

(ii) Patients who are resistant to the psychologic aspects of pain management and need a more technologic, concrete method of pain relief.

(iii) Patients who are too low in functioning where they need a machine to help them relax.

(iv) Biofeedback is done by attaching electrodes to a patient that monitor usually muscle tension or heart rate and make noise when the patient relaxes, thus providing concrete positive feedback that "pain" is being relieved, especially when this is associated with anxiety.

e. Modeling. This is done by having a patient imitate behavior of a model to obtain a reduced level of pain; this, hence, uses the positive reinforcement of conforming to a model.

III
Pharmacotherapy

18 Neuroleptic Antipsychotic Medications

I. **Introduction.**

A. **History.** The first drug used as an antipsychotic was reserpine. The first phenothiazine used in psychiatry was chlorpromazine. It was being used to potentiate anesthesia when Laborit recognized its unique psychotropic effects in 1952.

B. **Terminology.** For the most part, antipsychotic medications have been *neuroleptic* medications. "Neuroleptics" are a broad chemical class of medications that, in contrast to CNS depressants, are sedatives that do not produce impairment of sensorium, intellect, coordination, or reflexes. These neuroleptics have *neurotoxic* effects, which include extrapyramidal side effects (EPS), akathisia, and other parkinsonian side effects. In more recent years, drugs have been developed with antipsychotic action that are not neuroleptics. One such agent available in Europe is *clozapine* which is a dibenzodiazepine antipsychotic. It has minimal dopamine-blocking activity and minimal, if any, anticholinergic activity. It has a very low, if any, incidence of tardive dyskinesia, but it requires close follow-up with weekly CBCs to monitor for agranulocytosis.

II. Mechanisms of action.

A. The neuroleptics are believed to act primarily by *dopamine blockade* at postsynaptic receptors.

B. They also produce α-adrenergic blockade, which may explain their hypotensive action (particularly for the low-potency neuroleptics).

C. They have *anticholinergic* action by blocking the muscarinic receptor (greatest with the low-potency neuroleptics).

D. There are a variety of other less prominent actions: blockage of norepinephrine reuptake, and blockage of serotonin and histamine receptors.

III. Treatment uses.

A. Psychiatric conditions.

1. **Functional psychoses.** The antipsychotics are used in the *treatment of psychoses* seen in schizophrenia, mania, and depression.

2. **Organic psychiatric disorders.** These medications may be used to treat the agitation seen in delirium or dementia. However, the *anticholinergic* CNS toxicity may actually worsen cognitive status.

They may be used to treat the psychosis seen in amphetamine psychosis or alcoholic hallucinosis. They do not cross-react with sedative-hypnotics and so do not help in treating withdrawal symptoms directly. Because they may lower seizure threshold they should be used cautiously in patients experiencing withdrawal.

3. **Target symptoms.** Various *target symptoms* for which neuroleptic medications are sometimes used are listed on Table 18–1. This includes severe anxiety, which may be present in a variety of psychiatric disturbances. Included in this list are *"positive"* symptoms of schizophrenia (e.g., hallucinations, delusions) as well as what

are regarded as *"negative" symptoms* of schizophrenia (e.g., apathy, social withdrawal), which are "negative" by virtue of their representing primarily an absence of an attribute normally present (e.g., motivation, energy, sociability). In general these medications have their *main action on correcting the positive symptoms*, and may do little for the negative symptoms.

4. **Thought disorganization and formal thought disorder.** *Thought disorder* is another sign of psychosis for which antipsychotics are indicated. The most flagrant forms of thought disorder are *hallucinations*, and *delusions* are another major indication for antipsychotics. A partial list of various forms of thought disorder is presented in Table 18–2. At times, neuroleptics are used to help with the thought and affective disorder seen in people with severe personality disorders.

5. These medications are used in the acute management of *aggression* and severe *agitation*.

B. **Movement disorders.** The neuroleptics have found use in treatment of Tourette's syndrome, hemiballism, and Huntington's disease. In Tourette's, low doses of haloperidol, 0.5–1.5 mg t.i.d., usually suffice.

C. **Nonpsychiatric uses.** These include treatment of (1) nausea and vomiting; (2) intractable hiccups; (3) pruritus; and occasionally (4) pain syndromes.

IV. **Classification and description of neuroleptics.**

A. **Introduction.** The neuroleptics medications are divided into a number of chemical classes, which are presented in Table 18–3. This table includes the most commonly used neuroleptic medications in the United States.

Aside from potency, these medications are primarily distinguished by their side effect profile. This profile is indicated in Table 18–4 in terms of the most common problematic side effects: *sedation, anticholinergic effects, hypotension,* and *extrapyramidal* effects. For aid in prescribing these medications, Table 18–5 presents how these medications are formulated.

TABLE 18–1.

Target Symptoms for Neuroleptic Medications*

Agitation	Ideas of persecution
Aggressiveness	Inappropriateness
Anxiety	Incoherency
Apathy (or emotional flattening or blunting)	Indifference to environment
	Insomnia
Assaultiveness	Irrelevancy
Bizarre thinking or speech	Lack of insight
Catatonic motor behavior	Mannerisms or facial grimaces
Combativeness	Motor retardation
Confusion	Negativism
Defective judgment	Paranoid ideation
Delirium	Poor appetite
Delusions	Poor concentration
Deterioration of social habits	Pressure of speech
Difficulty in relating (poor rapport)	Resistiveness
	Slowed speech
Disorientation	Social withdrawal (seclusiveness)
Elation	Somatic concern
Excitement	Suicidal tendencies
Feelings of unreality	Suspiciousness
Flight of ideas	Tension
Grandiosity	Thought disorganization (see Table 18–2)
Guilt feelings	Uncommunicativeness
Hallucinations	
Homicidal ideation or behavior	
Hostility	Uncooperativeness
Hyperactivity	Unusual thought content
Irritability	Withdrawal from reality

*Adapted from Mason AS, Granacher RP: Clinical Handbook of Antipsychotic Drug Therapy. New York, Brunner/Mazel, 1980.

TABLE 18–2.

Examples of Thought Disorder*

Contamination	On the Rorschach form Card I, a patient stated: "A butterfly holding the world together because I see on both sides patterns of a map."
Incoherence	"I don't quite gather. I know one right and one left use both hands but I can't follow the system that's working."
Neologisms	A patient reports that he was "accused of mitigation."
Illogical thinking	A patient gave her family an IBM card she punched in order to overcome communication difficulties.
Loosening of associations	"I'm tired. All people have eyes. Do you have glasses? I'm thirsty, can I have a glass of water?"
Poverty of content	"Well er...not quite the same as, er...don't know quite how to say it. It isn't the same being in the hospital as er...working er...the job isn't quite the same, er..."
Condensation	(E): What does this saying mean: "One swallow doesn't make a summer."?

(Continued.)

	(S): "You can't enjoy everything in life just tasting the fruit one time."
Idiosyncratic word usage	"I have menu three times a day."
Clangs associations	On asking a patient the meaning of travesty, he reports: "I think of the treasure and the dynasty."
Concreteness	On asking a patient in what way are an orange and a banana alike, he reports that "you peel them."
Overinclusion	On asking the similarity between an orange and a banana, he reports: "They come from the earth."

*Adapted from Davis J, et al: Neuroleptics and psychotic disorders, in Coyne JT, Enna SJ (eds): Neuroleptics: Neurochemical, Behavioral, and Clinical Perspectives. New York, Raven Press, 1983.

TABLE 18–3.
Neuroleptic Medications: Potency and Dosages*

Chemical Group Generic Name (Trade Name)	Relative Potency	Approximate Equivalent Dose (mg/day)	Usual Adult Dosages	
			Oral (mg/day)	Single IM
Phenothiazines				
Aliphatic				
Chlorpromazine (Thorazine) (g)†	Low	100	100–1500	25–100
Piperidine				
Mesoridazine (Serentil)	Low	50	50–400	25
Thioridazine (Mellaril) (g)	Low	100	100–800	NA
Piperazine				
Fluphenazine (Prolixin, Permitil)	High	2–3	2–20	1.25–2.5 (of HCl)
Trifluoperazine (Stelazine) (g)	High	3–5	5–50	1–2
Perphenazine (Trilafon)	Med	5–10	8–65	5–10

Thioxanthenes				
Chlorprothixene (Taractan)	Low	100	75–600	25–50
Thiothixene (Navane)	High	3–5	5–60	2–6
Butyrophenones				
Haloperidol (Haldol)	High	2–3	2–20	2.5–5
Droperidol (Inapsine)	High	1–2	NA	5–10 IM / 5–100 IV
Dihydroindolones				
Molindone (Moban)	Med	10	50–225	NA
Dibenzoxazepines				
Loxapine (Loxitane)	Med	10–15	50–250	12.5–25
Diphenylbutylpiperidines				
Pimozide (Orap)	High	1–2	1–20	NA

*Adapted from Baldessarini[1] and Mason and Granacher.[9]
†(g) = generic form available; NA = not available.

TABLE 18–4.
Neuroleptic Medications: Side Effect Profiles*†

Chemical Group Generic Name (Trade Name)	Sedation	Anticholinergic	Hypotension	Extrapyramidal
Phenothiazines				
Aliphatic				
Chlorpromazine (Thorazine) (g)	+++	+++	Oral ++ IM +++	++
Piperidine				
Mesoridazine (Serentil)	++	++	++	+++
Thioridazine (Mellaril) (g)	+++	++	++	+
Piperazine				
Fluphenazine (Prolixin, Permitil)	+	+	+	+++
Trifluoperazine (Stelazine) (g)	+	+	+	+++
Perphenazine (Trilafon)	++	+	+	++

Drug	Sedation	Hypotension	Anticholinergic	Extrapyramidal
Thioxanthenes				
Chlorprothixene (Taractan)	+++	++	++	++
Thiothixene (Navane)	+	+	+	+++
Butyrophenones				
Haloperidol (Haldol)	+	+	+	+++
Droperidol (Inapsine)	+++	+	+/−	+
Dihydroindolones				
Molindone (Moban)	++	++	0	+
Dibenzoxazepines				
Loxapine (Loxitane)	++	++	+	++
Diphenylbutylpiperidines				
Pimozide (Orap)	+	+	+/−	+++

*Adapted from Baldessarini RJ: Chemotherapy in Psychiatry: Principles and Practice. Cambridge, Mass, Harvard University Press, 1985.
†Rated as follows: 0 = rare; + = mild; ++ = moderate; +++ = severe; +/− = equivocal.

TABLE 18–5.

Neuroleptic Formulary*†

Chemical Group Generic Name (Trade Name)	Available Formulations
Phenothiazines	
Aliphatic	
Chlorpromazine (Thorazine) (g)	Tabs: 10, 25, 50, 100, 200; SR: 30, 75, 150, 200, 300; Syrup: 10 mg/5 mL; Conc: 30 and 100 mg/mL; PR: 25 and 100; Amps: 25 mg/1 mL, 50 mg/2 mL; Vials: 10 mL of 25 mg/mL
Piperidine	
Mesoridazine (Serentil)	Tabs: 10, 25, 50, 100; Conc: 25 mg/mL; Amps: 25 mg/mL
Thioridazine (Mellaril) (g)	Tabs: 10, 15, 25, 50, 100, 150, 200; Conc: 30 mg/mL, 100 mg/mL; CS: 25 and 100 mg/5 mL
Piperazine	
Fluphenazine (Prolixin, Permitil)	Tabs: 1, 2.5, 5, 10; Conc: 5 mg/mL; Elix: 2.5 mg/5 mL; Vials: 2.5 mg/mL (HCl); Vials: 25 mg/mL (enanthate); Syringes and vials: 25 mg/mL (decanoate)

(Continued.)

Trifluoperazine (Stelazine) (g)	Tabs: 1, 2, 5, 10; Conc: 10 mg/mL; Vials: 10 mL of 2 mg/mL
Perphenazine (Trilafon)	Tabs: 2, 4, 8, 16; SR: 8 mg; Conc: 16 mg/5 mL; Amps: 5 mg/mL
Thioxanthenes	
Chlorprothixene (Taractan)	Tabs: 10, 25, 50, 100; Conc: 100 mg/5 mL; Amps: 25 mg/2 mL
Thiothixene (Navane)	Caps: 1, 2, 5, 10, 20; Conc: 5 mg/mL; Amps: 4 mg/2 mL, 5 mg/mL
Butyrophenones	
Haloperidol (Haldol)	Tabs: 0.5, 1, 2, 5, 10; Conc: 2 mg/mL (lactate); Amps: 5 mg/mL (lactate); Vials: 10 mL of 5 mg/mL (lactate); Amps: 50 mg/mL (70.5 mg of decanoate form)
Droperidol (Inapsine)	Amps: 1, 2, 5, 10 mL of 2.5 mg/mL
Dihydroindolones	
Molindone (Moban)	Tabs: 5, 10, 25, 50, 100; Conc: 20 mg/mL
Dibenzoxazepines	
Loxapine (Loxitane)	Caps: 5, 10, 25, 50 (succinate); Conc: 25 mg/mL (HCl); Amps: 50 mg/mL (HCl); Vials: 10 mL of 50 mg/mL (HCl)

(Continued.)

TABLE 18–5 (cont.)

Diphenylbutylpiperidines
    Pimozide   Tabs: 2
      (Orap)

*Adapted from Baldessarini RJ: Chemotherapy in Psychiatry: Principles and Practice. Cambridge, Mass, Harvard University Press, 1985.

†Dosages given in milligrams; (g) = generic available; different forms in parentheses: oral: Tabs = tablets, Caps = capsules, Elix = elixir, Conc = concentrate, CS = concentrated suspension, SR = sustained release; suppository: PR = per rectal suppository; injection: Amps = ampules.

B. Dosage. Table 18–3 includes the usual adult dose for each neuroleptic. Extreme dosage ranges are occasionally exceeded cautiously and only when other appropriate measures have failed. Doses for *elderly patients* are typically one-half to one-third the usual daily adult oral dose.

C. Equivalent doses. These medications are loosely divided into those of high, low, and medium *potency* (which refers inversely to the relative dosage of medication to achieve the same effect). The chart indicates this relative potency as well as a more quantitative comparison of the Approximate Equivalent Dose, in which 100 mg of chlorpromazine is used as a reference. While the tabulated drugs vary by more than 100-fold in potency, they are very similar in their clinical efficacy when used at equivalent doses. *Do not confuse equivalent doses with therapeutic dose levels.*

The data for equivalent doses are summarized as averages from several sources, some of which vary greatly. These numbers are only an approximate guide, and the *dosage for each patient must be established by clinical response*. In switching from high doses of one agent to a dissimilar one, it is well to proceed gradually over several days to decrease the risk of side effects from the newly introduced drug.

There are some general attributes that distinguish high- from low-potency neuroleptics in terms of their side effect profile. In comparison with high-potency neuroleptics, the low-potency neuroleptics have, in general, fewer extrapyramidal side effects, more sedation, more hypotension, and more anticholinergic side effects.

D. **Depot neuroleptics.**

1. **General comments.** These injectable, long half-life neuroleptics may require weeks to months to achieve a steady-state level in the patient. Therefore, supplementation with an oral neuroleptic will often be necessary in the first few weeks of treatment with depot neuroleptics. The oral supplementation can be gradually tapered and discontinued if the patient's symptoms remain well controlled over the ensuing weeks. Any increase in psychotic symptoms just before the next injection should be noticed, and would suggest the dose is too low or the time interval too long.

2. **Fluphenazine (Prolixin).**

a. **Fluphenazine ethanoate.** Injectable fluphenazine esters are commonly used in doses of 12.5–50 mg intramuscularly every 1 to 4 weeks. The enanthate (derived from a 7-carbon fatty acid) typically acts for 2 weeks.

b. **Fluphenazine decanoate.** This is currently the *more popular form*. The decanoate (an ester of a 12-carbon carboxylic acid) acts for up to 3 weeks. As an approximate equivalence, 25 mg (1 mL) of intramuscular fluphenazine decanoate *every 2 weeks* resembles in effectiveness about 10 mg of fluphenazine hydrochloride (orally) per day (or 500 mg of chlorpromazine), but oral-to-depot conversion must be individualized. Dosages range from 1.25 mg (0.05 mL) to 75 mg (3 mL); 12.5 mg (0.5 mL) is often sufficient.

3. **Haloperidol decanoate (Haldol decanoate).** The decanoate ester of haloperidol is also available and is given *every 3 or 4 weeks* in intramuscular doses of 20 times the daily oral dose.

E. **Other neuroleptics.**

1. **Droperidol** (Inapsine) is an extremely potent, short-acting neuroleptic, used as a preanesthetic or coanesthetic agent intramuscularly or intravenously. Only parenteral forms are available in the United States. It has powerful antipsychotic-sedative effects that are useful in *psychiatric emergencies*. Sedative effects are short lasting (approximately 6 hours). It can be administered as 1–10 mg IM (larger doses not recommended because of large volume), or IV (slow push) for *highly agitated* patients using up to 100 mg titrated to sedation.

2. **Pimozide** (Orap) is a potent diphenylbutyl-piperidine currently recommended only for *Tourette's syndrome* (severe tics and involuntary vocalizations) in patients older than 12 years. It is an effective antipsychotic and has been used in schizophrenia as well. Its half-life after oral doses is several days. It should be discontinued if ECG changes indicate depressed conduction (QT > 500 msec).

3. **Antiemetics.** Prochlorperazine (Compazine), thiethylperazine (Torecan), and promethazine (Phenergan), while having typical neuroleptic (and some antipsychotic) effects, are mainly used as antiemetic agents. The dose of *Compazine* as an antiemetic is 5–10 mg PO, every 6 to 8 hours, 5 to 10 mg IM every 4 to 6 hours, or 25 mg bid PRN. These drugs can produce the usual major side effects of neuroleptics, although much less frequently.

4. **Uncommon antipsychotics.** Other agents that are not commonly used or are less effective in the treat-

ment of psychoses are not included in Table 18–3. For example, butaperazine (Repoise), carphenazine (Proketazine), mepazine (Pacatal), promazine (Sparine), piperacetazine (Quide), actophenazine (Tindal), and thiopropazate (Dartal).

V. **Pharmacokinetics.** These drugs are variably absorbed when given orally. The peak plasma level is 2–4 hours after the oral dose. Plasma concentration is detected 15 to 30 minutes after an IM dose. Blood levels are higher after an IM dose such that usually one-third or one-fourth of the oral dose is given IM for the same effect.

Most *half-lives* are around 20 hours, with a range from 10 to 40 hours. This often permits once-a-day dosing after the patient's condition is stable and he is acclimated to the side effects. Most neuroleptics are degraded in liver by oxidation, conjugated with glucuronic acid, and excreted in the urine. *Age greatly affects metabolic rate.* *Blood levels* are still not used clinically, due to wide interindividual variation, and limited proof of clinically useful correlation with effect. Also some agents have numerous active metabolites.

They are all lipophilic and bind tightly to plasma proteins. They cross the placenta and are transported in human milk. No teratogenic effects are known, but it is best to avoid medications in pregnant or nursing women. They are not dialyzable.

VI. **Methods of prescribing.**

A. **Acute treatment of psychotic agitation.** Psychotic and aggressive symptoms may require acute intervention for the protection of staff and patients. Both psychopharmacologic and physical interventions should be considered.

1. **Psychopharmacologic interventions.**

a. **Rapid neuroleptization.** Any antipsychotic that can be administered can be used with frequent dosing until behavior is controlled while patient is carefully monitored and evaluated for response and side effects.

For example, 5–10 mg (IM; or orally if the patient is cooperative) of a high potency neuroleptic given every 30 to 60 minutes until target symptoms respond. With chlorpromazine one can use 25–50 mg IM every hour, watching for hypotension. For extremely agitated patients droperidol IV may be used by slow IV push up to 100 mg (usually the dose is titrated to sedation). Rapid administration of neuroleptics is *controversial*, and should only be carried out with frequent checks of the patient (every 15 minutes), including vital signs.

b. **Sedatives.** Sedatives such as benzodiazepines (for example, clonazepam for manic psychosis) and sodium amytal IM can be used to help control aggression and agitation.

2. **Physical interventions.** Physical restraints may be necessary in cases of extreme agitation, especially when physical injury is highly probable.

B. **Maintenance treatments.** The great majority of patients respond well to institution of a *maintenance dose* of neuroleptic medication. The dose can be judiciously titrated up or down (depending on the severity and response of symptoms and side effects). The dose will probably need to be adjusted over time, since with resolution of psychotic agitation less neuroleptic may be needed and sensitivity to sedation may increase. Start with divided doses. After several weeks, tolerance to many side effects often develops so that a dose every evening will suffice. An adequate drug trial should go for at least 4 weeks if possible. For some patients the full effect of the medication may take several months. Criteria for *termination* and recommended length of treatment are controversial, and depend on many factors including diagnosis. The *costs and benefits* should be considered and documented. In *schizophrenia*, consider continuing medication for at least 6 months after improvement, and possibly considerably longer for prophylaxis.

VII. Side effects.

A. Acute extrapyramidal effects; side effects (EPS).

These are some of the *most common* side effects. They are generally more common with the high-potency neuroleptics. The most common are *acute dystonia, parkinsonism,* and *akathisia*. Table 18–6 reviews the clinical features, period of risk, and treatment of these complications. Table 18–7 reviews the agents used to treat these acute extrapyramidal reactions. The most commonly used such agent are *anticholinergic* agents. Additional agents used include amantadine, propranolol, and clonidine. Included in the table is the usual daily dose, how the dose is usually divided, and how the medications are formulated. Since the half-lives of these medications is less than those of neuroleptics, they need to be given more frequently.

The agents listed in Table 18–7 are commonly given orally in two or three divided doses. Of the medications listed both for treatment and prophylaxis the most common ones used are Cogentin, Artane, Akineton, and Benadryl. Diphenhydramine and orphenadrine are antihistaminic (sedating) and antimuscarinic; ethopropazine is a strongly anticholinergic phenothiazine.

Some extrapyramidal reactions resistant to treatment with a single agent may require the application of a second medication (e.g., addition of amantadine to an anticholinergic in treating neuroleptic-induced parkinsonism).

1. **Acute dystonias.** These are often treated with benztropine (Cogentin) 2 mg or diphenhydramine (Benadryl) 25 or 50 mg. While they can be given orally, to facilitate quick termination of the dystonia they are given IM or IV. For benztropine, IM acts as quickly as IV.

2. **Prophylactic treatment.** It is recommended that

TABLE 18–6.
Extrapyramidal and Parkinson Side Effects of Neuroleptic Medications*†

Reaction	Features	Period of Maximum Risk	Proposed Mechanism	Treatment
Acute dystonia	Spasm of muscles of tongue, face, neck, and back; may mimic seizures; is not hysteria	1–5 Days	Dopamine excess ?; acetylcholine excess ?	Antiparkinsonism agents are diagnostic and curative (IM or IV, then PO)
Parkinsonism	Bradykinesia, rigidity, variable tremor, mask-like facies, shuffling gait, dysphagia	5–30 Days (may persist)	Dopamine blockade	Antiparkinson drugs; try low-potency drug; dopamine agonists risky ?
Akathisia	Motor restlessness; patient may experience anxiety or agitation	5–60 Days (commonly persists)	Unknown	Lower dose; try low-potency drug; low-dose propranolol; antiparkinson agents or ben-

"Rabbit" syndrome	Perioral tremor (late parkinsonism variant ?); usually reversible	Mo or yr	Unknown zodiazepines may help Antiparkinsonism agents; reduce dose of neuroleptic
Akinesia (akinetic mutism)	Waxy flexibility, poverty of speech and movement, posturing; sometimes mistaken for true catatonia and treated inappropriately with increase of antipsychotics	1–4 Wk	Unknown Reduce dosage of antiparkinson agent

*Adapted from Baldessarini RJ: Chemotherapy in Psychiatry: Principles and Practice. Cambridge, Mass, Harvard University Press, 1985.
†Antiparkinsonism agents are presented elsewhere and are typically anticholinergics.

TABLE 18-7.
Agents Used to Treat Neuroleptic Extrapyramidal Effects and Parkinson Side Effects*

Generic Name (Trade Name)	Usual Daily Dose (mg)	Divided as Times/Day	Available Formulations
Anticholinergic agents			
Benztropine (Cogentin) (g)	1–6	1–3	Tabs: 0.5, 1, 2; Amps: 2 mL of 1 mg/mL
Biperiden (Akineton)	2–10	1–4	Tabs: 1; Amps: 1 mL of 5 mg/mL
Diphenhydramine (Benadryl) (g)	25–200	1–4	Caps: 25, 50; Elixir: 12.5 mg/5 mL; Amps, Vials, or Syringes: 10 or 50 mg/mL
Ethopropazine (Parsidol)	50–200	1–3	Tabs: 10, 50
Orphenadrine (Norlex, Disipal) (g)	50–300	1–3	Tabs: 50, 100; Amps:

Procyclidine (Kemadrin)	5–30	1–4	Tabs: 5
Trihexyphenidyl (Artane) (g)	5–15	1–4	Tabs: 2, 5; Elixir: 2 mg/5 mL
Atypical agents			
Amantadine (Symmetrel) (g)	100–300	1–3	Caps: 100; Syrup: 50 mg/5 mL
Propranolol (Inderal) (g)	20–120	1–4	Tabs: 10, 20, 40, 60, 80, 90; Amps: 1 mg/mL
Clonidine (Catapres) (g)	0.2–0.8	1–3	Tabs: 0.1, 0.2, 0.3; Transdermal: approx 0.1, 0.2, or 0.3 mg/day

*Adapted from Baldessarini[1] and Lydiard et al.[8]
†Dosage forms: Tabs = tablets; Caps = capsules; Amps = ampules; Syringes and vials also for parenteral administration; (g) = also available in generic form.

extrapyramidal effects be prevented with these agents in: (1) patients with a history of prior extrapyramidal side effects on the same or similar neuroleptic; (2) patients at high risk for extrapyramidal side effects; young men are felt to be at higher risk for acute dystonia; and (3) patients with whom your therapeutic alliance is shaky, and for whom an adverse reaction, like a dystonic reaction, may lead them to become noncompliant with treatment.

3. **Atypical agents.**

a. **Amantadine** is not an anticholinergic, and may thus be used to avoid this extrapyramidal effects. Amantadine can be used for parkinsonism, catatonia, or akathisia, but is relatively expensive and may lose effectiveness within a few weeks. It may be dopaminergic. Overdoses may respond to physostigmine, even though amantadine is not strongly anticholinergic.

b. **Propranolol** in low doses with little cardiovascular effect appears to be selective against akathisia (other β-adrenergic antagonists are less effective). With increasing doses of propranolol to treat extrapyramidal effects, one must remember that with some of the neuroleptics there may be an additive effect on producing hypotension. Similarly *clonidine*, which may be effective for akathisia, carries a high risk of producing hypotension.

4. **Toxicity.** Note that most of these agents, on excessive dosing, can induce cerebral intoxication that may look like an exacerbation of the psychosis. Such *anticholinergic delirium* or psychoses are more common in the elderly. There are risks of using anticholinergics in patients with prostrate obstruction, closed-angle glaucoma, or paralytic ileus.

B. **Tardive dyskinesia.**

1. **Definition and description.** Tardive dyskinesia involves abnormal *oral-facial* and possibly limb, body, or respiratory choreiform, athetotic, and, occasionally,

dystonic movements. The period of risk begins *after 6 months* of being on a neuroleptic. This is why the dystonias are named "tardive." The incidence is 15% to 20% after prolonged neuroleptic exposure. It may temporarily worsen when the neuroleptic is stopped (*"withdrawal dyskinesias"*), but then frequently improves with time. It can sometimes be irreversible, especially in the elderly. For the most part, once tardive dyskinesia is detected it is not progressive. The risk is higher in the elderly and with patients with affective illness. It is presumed to relate to compensatory *supersensitivity to dopamine*, subsequent to the dopamine blockade from the neuroleptic. *Prevention* is the best management as most treatment is unsatisfactory. For many there is a slow spontaneous remission if the neuroleptic is stopped.

2. **Differential diagnosis.** There are many other neurologic problems that mimic tardive dyskinesia. The differential diagnosis is provided in Table 18–8. The table indicates which of these disorders have a familial pattern and which are associated with psychiatric symptoms, and provides comments about these disorders.

Note that in most cases the psychiatric history, exposure to neuroleptics, and pattern of symptoms are strongly indicative of tardive dyskinesia. Most of the alternatives are either rare or clearly indicated by the history and examination. Spontaneous dyskinesias, especially of tongue and jaw, sometimes seen in the elderly can be confused with tardive dyskinesia unless systemic choreic-dystonic symptoms are also present.

3. **Prevention.**

a. *Restrict neuroleptics* for serious indications only. Consider using clonazepam for control of agitation in manic patients. Obtain *informed consent* by discussing with patient and family. *Document* need for continued neuroleptic medication.

b. Use of *minimal effective dose for shortest time.*

TABLE 18–8.
Differential Diagnosis for Tardive Dyskinesia*

Alternative Disorder	Familial	Psychiatric Features	Specific Findings
Transient dyskinesias on neuroleptic withdrawal	0	+	Recent neuroleptic treatment
Stereotyped mannerisms of schizophrenia	?	+	Psychiatric history; characteristic movements, not choreic
Oral dyskinesias of the elderly (e.g., Miege's syndrome)	0	+/−	Miege's: progressive oral-mandibular dystonia with blepharospasm
Dental conditions, dentures	0	0	Dental history and examination
Torsion dystonia (dystonia musculorum deformans)	+	+/−	Early onset, progressive, no chorea
Focal dystonias (torticollis, mandibular dystonia, blepharospasm)	+/−	+/−	Dystonic rather than choreic
Tourette's syndrome; focal "tics"; "habit" spasm	+/−	+/−	Vocalizations prominent, rarer in tardive dyskinesia
Huntington's disease	+	+	Dominant inheritance; chorea early, dementia late; CT scan (caudate atrophy late)
Heavy metal intoxication (manganese, selenium)	0	+	Mining, industrial exposure; assays for specific metal
Wilson's hepatolenticular degeneration	+	+/−	Serum Cu < 80 µg/dL, ceruloplasmin < 20 µg/dL; urine Cu > 100 mg/dL; ophthalmic, hepatic, renal symptoms

Condition			Evaluation
Calcifications of basal gangalia (e.g., Fahr's syndrome	+/−	0	Skull x-ray
Rheumatic chorea (Syndenham's; St. Vitus' dance)	0	0	Recent streptococcal infection
Residua of encephalitis or anoxic damage	0	+/−	Specific history; EEG
Neural aspects of systemic, metabolic, or inflammatory disorders	0	+/−	Tests for specific diagnoses, including hepatic, renal, hyperthyroid, hypoparathyroid, hypoglycemic, inflammatory
Dopamine agonist excess	0	+/−	Recent exposure to levodopa, bromocriptine, amphetamine
Other drug intoxications	0	+/−	Phenytoin, lithium, antidepressants
Cerebral neoplasm (especially basal ganglia, thalamus)	0	+/−	Focal neural symptoms, CT scan, EEG
Lithium tremor (9–12 cps), an accentuated action tremor	0	+	Lithium treatment
Parkinsonian tremor (6–8 cps), occurs at rest, decreased by anticholinergics; both are regular	+	+/−	May also be caused by neuroleptics
Rabbit syndrome is an oral parkinsonian tremor sometimes associated with antipsychotic treatment	+	+	May also be caused by neuroleptics

*Adapted from Baldessarini[1] and Lydiard et al.[8]
†+ = usually present; +/− = variable; ? = uncertain.

c. Particular care in patients at higher risk: patient over 50 years old (particularly women), edentulous patients, and patients with organic brain damage.

d. Occasional brief "drug holidays" to expose covert tardive dyskinesia and identify at-risk patients in whom early withdrawal is given priority.

e. *Early detection* maximizes chances of recovery. Early signs are often detected in the tongue. Observe the tongue retracted in the open mouth. Look for vermicular movements. Conduct this examination and others to look for tardive dyskinesia regularly every few months, if not monthly.

4. **Treatment.**

a. Gradually *withdraw* the neuroleptic. Worsening before improvement is to be expected. Reversibility can only be ascertained after drug-free period of at least 6 months.

b. If neuroleptic withdrawal is clinically unjustifiable, then *dose reduction* is the next best strategy.

c. Withdrawal of any anticholinergic medication may help.

d. In cases in which tardive dyskinesia is irreversible in the presence of neuroleptic withdrawal or reduction, consider instituting:

(1) Trial of benzodiazepine (such as clonazepam). Innocuous and may evoke some improvement.

(2) Trial of cholinomimetic (such as deanol or lecithin). Fairly innocuous. Published data suggest efficacy, but double-blind trial awaited.

(3) Vitamin E is suggested by newer research to possibly have some benefit.

(4) Trial of tetrabenazine 100–150 mg/day. May allow reduction in dose of other neuroleptics without loss of antipsychotic effect, while ameliorating dyskinesia. Danger of subsequent breakthrough and risk of depression.

(5) Trial of lithium for 1 to 2 months.

(6) Trial of reserpine, 2–4 mg/day (a dopamine-depleting agent).

C. **Non-extrapyramidal CNS side effects of neuroleptics.** These are presented in Table 18–9 with their clinical features, period of risk, and treatment, as well as a list of the common neuroleptics that cause them. Mention should also be made of sedation. For many patients tolerance to the sedative effect develops over days to weeks.

D. **Peripheral side effects of neuroleptic medications.** These are presented in Table 18–10. Additional comments:

1. Mellaril causes **pigmentary retinopathy** in doses exceeding 800 mg/day. Other low-potency drugs are implicated.

2. **Dry mouth.** A common complaint to which some tolerance may develop. Can advise sugarless gum or artificial saliva.

3. **Orthostatic hypotension.** Some degree of tolerance may develop after several weeks. Acute management is to have person lie down, and give them fluids. If severe, metaraminol or norepinephrine can be given. Avoid β-adrenergic agents (like isoproterenol or epinephrine) because with the α-adrenergic blockade there may be further decrease in blood pressure.

4. Most allergic **rashes** are transient. Usually this can be solved by simply changing the drug, as there is little cross-sensitivity. If the original drug is stopped, it can often be restarted without recurrence of the rash. Serious exfoliative dermatitis is very rare.

5. **Nasal stuffiness.**

6. Skin problems include **photosensitivity** with increased sensitivity to sunburn, particularly with low-potency drugs. With phototoxicity, only a few minutes of sunlight can cause a reaction. With prolonged use of low-potency medication at high dose, some patients

TABLE 18–9.
Non-extrapyramidal CNS Side Effects of Neuroleptics*

Syndrome	Features	Period of Maximum Risk	Proposed Mechanism	Treatment	Common Offenders
Central anticholinergic syndrome	Toxic psychosis (delirium)	Weeks	Central anticholinergic excess	Recognize early; don't confuse with exacerbation of "functional" psychosis; consider physostigmine test for diagnosis; stop or decrease anticholinergic, antiparkinsonian, antidepressant, and antipsychotic agents	Mellaril; thorazine; low-potency agents > others; caution in elderly and organically impaired
Neuroleptic malignant syndrome ("lethal catatonia")	Change in mental status; autonomic instability of vital signs in any combination (pulse, BP, temperature, respiration, +/− diaphoresis); ri-	Unpredictable, can occur idiosyncratically even after years of neuroleptic treatment	? Hypothalamic interference with temperature and vital signs regulation	Early detection; any 1 or more of the features listed (especially vital signs and mental status) should alert staff; stop neuroleptic; antipar-	All agents

Effect	Symptoms	Mechanism	Treatment	Agents
	gidity, increased CPK; myoglobinemia; lethal in 20%; syndrome develops over 24–72 hr		kinsonism agents usually fail; bromocriptine often helps; dantrolene variable; parenteral benzodiazepines sometimes help; general supportive care crucial (usually ICU setting)	
Temperature dysregulation	Hyperthermia, hypothermia	Affected by environmental temperature extremes and activity level	? Peripheral interference with temperature regulation	Stop drug; rule out "lethal catatonia"; cooling techniques, massage; other supportive treatment for hyperthermia	All agents
Decrease in seizure threshold	Seizure activity is rare	Weeks	? Anticholinergic	Minimize dose; slowly increase if necessary; anticonvulsants	Thorazine; promazine; low-potency agents > others, especially at high or rapidly rising dosage; Moban and piperazines least

*Adapted from Baldessarini[1] and Lydiard et al.[8]

TABLE 18-10.
Peripheral Side Effects of Neuroleptic Medications*

Body System	Clinical Features	Period of Maximum Risk	Proposed Mechanism	Treatment	Common Offenders and Comments
Autonomic Nervous System					
A. Cardiovascular	Dizziness, syncope, postural hypotension	Day-weeks	α-adrenergic blockade	Decrease dose; support hose	Thorazine; thioridazine; low-potency agents > others
B. Gastrointestinal	Nasal congestion, dry mouth, constipation, absent bowel sounds can progress to paralytic ileus	Day-weeks	Anticholinergic	Decrease dose; decrease or stop concomitant anticholinergic effect, stool softeners	Thorazine, Mellaril
C. Genitourinary	Urinary hesitancy, urinary retention, impaired erection, ejaculatory disturbance (absent, delayed, retrograde), priapism	Day-weeks	Anticholinergic; multiple autonomic effects	Decrease dose; decrease or stop concomitant anticholinergic medications	Low potency agents > other agents; caution in elderly, especially males with enlarged prostates

Antipsychotics

D. Vision					
Opthalmologic	Blurred vision	hours-Days	Anticholinergic	Decrease anticholinergic agents; pilocarpine eye drops	Tolerance usually develops
	Precipitation of narrow-angle glaucoma	Weeks-months (rare)	Anticholinergic	Immediate medical treatment	
	Pigmentary retinopathy	Years	Drug-melanin interaction in retina	Avoid > 800 mg thioridazine; switch to high-potency nonphenothiazine	Thioridazine > other phenothiazines
	Lens and corneal opacities	Years	Drug-protein interaction	Switch to high-potency nonphenothiazine	Chlorpromazine in high doses
Cardiac	ECG effects: ST-segment depression, T-wave flattening, notching, and inversion; increased PR interval; increased QRS duration; increased QT interval; sinus tachycardia	Days	Quinidine-like effect	Discontinue medication if clinically indicated.	Low-potency agents > others, especially thioridazine; avoid in patients with cardiac disease; clinical significance of ECG changes uncertain
			Anticholinergic	Decrease or stop anticholinergics	

(Continued.)

TABLE 18–10 (cont.)
Peripheral Side Effects of Neuroleptic Medications*

Body System	Clinical Features	Period of Maximum Risk	Proposed Mechanism	Treatment	Common Offenders and Comments
Allergic					
A. Dermatoses	Ulticarial, maculopapular, petechial, edematous eruptions	Days–weeks	Drug protein complexes formed in skin	Stop medication	Phenothiazines, especially thorazine
Systematic photosensitivity	Severe sunburn	Depends on exposure	Allergic	Prevent by using sunscreens	Phenothiazines, especially thorazine
B. Agranulocytosis	Unexplained sore throat, fever and malaise; incidence: 1:4,000–10,000; fatalities associated with concurrent illness	Weeks–months	Unknown	Stop medication; reverse isolation; antibiotics; supportive care	Thorazine, promazine, rare cases other phenothiazines; never proven to occur in nonphenothiazines
Leukopenia	Lowered WBC count	Weeks–months	Unknown	Benign; usually is transient	More with low-potency agents

Antipsychotics

C. Hepatotoxicity, jaundice, elevated liver enzymes	Jaundice followed in 1–7 days by fever, nausea, right upper quadrant pain, malaise	Days-weeks	Idiosyncratic	Stop drug; switch to another class if continued treatment urgent	More with low-potency agents
Metabolic and endocrine	Galactorrhea, irregular menses or amenorrhea; gynecomastia	Weeks-months	Prolactin elevation	In females rule out pregnancy; decrease dose.	All agents
	Decreased libido	Weeks-months	Hypothalamic	Decrease dose	May be > with thioridazine in men
	Polydipsia, edema (? same mechanism)	Days-weeks	Inappropriate ADH secretion	Rule out SIADH	
	Weight gain	Weeks-months	? Hypothalamic	Restrict caloric intake; increase exercise; decrease dose	Most with low-potency agents; least with Moban

*Adapted from Baldessarini[1] and Lydiard et al.[8]

develop blue-gray skin **discoloration** especially in sun-exposed areas.

E. **Sudden death.** There have been occasional reports of **sudden death** in previously healthy patients receiving antipsychotic medication. Hypothetical explanations include asphyxiation, cardiac arrhythmias, aspiration from impaired swallowing, and dystonic strangulation. A recent review by Leber (1981) questions the evidence for any greater risk of sudden death in patients on neuroleptics.

F. **Drug interactions.** A list of important *drug interactions* with the antipsychotics is presented in Table 18–11.

G. **Summary of important side effects.** Discussion of these considerations should be included in the *informed consent* protocol.

1. Review the common extrapyramidal side effects (including acute dystonia), anticholinergic, orthostatic hypotension, and sedative side effects. The latter would prohibit operation of heavy machinery and, possibly, driving.

2. Review the risks of tardive dyskinesia.

3. Inform the person that if they develop cold symptoms (sore throat, malaise) they must see a physician and get a CBC immediately, to rule out agranulocytosis.

4. Warn the person about photosensitivity and risks of sunburn.

5. Ask about symptoms or family history of closed-angle glaucoma (history of eye pain, blurring, or halos).

6. If person needs long-term low-potency medication, get yearly opthalmologic examinations to evaluate for ocular pigmentation.

7. Warn women of potential galactorrhea and possible breast engorgement. This also happens in males in rare instances. While there is no evidence that neu-

roleptics contribute to breast cancer, because of the prolactinemia that neuroleptics produce, you may decide not to give them to women with a personal or family history of breast cancer.

VIII. **Overdose.** All of these drugs have a high therapeutic ratio: lethal dose/therapeutic dose. Deaths from overdose are rare. Intervention includes pumping the stomach even if there has been an appreciable time delay, as the anticholinergic effects may delay gastric emptying. Ipecac may not work due to anti-emetic effects (particularly in low-potency drugs). Use activated charcoal. The major danger is from hypotension and arrhythmias, so support blood pressure. As antipsychotics can have quinidine-like effects, if you need to treat arrhythmias produced by the overdose avoid quinidine or other type I antiarrhythmic agents.

IX. **Withdrawal.** While neuroleptics are not addicting, discontinuation of neuroleptics may lead to anticholinergic rebound and other withdrawal effects which include: abdominal cramps, diarrhea, increased salivation, insomnia, nightmares, nausea, vomiting, and muscle discomfort. There may be withdrawal dyskinesias, or the unmasking of tardive dyskinesias. If these drugs are to be stopped it is best to gradually lower the dose, such as by 5% to 10% per day.

TABLE 18–11.

Important Drug Interactions With Antipsychotic Medications*

Agent	Possible Effect
Anesthetics	Potentiate hypotension
Antacid	Decrease absorption of antipsychotic
Anticholinergics	Decrease absorption
Anticoagulants	Increase bleeding time
Anticonvulsants	Increase anticonvulsant levels, effect on seizures variable; decrease neuroleptic levels
Antidepressants	Increase tricyclic and neuroleptic levels, additive hypotension effects
Antihypertensives	Generally potentiates hypotension
α-methyldopa	May potentiate hypotension; ? organic brain syndrome with haldol
β-blockers (propranolol)	Potentiate hypotension
Clonidine	Variable
Diuretics and smooth-muscle blockers	May potentiate hypotension
Guanethidine	Antagonizes antihypertensive effect
Barbiturates	
Chronic use	Decrease antipsychotic level
Acute use	Increase CNS depressant effect
Digitalis	Thioridazine may nullify inotropic effect

(Continued.)

Estrogens	May increase antipsychotic blood level
Levodopa	Mutual antagonism
Lithium	Possible toxic synergism, ? decreased chlorpromazine levels
Narcotics	Potentiate analgesia, increased respiratory depression
Oral hypoglycemics	Variable
Pressor agents	
α-agonists (norepinephrine)	Antagonize pressor effect
β-agonists (isoproterenol)	Marked hypotension
Quinidine	May potentiate cardiac effect
Sedative-hypnotics	Additive CNS depressant effects
Tegretol	Decreases plasma levels of Haldol and possibly all neuroleptics

*Adapted from Lydiard RB, Carman JS, Gold MS: Antipsychotics: Predicting effect/maximizing efficacy, in Gold MS, Lydiard RB, Carman JS (eds): Advances in Psychopharmacology: Predicting and Improving Treatment Response. Boca Raton, Fla, CRC Press, 1984.

REFERENCES

1. Baldessarini RJ: *Chemotherapy in Psychiatry: Principles and Practice* (revised and enlarged edition). Cambridge, Mass, Harvard University Press, 1985.
2. Baldessarini RJ: Drugs and the treatment of psychiatric disorders, in Gilman AG, Goodman LS, Rall TW, et al (eds): *Goodman and Gilman's the Pharmacological Basis of Therapeutics,* ed 7. New York, Macmillian Publishing, 1985.
3. Bassuk EL, Schoonover SC, Gelenberg AJ, (eds): *The Practitioner's Guide to Psychoactive Drugs,* ed 2. New York, Plenum, 1983.
4. Davis J, Janicak P, Linden R, et al: Neuroleptics and psychotic disorders, in Coyne JT, Enna SJ (eds): *Neuroleptics: Neurochemical, Behavioral, and Clinical Perspectives.* New York, Raven Press, 1983.
5. Haase H-J, Janssen PAJ: *The Action of Neuroleptic Drugs,* ed 2. New York, Elsevier, 1985.
6. Klein DF, Gittleman R, Quitkin F, et al: *Diagnosis and Drug Treatment of Psychiatric Disorders: Adults and Children,* ed 2. Baltimore, Williams & Wilkins, 1980.
7. Leber P, Sudden death as a risk of neuroleptic treatment: A continuing controversy. *Psychopharmacol Bull* 1981; 17:6.
8. Lydiard RB, Carman JS, Gold MS: Antipsychotics: Predicting response/maximizing efficacy, in Gold MS, Lydiard RB, Carman JS (eds): *Advances in Psychopharmacology: Predicting and Improving Treatment Response.* Boca Raton, Fla, CRC Press, 1984.
9. Mason AS, Granacher RP: *Clinical Handbook of Anti-Psychotic Drug Therapy.* New York, Brunner/Mazel, 1980.

19
Antidepressants

Antidepressants can be classified into two major groups by their mode of action: (1) heterocyclics and (2) monoamine oxidase inhibitors (MAOIs).

I. **Heterocyclics.**

A. **Structural classification.**

1. Tricyclics.

a. Tertiary amines.

(i) Amitriptyline.

(ii) Imipramine.

(iii) Trimipramine.

(iv) Doxepin.

b. Secondary amines.

(i) Desipramine.

(ii) Nortriptyline.

(iii) Protriptyline.

2. Second-generation antidepressants.

(i) Trazodone.

(ii) Amoxapine.

(iii) Maprotiline.

B. **Mechanism of action.** Originally, the heterocyclic mechanism of action was thought to be an increased availability of norepinephrine or serotonin created by a blunting reuptake into presynaptic neurons. Tertiary amines were thought to block predominantly serotonin and secondary amines predominantly norepinephrine. It now appears that the action is more complex and that down-regulation of adrenergic receptors may play a major role in an antidepressant effect.

It is now recognized that most antidepressants have effects on both norepinephrine and serotonin and, furthermore, have capacities to block several types of receptors, including H_1- and H_2-receptors, α_1- and α_2-adrenergeric receptors, and muscarinic receptors. Blockade of these receptors correlates with a range of side effects.

C. **Side effects.** Side effect profiles vary among antidepressants and are often the key factor in the choice of a drug. The most common side effects are as follows.

1. Sedation—correlates with histamine receptor blockade.

2. Anticholinergic effects—dry mouth, blurry vision, constipation, and urinary hesitancy; correlates with muscarinic blockade.

3. Orthostatic hypotension—related to a complex interaction of receptor and reuptake blockades.

See Table 19–1 for a ranking of these effects for each drug. Other side effects include the following types.

4. Cardiac effects.

a. Increased heart rate.

b. Slowed conduction from bundle of His through bundle branches and Purkinje fibers, i.e., type I antiarrhythmic effects.

c. Electrocardiographic (ECG) changes.

(i) Prolonged PR, QRS, and QT_c intervals.

TABLE 19-1.
Ranking of Drug Effects

Drug	Sedation	Anticholinergic Effects	Orthostasis
Amitriptyline (Elavil, Endep)	High	High	Medium
Doxepin (Sinequan, Adapin)	High	Medium-low	Medium
Trazodone (Desyrel)	High-medium	Very low	Low
Maprotiline (Ludiomil)	Low	Low	Low
Imipramine (Tofranil, Presamine)	Medium	Medium	High
Nortriptyline (Aventil, Pamelor)	Low	Medium	Low
Amoxapine (Asendin)	Low	Medium	
Desipramine (Norpramin, Pertofrane)	Low	Low	Low

(ii) T wave flattening.

d. Cardiac function—current techniques have not demonstrated decreased cardiac function even in patients with heart failure, though in vitro studies have suggested negative inotropic and chronotropic effects.

e. Suggested cardiac monitoring.

(i) Baseline ECG in patients aged older than 40 years or in those patients with a history of mitral valve prolapse or arrhythmia.

(ii) Follow-up ECGs after dose is increased in patients with susceptible conduction systems.

(iii) Cardiology consultation in patients with heart failure or conduction defects.

5. Other side effects—general.

a. Tremor and myoclonic jerks.

b. Sweating.

c. Impotence.

d. Gastrointestinal (GI) disturbance—constipation.

e. Weight gain.

f. Seizures.

g. Dry mouth—most common.

h. Blurred vision.

6. Other side effects—specific drugs.

a. Priapism—trazodone.

b. Extrapyramidal syndromes and tardive dyskinesia possible with amoxapine, which can be metabolized to loxaprine succinate (Loxitane), a neuroleptic.

c. Maprotiline—seizures.

D. **Selection of antidepressant.** This should be based on the following in this order:

1. Personal history of positive response.

2. Family history of positive response.

3. Side effect profile, e.g., a sedating drug for a patient with initial insomnia, drugs with low orthostatic and anticholinergic effects for the elderly, or a drug such as trazodone with low overdose toxicity for suicidal patients.

4. Methylphenidate (Ritalin) trial—a onetime oral dose of 15 mg of methylphenidate may be administered, with a depression rating scale given just before and 2 hours after the dose. A marked but transient improvement in mood suggests a possible response to imipramine or desipramine, while no effect or a worsening of mood suggests the use of nortriptyline or amitriptyline.

E. **Dosing.** Inadequate dosing is a common cause of therapeutic failure.

1. **Method.** Therapy may be begun with a low-unit dose; every 2 to 4 days, the dose may be increased until (1) a distinct response is noted, (2) side effects preclude a further increase, or (3) a maximum is reached (see Table 19–2). For elderly, debilitated, or medication-sensitive patients, the doses should be halved.

2. **Metabolism.** All of the antidepressants are rapidly absorbed when taken orally. They are metabolized in the liver and excreted in the kidney. They may be taken once a day, except for trazodone, which has a short half-life and may be given in two to three divided doses.

3. **Drug levels.** Levels are available for several of the heterocyclics. However, nortriptyline and imipramine are the only drugs for which a correlation of level with clinical effect has been clearly demonstrated. For nortriptyline, there is evidence of a therapeutic window from 50 to 150 ng/mL. For imipramine, the range of 180 to 225 ng/mL is the threshold for the combination of imipramine and desipramine levels. Since different laboratories have different standards, the norms of one's

TABLE 19–2.

Low-Unit and Maximum Dose Drug Therapy

Drug	Unit Dose, mg	Maximum Dose, mg
Imipramine	50	300
Amitriptyline	50	300
Trimipramine	25	150
Doxepin	50	400
Nortriptyline	25	150
Desipramine	50	300
Protriptyline	10	60
Trazodone	100	600
Maprotiline	50	150–200 in females, 200–250 in males
Amoxapine	100	600

own laboratory should be followed. Levels for other antidepressants are useful only when they are very high or very low.

4. **Continuing medication.** Once a patient has an adequate level or maximum dosing, the drug must be continued at least 4 to 6 weeks for an adequate trial. There is evidence that patients continue to demonstrate a response up to 8 weeks after the initiation of therapy.

If the patient does respond, most clinicians continue the medication for 6 to 12 months. The drug may be slowly tapered during several weeks. Sudden cessation of the drug may result in cholinergic rebound, especially with imipramine and amitriptyline. Symptoms usually consist of the following types:

GI: Nausea, vomiting, diarrhea, and gastric distress.

Central nervous system: Vivid dreams, anxiety, and frequent awakenings.

Genitourinary: Frequent urination and increased sexual desire and fantasies.

F. **Tricyclic overdose.** This is a common and serious occurrence.

1. A marked interpersonal variation in metabolism makes widely varying doses lethal. The lethal dose for 50% of a population is approximately 35 mg/kg, and greater than 50 mg/kg is usually fatal. A common rule of thumb for a fatal overdose is seven to ten times the daily dose. It is wise to prescribe less than that for a suicidal patient at a time.

2. Central nervous system effects include confusion, myoclonic jerks, seizures, and coma.

3. Cardiovascular effects are frequently most lethal. These include hypertension, hypotension, tachycardia, ventricular arrhythmias, and conduction defects. A QRS interval of greater than 100 ms correlates with a severe overdose and plasma levels of over 1,000 ng/mL (although this QRS interval is also found in 25% of normal subjects). Since tricyclics act as type I antiarrhythmics, it is important not to use these antiarrhythmics for treatment of an overdose.

4. Delayed complications, including a lapse into coma or late arrythmias, are sometimes seen.

II. **Monoamine oxidase inhibitors (MAOIs).**

A. **Classification.**

1. Hydrazines.

a. Phenelzine (Nardil).

b. Isocarboxazid (Marplan).

2. Nonhydrazines.

a. Tranylcypromine (Parnate).

B. **Mechanism.** These second-line, but effective, antidepressants inhibit MAO, the enzyme present in many tissues that oxidizes norepinephrine, serotonin, dopamine, and tyramine.

TABLE 19-3.

Detailed Instructions for Patients Regarding MAOIs, Diet, and Medication Restrictions*

Instructions

Food and beverages to avoid:
  Cheese (cottage and cream cheese OK)
  Red wine, beer, sherry, vermouth, brandy, liqueurs (white wine and distilled liquor OK although distilled liquor will produce rapid intoxication with phenelzine [Nardil])
  Yeast or protein extracts (sometimes present in soups or stews)
  Broad beans, fava beans, or Chinese pea pods (includes Italian green beans)
  Banana peels
  Any proteins that are not fresh or freshly frozen or canned (includes game meats, sausage, bologna, pepperoni, salami, corned beef, lox, pâté)
  Liver
  Pickled or smoked fish (e.g., herring)
  Canned or overripe figs

Foods and beverages to be used in moderation:
  Caffeinated beverages, such as coffee, tea, and cola
  Chocolate
  Other alcoholic beverages
  Avocados
  Soy sauce
  Yogurt and sour cream (eat reputable brands only)
  Other fruits and banana pulp

Medications to avoid (very important):
  Meperidine (Demerol)
  Cough medicines that contain dextromethorphan (e.g., guaifenesin [Robitussin-DM])
  Cold tablets or drops
  Nasal decongestants/sinus tablets/hay fever medication

(Continued.)

Weight-reducing preparations/"pep pills"
Appetite suppressants
Asthma inhalants
Other antidepressants (except with caution as outlined)
Epinephrine in local anesthetics
Cocaine/amphetamines/Methylphenidate (Ritalin)

MAOIs = monoamine oxidase inhibitors.

C. Side effects.

1. Acute hypertension can occur following ingestion of tyramine in food or pressor amines in drugs.

a. This is the most well-known side effect; in practice, it is quite rare.

b. The usual symptom is a severe pulsating or throbbing headache.

c. Instructions for patients are to take no drugs, including over-the-counter medications, without consulting a physician and to follow a low-tyramine diet (see Table 19–3 for details).

d. Patient may be given 10 mg of nifedipine, to be taken sublingually should a sudden severe headache develop; the patient should go to an emergency room if the headache continues.

2. Sudden death has occurred with meperidine (Demerol), other synthetic narcotics, and dextromethorphan in patients receiving MAOIs.

3. Orthostatic hypotension is the most common side effect and is severe in 5% to 10% of patients. This may abate over time. It may be treated with salt tablets or fluorinef.

4. Other side effects.

a. Sedation.

b. Agitation.

c. Dry mouth.

d. Anorgasmia/impotence.

e. Weight gain.

D. **Indications.**

1. The MAOIs can be used as second-line drugs for depressions resistant to heterocyclic treatment.

2. There is anecdotal evidence of special effectiveness for "atypical" depressions characterized by overeating, oversleeping, and anxiety.

3. The MAOI may be used in combination with heterocyclics provided that the MAOI is added to the heterocyclic, or they are started together at a low dose. There is the potential for hyperpyrexia in adding a heterocyclic to an MAOI.

E. **Dosing.** Therapy should be started with a unit dose and increased by a unit dose every 3 days until a maximum is reached or side effects are limiting (Table 19–4).

TABLE 19–4.

Dosing Schedule for MAOIs*

Drug	Unit Dose, mg	Maximum Dose, mg
Phenelzine	15	90
Isocarboxazid	15	90
Tranylcypromine	10	60

*MAOIs = monoamine oxidase inhibitors.

20
Lithium and Other Antimanic Agents

Lithium is used primarily for the treatment of affective disorders, particularly bipolar disorder. Various potential alternatives to lithium are now being used. Below are guidelines to the clinical use of lithium and the other antimanic agents.

I. **Lithium.**

A. **Description.** Lithium, a monovalent cation, has been used in treating thousands of patients with bipolar disorder and has been proved to be effective for treating acute mania and for the prophylaxis of recurrent affective episodes. Despite lithium's proven efficacy, its mechanism of action remains unclear.

B. **Indications.**

1. Definite indications.

a. Acute mania: Lithium is the drug of choice, but an adjunctive antipsychotic agent is used for behavioral control before lithium's onset of action. Lithium's effect in this state often takes 7 to 10 days.

b. Bipolar prophylaxis: Maintenance lithium therapy is indicated in any of the following situations.

(i) Two or more bipolar affective episodes in 2 years.

(ii) More than three lifetime bipolar affective episodes.

(iii) High risk of morbidity or mortality if symptoms recur.

(iv) Note: Maintenance lithium therapy is not usually indicated after a single, uncomplicated, affective episode.

c. Bipolar depressive states: Lithium may be used alone or in conjunction with either a heterocyclic antidepressant or a monoamine oxidase inhibitor (MAOI) to prevent "switching" into mania due to the antidepressant. In cases of moderate depression, lithium alone may be sufficient.

d. Treatment refractory unipolar depressions: Lithium, in combination with other antidepressant agents, is often helpful when patients fail to respond to more conventional somatic therapies. Hence, lithium is often added to existing dose schedules that may include tricyclics, MAOIs, and thyroid hormones.

2. Other possible uses.

a. Schizoaffective disorder: Lithium may be used in conjunction with neuroleptics for treating this disorder.

b. Schizophrenia: Lithium may be useful in treating some refractory patients. However, it may make some schizophrenics worse.

c. Recurrent unipolar depressions: Lithium may be useful in preventing depressive relapse.

3. Controversial uses: Lithium has been reported to be effective for treating several other conditions, such as cyclothymia, premenstrual syndrome, borderline personality disorder, and post-traumatic stress disorder. However, these claims are not well substantiated.

C. **Pharmacokinetics.**

1. Absorption: Orally administered doses are almost completely absorbed.

2. Excretion: 99% is via kidneys, and it is prolonged by impaired renal function.

3. Peak serum levels: These occur 1 to 3 hours after ingestion in normal subjects for lithium carbonate and 5 to 6 hours for slow-release preparations.

4. Half-life: 18 hours for normal subjects, increasing to ≥36 hours in the elderly.

5. Steady state: 5 days in young normal subjects, increasing to 7 days in the elderly.

D. **Precautions.**

1. Situations arise in which lithium should be used only when the benefits clearly outweigh the risks. These conditions, the potential problems, and general measures to avoid these problems are listed in Table 20–1. In many cases, electroconvulsive therapy (ECT) or other pharmacologic agents (e.g., neuroleptics) may be safer alternatives.

2. Situations in which lithium can be used but which require close monitoring of side effects and lithium levels are listed in Table 20–2 along with the problems that may arise. Generally these conditions necessitate smaller doses with careful titration of the doses.

E. **Treatment guidelines.**

1. Pretreatment evaluation.

a. Complete blood cell count (CBC).

b. Electrolyte levels.

c. Blood urea nitrogen (BUN) and creatinine levels.

d. Routine urinalysis.

e. Thyroid studies.

f. Electrocardiogram (ECG) and physical examination if the patient has significant medical problems or is over 40 years old.

2. Initiation of treatment: When a patient is moderately to severely manic, adjunctive therapy with a high-potency neuroleptic is common. Neuroleptics act much more quickly than lithium in calming behavior.

TABLE 20–1.

Conditions in Which Lithium Use Poses Significant Risk

Condition	Potential Problem	Management Approach
Pregnancy (especially 1st trimester)	Increased risk of fetus developing of tetralogy of Fallot	Avoid lithium in 1st trimester, ECT or neuroleptics are safer, general counseling, consider abortion if lithium used
Breast-feeding	Lithium toxicity in infant from lithium excreted in breast milk	No breast-feeding with lithium, provide formula feeding
Sick sinus syndrome	Cardiac arrest reported	Consider pacemaker placement, consider ECT or neuroleptics
Postmyocardial infarction	Potential for dysrhythmias	Slow-dose increases, frequent ECG monitoring, hold lithium and consider neuroleptics
Altered fluid and electrolyte status	Potential for lithium toxicity	
Labor and delivery	Lithium toxicity in mother due to fluid shifts, lithium toxicity in infant	Reduce dose by 50% in last week of pregnancy, discontinue lithium at onset of labor

Lithium can be started with the neuroleptic or held until the patient is cooperative enough to take oral medications.

There are at least two methods for starting lithium, with the choice depending on the severity of illness.

a. Test dose method: The procedure is described in Table 20–3. Check serum levels three times per week for the first two weeks until the dose, serum level, and clinical status are stable.

b. Step increase method.

(i) Initiate at low dose (e.g., 300 mg po bid).

(ii) Check serum level at steady state (5 to 7 days later).

(iii) If serum levels are insufficient, increase the dose and recheck serum levels when steady state is reached.

(iv) Levels may rise as the mania abates. Once the level and dose have been stable for 3 weeks, check the level every month for the first few months. If no prob-

TABLE 20–2.

Conditions in Which Lithium Use Poses Significant Risk

Condition	Potential Problem
Renal insufficiency	Delayed excretion increases half-life and increases risk of developing toxic levels
Advanced age	Side effects and therapeutic response often at lower doses, increased serum levels at usual therapeutic doses secondary to diminished renal function
Organic brain syndromes	Side effects, especially cognitive changes are more likely

TABLE 20–3.
Method of Predicting Initial Dosage Regimen of Lithium Therapy*

Procedure:

The patient is given a loading dose of lithium carbonate, 600 mg by mouth (po), at 8 A.M. on day 1.

Precisely at 8 A.M. (or exactly 24 hr following the loading dose) on day 2, blood is drawn and a serum lithium determination made. The morning dose of lithium must be held until blood is drawn.

The resulting serum lithium value is entered into the table below to predict the dosage regimen.

Determination of dosage regimen:

Serum Lithium, mEq/L (24 hr Following 600-mg Loading Dose)	Dosage Regimen to Maintain 0.6–1.2–mEq/L Lithium Level[†]
0.24–0.30[‡]	300 mg bid
0.20–0.23	300 mg tid
0.15–0.19	300 mg qid
0.10–0.14	600 mg tid
0.05–0.09	900 mg tid
0.05	1200 mg tid

*From Cooper TB, Simpson GM: The 24-hour lithium level as a prognosticator of dosage requirements. Am J Psychiatry 1978; 133:440-443.
[†]bid = twice daily; tid = three times daily; qid = four times daily.
[‡]For serum levels above 0.30 mEq/L, lithium should be administered with caution, and further patient evaluation is advised.

lems arise, check levels every 4 to 6 months. The level, in all cases, is checked 12 hours after the last dose.

3. Dosing: Lithium is generally given in two to four

doses per day. Fewer daily doses may increase some side effects but may also improve compliance and minimize the risk of nephrotoxicity.

4. Serum levels: The levels suggested in Table 20–4 are general guidelines. Dosages need to be titrated for an individual patient's tolerance of and response to lithium.

5. Maintenance therapy laboratory studies.

a. Lithium level every 4 to 6 months.

b. Thyroid-stimulating (TSH) level every 12 months.

c. BUN and creatinine levels every 12 months. If complications (such as severe side effects, altered fluid and electrolyte status, renal disease, dose change, weight change, mood change, or on beginning diuretics) arise during treatment, a lithium level should be checked promptly while appropriate evaluation of the complication is undertaken.

F. **Adverse effects.**

1. Table 20–5 lists the effect that lithium may have on common laboratory values.

2. Side effects: Most side effects are dose related. Patient and physician should be aware of them in advance and discuss them if they occur. Side effects occur in 88% of patients, are often unpleasant to the patient, and are the most common cause of noncompliance with

TABLE 20–4.

Suggested Serum Lithium Levels for Various Conditions

Condition	Suggested Serum Level, mEq/L
Mania	1.0–1.6
Bipolar prophylaxis	0.6–1.0
Other disorders	0.6–1.0

TABLE 20–5.
Possible Effects of Lithium on Laboratory Values

Laboratory Value	Possible Effect of Lithium
White blood cells (WBCs)	Increased count
Serum glucose	Increased level
Serum magnesium	Increased level
Serum potassium	Decreased level
Serum uric acid	Decreased level
Serum thyroxine	Decreased
Serum cortisol	Decreased A.M. levels
Serum parathyroid hormone	Increased level due to adenoma
Serum calcium	Increased level due to increased parathyroid hormone level
Serum phosphorus	Decreased level due to increased parathyroid hormone level

TABLE 20–6.
Side Effects of Lithium and Their Management*

Side Effect	Management
Gastrointestinal complaints	Give lithium after meals, give smaller doses more often, try slow-release preparation, lower the dose
Tremor	Lower the dose, give propranolol (40–100 mg/day), consider adding a benzodiazepene
Polyuria/diabetes insipidus	Try slow-release preparation, lower the dose, add amiloride (5–10 mg/day), careful monitoring of lithium levels

Acne	Benzoyl peroxide (5%–10%) topical solution, erythromycin (1.5%–2%) topical solution
Muscular weakness, fasciculations, headaches	Usually resolve with first few weeks of treatment
Hypothyroidism	Levothyroxine (0.05 mg qd), follow TSH level and increase to 0.2 mg qd as needed
T wave inversion	Benign, no treatment needed
Cardiac dysrhythmias	Usually must discontinue lithium
Psoriasis, alopecia areata	Dermatology consult, reversible if lithium stopped
Weight gain	Difficult to treat, diet, may be partially reversible if lithium stopped
Edema	Consider spironolactone (50 mg po qd); *if severe*, monitor lithium levels; resolves when lithium stopped
Leukocytosis	Benign, no treatment needed

qd = every day.

---

lithium. Many side effects are treatable, and many resolve with time. The most common side effects are thirst, polyuria, tremor, ataxia, lethargy, gastrointestinal complaints, weight gain, edema, and hypothyroidism. Table 20–6 lists side effects of lithium with their management.

G. Drug interactions with lithium are listed in Table 20–7.

TABLE 20–7.

Drug Interactions With Lithium*

Drug	Potential Interaction
Psychotropics	
Heterocyclic antidepressants	Enhanced antidepressant effects
Phenothiazines	Increase cellular uptake of lithium that may increase risk of lithium toxicity
Amphetamines	Lithium blocks amphetamine-induced highs and anorexia
Butyrophenones	High doses of lithium and haloperidol (Haldol) should be avoided because of possible toxicity
Diuretics	
Thiazides/ethacrynic acid	Enhanced sodium excretion, leading to increased serum lithium concentrations
Furosemide, triamterene, spironolactone	Same as for thiazides but to lesser degree
Mannitol, urea, acetazolamide	May enhance lithium excretion
Salts	
Sodium bicarbonate, sodium chloride	Increased lithium excretion secondary to increased sodium level
Potassium iodide	Acts synergistically with lithium to decrease T_4 level

(Continued.)

NSAID, indomethacin, phenylbutazone	May increase lithium levels
Neuromuscular blockers	Lithium prolongs neuromuscular blockade
Depolarizing (succinylcholine)	
Nondepolarizing (pancuronium)	Same as for depolarizing agents
Aminophylline	Enhances lithium excretion
Others	
Methyldopa	May increased lithium level
Tetracycline	May increase lithium level
Digoxin	Lithium may exacerbate digoxin intoxication by decreasing intracellular potassium stores

*T_4 = thyroxine; NSAID = nonsteroidal anti-inflammatory drug.

Early studies suggesting a toxic interaction between lithium and haloperidol have not been substantiated by later, more rigorous studies.

H. Table 20–8 lists the causes, assessment, and treatment of lithium intoxication. It should be noted that signs and symptoms are the most important factors for monitoring intoxications.

II. **Alternative antimanic agents.** Up to 30% of patients with bipolar disorder are refractory to or intolerant of lithium. Numerous agents are being tried as alternatives to lithium. At this point, carbamazepine and ECT are the only clinically applicable alternatives. The other agents are still considered to be experimental.

TABLE 20–8.

Approach to Lithium Intoxication

Causes	Dehydration
	Sodium depletion
	Diuretics
	Renal disease
	Overdose
Assessment	Early signs and symptoms
	Nausea, vomiting, diarrhea, dysarthria, lethargy, coarse tremor
	Late signs and symptoms
	Ataxia, obtundation, seizure, coma, death
	Laboratory evaluation
	Serum lithium level (levels between 2–4 mEq/L associated with severe toxicity, levels ≥4 mEq/L are potentially fatal)
	Electrolyte levels
	BUN, creatinine levels
	ECG
Treatment	Discontinue lithium
	Basic supportive medical care
	IV saline diuresis ≥5 L/day
	IV aminophylline, urea, or mannitol has not been proved to be more effective than saline diuresis
	If intoxication is severe or refractory to initial treatment, consider peritoneal or hemodialysis

IV = intravenous.

A. Carbamazepine.

1. Description: Originally used as an anticonvulsant, it has been found to be effective for acute mania, as well as for prophylaxis against bipolar episodes.

2. Indications.

a. Acute mania: Carbamazepine is used, either with or without lithium or neuroleptics, in treating patients who are unresponsive or partially responsive to lithium. The response is rapid, similar to that seen with neuroleptics. Patients with more severe mania, more severe psychosis, or rapid cycling may be more likely to respond.

b. Bipolar prophylaxis: Carbamazepine appears to be quite effective in treating some patients, with or without lithium.

c. Depression: A few studies suggest carbamazepine has mild antidepressant properties.

3. Pharmacokinetics.

a. Absorption: Absorbed rapidly after oral administration.

b. Half-life: 13 to 17 hours with long-term use.

c. Metabolism: Metabolized by the liver to a 10,11 epoxide that may be the substance responsible for an antimanic effect; induces its own metabolism, causing serum levels to decline with long-term use.

d. Peak serum levels occur 2 to 6 hours after dosing.

4. Adverse effects.

a. Nausea, vomiting, sedation, diplopia, blurred vision, and ataxia are the most common side effects. These effects correlate with dose and rate of increase of dose.

b. A maculopapular rash develops in 15% of patients and requires discontinuation of carbamazepine as it can progress to a severe, exfoliative dermatitis.

c. Leukopenia is common but is usually modest, transient, and clinically insignificant.

d. Aplastic anemia is a rare complication (occurs in approximately one in 30,000 patients receiving carbamazepine).

e. Hepatitis is likewise rare but can be fatal.

5. Treatment guidelines.

a. Pretreatment evaluation.

(i) CBC, differential, and platelet counts.

(ii) Liver function tests.

(iii) ECG and physical examination if patient has serious medical illness or is over 40 years old.

b. Initiation of treatment: Carbamazepine is started at low doses (i.e., 200 mg bid), and the dose is increased 200 mg every 3 to 4 days, as tolerated, to minimize side effects.

c. Dosing: The usual therapeutic dose ranges from 800 to 1,200 mg/day in three to four divided doses. Occasionally, patients require up to 2,000 mg/day. However, this dose range is reserved for patients who have shown a partial but incomplete response at lower doses. The optimal method to determine the dose is to increase the dose until limited by side effects or until therapeutic effect occurs.

d. Serum levels: Levels are not closely correlated to response, but often, patients respond when levels are between 6 and 12 mg/mL.

e. Maintenance therapy laboratory studies: This area is controversial because of the rare cases of aplastic anemia.

(i) Uncomplicated treatment: Check CBC and platelet counts every week for the first 2 months. Then, check CBC and platelet counts every 3 months.

(ii) Complicated treatment: If the patient develops

TABLE 20–9.

Guidelines for Discontinuing Carbamazepine Therapy

Indicator	Value
Total count WBC	$<3,000/mm^3$
Neutrophils, no.	$<1,500/mm^3$
Erythrocytes, no.	$<4.0 \times 10^6/mm^3$
Hematocrit	$<32\%$
Hemoglobin level	<11 gm/100 mL
Platelet count	$<100,000/mm^3$
Reticulocyte count	$<0.3\%$
Serum iron level	<150 mg/100 mL

a sore throat, malaise, fever, bruising, bleeding, or petechia, the physician should be notified immediately, and CBC and platelet counts should be checked. If symptoms of liver disease develop, check liver function test results.

    f. Guidelines for discontinuation of carbamazepine are listed in Table 20–9.

  6. Potential interactions between carbamazepine and other drugs are listed in Table 20–10.

B. **ECT:** ECT is effective for acute mania but is not often used because pharmacologic interventions have been proved to be so useful. ECT should be considered if the patient is unresponsive to or intolerant of medications or if the manic patient is acutely lethal.

C. **Valproic acid:** It appears to be effective in combination with lithium for treating acute mania but is not a good prophylactic agent in treating bipolar illness; however, supporting data are limited.

D. **Clonazepam:** It is effective in calming manic behavior. There is no apparent prophylactic or antidepressant value.

TABLE 20–10.

Interactions Between Carbamazepine and Other Drugs

Influence of other drugs on carbamazepine
  Increased carbamazepine levels
    Isoniazid
    Tranylcypromine
    Valproic acid (increased free carbamazepine in vitro)
    Propoxyphene
    Erythromycin
    Nicotinamide
    Cimetidine
  Decreased carbamazepine levels
    Phenobarbital
    Phenytoin
    Primidone
Influence of carbamazepine on other drugs
  Carbamazepine increases
  Escape from dexamethasone suppression
  Carbamazepine decreases the effects of
    Clonazepam
    Dicumarol
    Doxycycline
    Phenytoin
    Valproate sodium
    Theophylline
    Ethosuximide
    Warfarin
    Pregnancy tests

E. **Verapamil:** It has been reported to be effective in treating acute mania and for prophylaxis of bipolar episodes.

F. **Other potential agents.**

1. Adrenergic agents: Propranolol, clonidine.

2. Adenylate cyclase inhibitors: demeclocycline.

3. Cholinomimetics: Choline, lecithin, physostigmine.

4. Serotonergic agents: Tryptophan, fenfluramine.

5. Clorgyline.

6. Bupropion.

7. Spironolactone.

REFERENCES

1. Johnson FN (ed): *Handbook of Lithium Therapy*. Baltimore, University Park Press, 1980.
2. Mason AS, Granacher RP: Lithium therapy, in *Clinical Handbook of Antipsychotic Drug Therapy*. New York, Brunner/Mazel, Inc, 1980.
3. Lerer B: Alternative therapies for bipolar disorder. *J Clin Psychiatry* 1985; 46:309–316.
4. Post RM, Uhde TW: Clinical approaches to treatment resistant bipolar illness, in Hales RF, Francis AJ (eds): *APA Annual Review*, vol 6. Washington, DC, American Psychiatric Press, Inc, 1987.

21

Benzodiazepines

Below are the major features of this class of drugs.

I. **Central nervous system.**

A. For antianxiety agents, efficacy is established only for short-term use; there is a high-dependence and abuse potential.

B. Hypnotics decrease sleep latency; in usual dosages, they do not suppress rapid eye movement sleep but do diminish or eliminate stage 4 sleep. They have been used to treat night terrors that arise in stage 4 sleep. Their hypnotic efficacy has only been documented for short-term use (2 to 4 weeks).

C. Benzodiazepines raise the seizure threshold and are anticonvulsant. Diazepam is used to treat status epilepticus, and clonazepam treats petit mal epilepsy.

D. There is an endogenous benzodiazepine receptor in the brain. This is linked to the inhibitory neurotransmitter and an associated chloride channel gamma-aminobutyric acid (GABA). Benzodiazepines act to facilitate GABA-ergic synaptic transmission; their main functions are medicated by GABA-ergic synapses. Benzodiazepines inhibit cells by altering membrane permeability to chloride ions, thus facilitating GABA effects.

II. **Cardiovascular and respiratory systems.** There does not appear to be a significant depression of cardiovascular or respiratory function when the benzodiazepines are given in usual dosages by oral administration. However, depression of these systems may be significant in major or combined overdosages.

III. **Skeletal muscle.** Benzodiazepines have mild skeletal muscle relaxant properties; these occur due to their action on interneuronal transmission in the brain stem. There is no direct effect on muscle function.

IV. **Absorption, fate, and excretion.**

A. Pharmacokinetics: This varies considerably among the various preparations. As a general guideline, five times the half-life yields the steady-state concentration of the drug. Drugs with a long half-life accumulate in the body, causing drowsiness, sedation, memory impairment, and alteration of intellectual and psychomotor activity. This is especially common in the elderly. In addition, the appearance of withdrawal symptoms is related to the rate of elimination of the drug withdrawal, occurring later and/or being less severe in agents with a long half-life.

B. Metabolism: All benzodiazepines can be divided into two groups based on their metabolic pathway. The first group undergoes hepatic microsomal oxidation and subsequent glucuronic conjugation. Diazepam, clorazepate, halazepam, prazepam, and chlordiazepoxide are examples of this group. The second group undergoes glucuronide conjugation directly. Lorazepam, oxazepam, and temazepam are examples of this group. Those drugs that undergo hepatic metabolism form active metabolites that may accumulate and produce side effects. Obviously, drugs from this group should be avoided in patients with liver disease.

C. Alprazolam reaches a peak plasma concentration in 1 to 2 hours after administration; its half-life is from 4 to 6 hours. Metabolites have uncertain clinical activity.

D. Chlordiazepoxide is slowly absorbed and may take several hours to reach peak plasma levels; its half-life is 1 to 2 days. Active metabolites are formed. Excretion is via conjugation in the liver and then excretion by the kidneys.

E. Clorazepate: Therapeutic action is primarily by an active metabolite, nordiazepam.

F. Diazepam is rapidly absorbed, with peak plasma levels reached in 1 hour. Elimination is biphasic, with the rapid phase lasting 2 to 3 hours and a slow decay of 2 to 8 hours. Steady-state concentration is achieved in about 1 week. Active metabolites are formed. Excretion is predominantly via the kidneys.

G. Flurazepam given orally is rapidly absorbed. Peak serum levels occur 30 to 60 minutes after administration. Its half-life is about 2.3 hours. It has an active metabolite with a half-life of 47 to 100 hours. The metabolite reaches a steady state after 7 to 10 days of administration. It is metabolized by the liver and excreted in the urine.

H. Halazepam given orally reaches a peak serum level in 1 to 3 hours. Its half-life is about 40 hours; its active metabolite has a half-life of 50 to 100 hours.

I. Lorazepam given orally is rapidly absorbed, with a peak plasma level being reached in 2 hours after administration. Injectable lorazepam has a predictable pattern of absorption. When used, peak plasma levels are reached 60 to 90 minutes following injection. Its half-life following intravenous or intramuscular injection is about 16 hours. It is metabolized in the liver and excreted in the urine. With the injectable form, a steady state is reached in 2 days. The half-life of lorazepam is 12 hours; that of its primary metabolite is 18 hours.

J. Oxazepam reaches a peak plasma level in 4 hours and is excreted in the urine. There are no active metabolites.

K. Prazepam reaches a peak serum level in 6 hours; its mean half-life after repeated dosing is 70 hours. It is metabolized by the liver and excreted in the urine.

L. Temazepam reaches a peak serum level in about 2 to 3 hours after oral administration. Parent drug elimination is biphasic with half times of 30 minutes and 10 hours. There is no accumulation of metabolites. It is metabolized in the liver and excreted in the urine. A steady state is reached after 3 days of regular once a day administration.

M. Triazolam has a mean plasma half-life of 2.6 hours. It is rapidly absorbed after oral administration, with peak plasma levels being reached 1.3 hours after administration. There are no known active metabolites. It is metabolized in the liver and excreted in the urine.

V. **Tolerance and physical dependence.**

A. These occur with all members of this class of drugs. Habituation is common. Due to the long half-lives of many agents and conversions to active metabolites, withdrawal symptoms may not appear for up to a week after discontinuation of the drug. Withdrawal from short-acting agents may have an earlier onset and be more severe than those seen with long-acting agents. The advantage of short-acting agents is that they are rapidly cleared and have less of a risk of accumulation. Withdrawal symptoms may occur in patients who take therapeutic dosages for several months. It is most likely to occur if patients take benzodiazepines for more than 4 months, use a high dosage, and stop the drug abruptly after having used a short-acting benzodiazepine.

1. Dependence.

a. Psychologic, i.e., the feeling state of users that they need a certain dose to perform optimally. This is often accompanied by drug-seeking behavior.

b. Physical-biologic adaption to the drug effects, as demonstrated by the development of tolerance and withdrawal reactions.

c. After a course of treatment, patients may complain of a resurgence of the symptoms that they were initially treated for. These may, in fact, be withdrawal symptoms due to dependence. There is a group of patients who use benzodiazepines in clinically appropriate doses for long periods of time who have considerable trouble discontinuing their medication.

2. Tolerance: The effects of a given drug dose decrease over time and the original effects are only reproduced by an increase in the dose. These effects may be due to changes in drug metabolism or changes in receptor sites. Tolerance to the sedative side effects occurs rapidly (days). Tolerance to the therapeutic effects can occur during either long- or short-term administration. Cross-tolerance to other drug classes occurs (e.g., alcohol, barbiturates). This cross-tolerance is utilized in the management of alcohol withdrawal.

3. Withdrawal phenomena occur after drug ingestion has been discontinued. Possible responses on discontinuation as follows.

a. No patient difficulty with withdrawal—common if the drug is slowly discontinued.

b. An increase in symptoms may be due to a placebo effect, return of original symptoms (relapse), return of symptoms at a level higher than before treatment (rebound), or an abstinence response unrelated to the original condition. The severity of symptoms at various times can be documented using rating scales (e.g., Hamilton Anxiety Scale).

c. The withdrawal reaction can be suppressed by reinstitution of the discontinued medication.

4. Minor symptoms include anxiety, insomnia, irritability, nausea, palpitations, headache, muscle tension, tremor, and dysphoria. Agitation, tachycardia, diaphoresis, anorexia, depersonalization, numbness, photophobia, and hyperacusis are also common.

5. Severe symptoms include seizures, confusional states, abnormal perception of movement, muscle twitching, lowered perceptional threshold for sensory stimuli, and delirium.

VI. Toxic reactions and side effects.

A. Most commonly, this consists of drowsiness and ataxia. This is especially common in preparations with a long half-life. However, with long-term use, tolerance usually develops to the sedation.

B. Paradoxical reactions, including hostility and an increase in anxiety, have been reported.

C. Less common reactions have included weight gain, skin rash, nausea, headache, impairment of sexual function, vertigo, memory disturbances, and lightheadedness. Agranulocytosis and menstrual irregularities, including anovulation, are less common. A liver functon test result may become abnormal with extended use.

D. Overdosage is frequent, but serious sequalae are rare. Treatment is that of support for respiratory and cardiovascular function.

VII. Drug interactions.
Interactions are infrequent, except for the additive effect with other central nervous system depressants.

A. Cimetidine, isoniazid, propoxyphene, estrogen, propranolol, disulfiram, and ethanol all inhibit clearance of benzodiazepines.

B. Probenecid inhibits glucuronidation.

C. Concomitant use of scopolamine may result in increased sedation, hallucinations, and irrational behavior.

VIII. Preparations and dosage.

A. Drug selection: Many preparations are therapeutically similar. The first step in selection is patient diagnosis. For example, if a patient has a secondary anxiety disorder (as opposed to a primary anxiety disorder), treatment should be directed toward the primary disorder and not the anxiety. To treat dependency on the type of primary anxiety disorder (e.g., panic disorder), other drugs, such as tricyclics, may be useful. In patients suffering from generalized anxiety disorder, situational anxiety, and phobic disorder, benzodiazepines provide relief. In some cases of anxiety due to mild stress, medication may not be indicated.

1. Short-acting agents are often used to treat those patients in whom clearance is slow (e.g., the elderly) or when a hypnotic is desired that will be free of sedation on the next day. Some investigators suggest that acute, short-term problems are best treated with short-acting agents.

2. With long-acting agents, some investigators suggest that these drugs have an advantage in treating patients who have a chronic anxiety state and need proglonged therapy.

B. Alprazolam (Xanax) is given in 0.25-, 0.5-, and 1-mg tablets; usual daily antianxiety dosages range from 0.75 to 1.5 mg.

C. Chlordiazepoxide (Librium) is given in 5-, 10-, and 25-mg capsules; usual daily dosages range from 20 to 60 mg. Ampules of 100 mg are for intramuscular or intravenous use (see "Alcohol Withdrawal" section below).

D. Clorazepate (Tranxene) is given in 3.75-, 7.5-, and 15-mg capsules; usual daily antianxiety dosages range from 15 to 30 mg.

E. Diazepam (Valium) is given in 2-, 5-, and 10-mg tablets; usual daily antianxiety dosages range from 5 to 20 mg.

F. Flurazepam (Dalmane) is given in 15- and 30-mg capsules; usual hypnotic dosages range from 15 to 30 mg.

G. Halazepam (Paxipam) is given in 20- and 40-mg tablets; usual daily antianxiety dosages range from 80 to 160 mg.

H. Lorazepam (Ativan) is given in 0.5-, 1-, and 2-mg tablets; usual daily antianxiety dosages range from 2 to 6 mg.

I. Oxazepam (Serax) is given in 10-, 15-, and 30-mg capsules; usual daily dosages range from 30 to 90 mg.

J. Prazepam (Centrax) is given in 5-, 10-, and 20-mg capsules; usual daily antianxiety dosages range from 20 to 60 mg.

K. Temazepam (Restoril) is given in 15- and 30-mg capsules; usual daily hypnotic dosages range from 15 to 30 mg.

L. Triazolam (Halcion) is given in 0.125-, 0.25-, and 0.5-mg tablets; usual daily dosages range from 0.125 to 0.5 mg, as a hypnotic agent.

IX. **Therapeutic uses in psychiatry.**

A. Anxiety: The selection of an antianxiety drug is less of a problem than the initial decision to use one. Patient preference may need to be considered. There is little to guide one in the specific selection of a drug from this class. In fact, consistent differences between various benzodiazepine preparations in overall clinical efficacy have not been demonstrated. Symptoms and causes should dictate the dosage regimen. The selection of a particular agent is often based on the half-life and the presence of active metabolites. Due to the long half-lives of most of these drugs, arranging so that two thirds of the daily dose is taken at bedtime and the other third in two divided doses during the day, provides hypnotic and continuous antianxiety effect. The elderly and those patients with compromised hepatic function may be more sensitive to agents with long half-lives or in need of hepatic metabolism. Due to the development of tolerance and the frequently self-limited nature of anxiety, long-term courses are rarely indicated.

B. Alcohol withdrawal syndromes: A commonly used protocol is based on the use of chlordiazepoxide (Librium). The daily dosage should not exceed 300 mg. The patient is initially given 50 to 100 mg intramuscularly or intravenously; this is repeated every 2 to 4 hours, as necessary. Lower dosages (25 to 50 mg) should be used in treating the elderly or debilitated patients.

C. Hypnotic action: All benzodiazepines have hypnotic actions. Usually, flurazepam, temazepam, or oxazepam are used.

D. Depression: Alprazolam has been shown to be effective in the treatment of anxiety-related depressions and appears to be as good an antidepressant as amitriptyline or imipramine in the treatment of primary depressions. Clonazepam has been used to treat both unipolar and bipolar depressions.

E. Clonazepam and lorazepam (Ativan) have been found to be effective in the treatment of acute mania.

22

Stimulants

I. **Introduction.** This chapter will present the therapeutic use of the stimulant drugs methylphenidate, dextroamphetamine, and pemoline. There are a variety of uses for these agents, some of which are unconventional, due in part to the great idiosyncrasy in the response of some patients to stimulants.

II. **Attention deficit disorder with hyperactivity disorder (ADHD).** This is characterized by inattention, impulsivity, and overactivity. It occurs in up to 5% of schoolchildren. It is ten times more frequent in boys than girls. It needs to be distinguished from hyperactivity from other causes and from learning disabilities alone. Central nervous system–stimulant drugs are the drugs of choice in the treatment of ADHD, with 75% to 90% of patients responding favorably. The short-term benefit of stimulants in reducing impulsivity, aggression, and activity level, and in increasing concentration and classroom manageability has been well established. However, it is not clear whether the long-term outcome in terms of the ultimate level of functioning and achievement is enhanced. Usually, the stimulant is stopped when the child reaches puberty, although there is no reason to stop if the drug can be shown to be still beneficial. Certainly, there are adults with residual ADHD who benefit from stimulants. As

20% of people with borderline personality show symptoms suggestive of ADHD, this may be one special group that would benefit.

III. **Narcolepsy.** In narcolepsy, sleep attacks are largely prevented, and catalepsy is improved with stimulants. The dose of dextroamphetamine used varies from 5 to 60 mg/day.

IV. **Questionable, controversial, and other uses in adults.** Disease or mental retardation is sometimes treated with stimulants with mixed results.

Questionable uses of over-the-counter and prescription stimulants are to counter fatigue, enhance performance, and reduce weight. In dieting, it is unclear whether there is any long-term benefit, as weight is usually regained after the stimulant is stopped. If dextroamphetamine is used to help in weight reduction, the dose is 5 to 10 mg before each meal or a 10- to 15-mg spansule every morning. This use should be limited to a few weeks to prevent the development of dependence. Stimulants may be given to counter unwanted sedative effects of other medications, such as anticonvulsant drugs.

Stimulants have been used in treating reactive depressions and depression in medically ill patients. Here, the use is best limited to usually under 6 weeks. There is no established role for stimulants to treat chronic mild depressions or as the primary agents to treat major depressions. Use in medically ill depressed patients shows a favorable response in 75%, with only 7% of patients not tolerating the drug due to side effects. Stimulants have been used in a variety of medical conditions, including cardiac disease and hypertension.

The response is evident in 2 days. One can start with 5 mg of methylphenidate or dextroamphetaine, using twice daily to four times daily dosing. Rarely is more than 20 mg of methylphenidate required. The maximum dose for methylphenidate is usually 30 mg/

day and for dextroamphetamine, 15 mg/day. One specific application is to medical patients with conversion symptoms, which are presumed to be related to a depression. A very short course may be sufficient to help the patient over their current difficulty and to enhance their medical improvement.

Likewise, people with apathy and anergic problems and neurasthenic complaints may benefit, particularly if the problem is seen as transient. A very controversial use is to help correct the negative symptoms of schizophrenia, at the risk of aggravating or precipitating psychotic symptoms.

Treatment-resistant depressions may be responsive to combined drug therapy in which a stimulant is added to a tricyclic antidepressant (TCA), a monoamine oxidase inhibitor (MAOI), or even a combination of a TCA and an MAOI. While combining a stimulant with an MAOI goes against conventional wisdom and has the risk of leading to a hypertensive or hyperthermic crisis, this is, in fact, a very infrequent complication. In fact, the stimulant may counter orthostatic hypotension that otherwise would prevent the use of these antidepressants. Here, one would add the stimulant last, starting with a low dose, increasing gradually, and monitoring closely.

In geriatric populations, stimulants have been used alone or in combination with other antidepressants in the treatment of depression. Stimulants have few severe side effects and may be better tolerated in geriatric patients than other antidepressants. Up to 20% of these patients may not tolerate stimulants because they produce agitation, confusion, or aggression. The doses used are as defined above for reactive depression.

V. **General comments of side effects.** The following comments apply to all stimulant drugs and to their use in treating children and adults unless otherwise specified. In children, a reduced appetite and insomnia may initially occur in 30%. Usually, these diminish during

2 weeks. After 6 weeks of dosage adjustments, only 5% should have problems with persistent anorexia or insomnia that limits continuation. More rarely, sadness, touchiness, and crying spells may occur, but these too diminish over time. Usually, side effects are handled by lowering the dose and, later, by raising it gradually. To limit insomnia, generally, the last dose of stimulant is never given later than 4 P.M. Paradoxically, a few patients actually sleep better if given an evening dose. Of course, if insomnia remains a problem, diphenhydramine can be used as a hypnotic at bedtime. Ten percent of children may experience headache, abdominal cramps, or nausea.

In children, stimulants (except possibly pemoline) produce growth retardation. Growth rebound follows discontinuation, as long as this is permitted (as in summer vacation drug holidays) before epiphyses close. Height and weight records should be kept.

Stimulants can precipitate or aggravate psychotic symptoms (hallucinations) in susceptible people (e.g., acutely schizophrenic). It is unclear what risk patients with remitted schizophrenia have for this, but there is probably some risk. Hallucinations have been elicited in patients with *DSM III* diagnoses of borderline personality by stimulants.

In depression, stimulants can worsen the vegetative symptoms of anorexia, weight loss, and agitation. Some people paradoxically respond to stimulants with fatigue, listlessness, and dysphoria.

Problems with tachycardia or hypertension are rare, but vital signs should be monitored whenever the dose is increased. Even in patients with hypertension, tolerance usually develops to the pressor effect.

Stimulants can inhibit the metabolism of anticoagulants, anticonvulsants, TCAs, and phenylbutazone. If the patient is taking these medications, lowering the dose and monitoring blood levels would be appropriate. Stimulants may change insulin requirements. When stimulants are given with antihypertensives, one must realize that each can alter the effect of the other.

Additional side effects reported include dry mouth, irritability, excitation, increased motor activity, nausea, tremor, dizziness, palpitations, angina, cardiac arryhthmias, blurred vision, impotence, compulsive behavior, and allergic reactions. Seizures have been reported but are primarily limited to patients with a seizure history. Lowering the dose or adding anticonvulsants may permit continuation. Rarely, there is the appearance of tics, dyskinesias, or motor stereotypy.

This is usually limited to children with a history of tics or Tourette disorder. Paradoxically, some patients with Tourette disorder will improve with stimulants. There are isolated case reports of onset of obsessive-compulsive symptoms after months to years of taking stimulants; these symptoms may persist for months after the drug is stopped. There have been rare reports of hair loss, leukopenia, or anemia.

In conclusion, relative contraindications, particularly for children, are a child with mental retardation, a highly anxious child, or a child with tics. One should ask about any family history of tics or Tourette disorder. Absolute contraindications are if the medication produces an allergic reaction or psychotic symptoms. Glaucoma may be a contraindication.

Certainly, all of the stimulants have an abuse potential and can be addicting. Despite the concern that use of stimulants to treat ADHD will lead to drug abuse, there has been no evidence to substantiate this concern. Nonetheless, with adolescents, it is best to monitor their use and control their access to the medication. Further discussion of stimulant abuse and its symptoms will not be covered in this chapter. There is no evidence of any long-term negative effect of stimulant use on cognition.

VI. **Mechanism of action.** The stimulants are believed to work by both stimulating the release of catecholamines (norepinephrine, dopamine) and by blocking their reuptake.

VII. **Clinical guidelines.** This section will address the use of stimulants to treat children with attention deficit disorder with and without hyperactivity. Dose prescription for adults and for other applications was presented above. The timing of doses needs to be individualized. Most children get a twice daily dosing, but dose regimens, every morning and three times daily, are also used. One starts with a small dose and then pushes it up to optimal levels. One can increase the dose every 3 to 7 days. Occasionally, small supplemental doses, immediately on awakening or in the late afternoon or evening, are used. It is best to administer the medication with or after meals to limit anorexia and stomach cramps.

Because of a wide variation in children's behavior over time, at least 1 to 2 weeks are needed to assess fully the response at a new dose level. A full trial should continue for a month. Most side effects last only the first week. Initially, the child should be seen weekly, with documented reports from the school on his/her response to the medication. Weekend drug holidays are advised but not necessary if the child is too disruptive at home without the medication. This also applies to trying to stop the medication during summer vacation. At least every 6 to 12 months, the drug should be stopped for 2 weeks to see if it is still needed. It may take 2 weeks for the child to reach a new baseline after withdrawing from the stimulant. Usually, stimulants are stopped by the ages of 10 through 12 years as hyperactivity tends to improve around puberty, but there may be a manifest need to continue. A history of nonresponding should not prevent a repeated trial, as there are age-related changes in responsiveness.

VIII. **Specific stimulant medications.** See Table 22–1 for further specification of doses.

TABLE 22–1.
Dosing Information for Stimulants in Treatment of ADHD*

Drug [Age Limit]	Starting Dose, mg/Day	Increment by mg/Day	Interval Between Increases	Maximum Dose, mg/Day	Averge Dose, mg/Day	Average Dose, mg/kg/Day
Methylphenidate (Ritalin) [>6 yr]	5–10	5–10	3–7 days	60–80	20–30	1.0–2.0
Dextropamphetamine (Dexedrine)						
[3–5 yr]	2.5	2.5	3–7 days			0.15–0.50
[≥6 yr]	2.5–1.0	5.0	3–7 days	40	10–20	0.15–0.50
Pemoline (Cylert) [>6 yr]	18.75–37.5	18.75	1 wk	112.5	56.25–75	0.5–2.0

ADHD = attention deficit hyperactivity disease.

A. **Methylphenidate (Ritalin).** This is the drug of choice for children with ADHD who are older than 6 years of age. It is available in 5-, 10-, and 20-mg tablets, and a 20-mg slow-release (SR) formulation (remember SR pills should be swallowed whole and not chewed). Its clinical effect lasts 2 to 4 hours. The SR form is said to last 8 hours. An above 20-mg/day weight loss can become a problem.

B. **Dextroamphetamine (Dexedrine).** This can be tried if methylphenidate is ineffective. The clinical effect lasts 2 to 6 hours. Ten percent of children will become more hyperactive while they are taking this drug. This drug is not recommended for children younger than 3 years of age. There is no proven benefit for children between the ages of 3 and 5 years, but it is, at times, given. Many children will need only one morning dose. It is available in 5-mg tablets, Spansules of 5, 10, and 15 mg, and as a 5 mg/5 mL elixir.

C. **Pemoline (Cylert).** This is structurally different from the above drugs. It has similar pharmacologic actions without significant sympathomimetic activity. However, it is not as consistently effective as the other two stimulants. The half-life is around 12 hours. The onset of action is delayed, taking 2 to 6 weeks. One morning dose is sufficient. It may take 3 weeks for the initial transient side effects to abate. Because of the long half-life, one should wait at least a week before increasing the dose. As the drug is excreted by the kidney, caution should be observed in children with renal failure. The drug, which is metabolized in the liver, can produce reversible elevations in liver function tests results, as well as hepatitis and jaundice, all of which indicate that the drug should be stopped. The drug should not be given to patients with impaired hepatic function. Aspartate and alanine aminotransferase levels should be checked at regular intervals. As this drug has no euphoric effect, it can be used where there is particular concern about drug abuse. Use in children younger than 6 years of age has not been established. It is available in 18.75-, 37.5-, and 75-mg tablets.

23 | Extrapyramidal Symptoms, Neuroleptic Malignant Syndrome, and Their Treatment

I. **Definition and pathogenesis of extrapyramidal symptoms (EPSs).**

A. The term *extrapyramidal symptoms* (EPSs) refers to a group of symptoms or reactions induced by the short- or long-term use of antipsychotic medication. The term was presumably coined because many of the symptoms manifest themselves as skeletal muscle movements, spasms, or rigidity; yet, these symptoms are outside the control of the corticospinal (pyramidal) tract. The name is, however, somewhat misleading as some of the symptoms (e.g., akathisia) may not be motor problems at all. Also, several extrapyramidal symptoms may coexist in one patient and mask each other.

B. The antipsychotic (neuroleptic) medications work, it is believed, through their postsynaptic D2 dopamine receptor blockade action in the central nervous system, specifically in the limbic system. Dopamine blockade in the striatum is believed to cause EPSs, either directly by causing a dopamine-acetylcholine systems imbalance, or as is postulated to occur in tardive dyskinesia, by inducing postsynaptic dopamine receptor supersensitivity due to chronic blockade.

II. **Types of EPSs.**

A. **Acute dystonic reaction (ADR).** This is an acute, involuntary spasm or contraction of one or more skeletal muscle groups that generally develops over a matter of minutes. The most frequently involved groups are the muscles of the face, neck, tongue, or extraocular muscles, manifested as torticollis, speech dysarthrias, oculogyric crisis, and unusual posturing. An ADR is generally quite disturbing to the patient. It may be painful or may be even life threatening with symptoms, such as laryngeal or diaphragmatic dystonias. Acute dystonic reactions frequently occur within the first day or two of initiating treatment, but may occur anytime. They occur in approximately 10% of patients, more commonly in young males, and more often with high doses of the higher potency neuroleptics, such as haloperidol or fluphenazine. Acute dystonic reactions may be a major cause of neuroleptic noncompliance, since a patient's view of medication can be permanently tarnished by a distressing dystonic reaction.

B. **Akathisia.** This EPS is, by far, the most common. It probably occurs in the majority of patients treated with neuroleptic medication, particularly in the younger patient population. It consists of an inner feeling of restlessness, jitteriness or a desire to stay in motion. It has also been described as a sensation of muscular itching. Patients may complain of anxiety or difficulty with sleeping, which may be misinterpreted as a worsening of psychotic symptoms. Conversely, akathisia can cause an exacerbation of psychotic symptoms due to extreme discomfort. Obvious agitation, pacing, or other physical manifestations of akathisia may only be present in severe cases. Also, the akinesia seen in neuroleptic-induced parkinsonism may mask any objective signs of akathisia. Akathisia often appears shortly after starting neuroleptic medication, and patients will rightfully associate the discomfort that they feel with the medication, resulting in compliance problems. A more objective method of checking for akathisia, and how it may be responding to treatment, is to use the following questionnaire.

Please tell us how you feel by marking an X along the lines below:

1. Do you feel *irritable*?

Not at all	A little	Some	Quite a bit	A lot
1	2	3	4	5

2. Do you feel *tense*?

Not at all	A little	Some	Quite a bit	A lot
1	2	3	4	5

3. Do you feel *restless*?

Not at all	A little	Some	Quite a bit	A lot
1	2	3	4	5

4. Do you feel *jittery*?

Not at all	A little	Some	Quite a bit	A lot
1	2	3	4	5

5. Do you have difficulty with *sitting still*?

Not at all	A little	Some	Quite a bit	A lot
1	2	3	4	5

A total score should be noted and compared with subsequent scores obtained after adjustment of neuroleptic dose or anti-EPS medication.

C. **Parkinson syndrome.** This is another fairly common EPS that may start hours after the first dose of a neuroleptic or begin insidiously after years of treatment. Its manifestations include the following types.

1. Akinesia, which includes mask facies, paucity of spontaneous movement, decreased arm swing on walking, decreased blinking, and decreased swallowing, which may lead to drooling. In its milder forms, aki-

nesia may be evident only as a behavioral state with paucity of speech, diminished spontaneity, apathy, and difficulty with initiating normal activities, all of which may be mistaken for the negative symptoms of schizophrenia.

2. Tremor, particularly at rest, classically of the pill-rolling type. The tremor may involve the jaw, which is sometimes referred to as "rabbit syndrome." This may be mistaken for tardive dyskinesia, but it may be differentiated by its more rhythmic character, its tendency to involve the jaw rather than the tongue, and its response to anticholinergic medication.

3. Shuffling, stooped gait with en bloc turns, and loss of arm swing.

4. Muscular rigidity, particularly of the cogwheeling type.

D. **Tardive dyskinesia.** This syndrome consists of abnormal, involuntary, choreiform, jerky, ballistic, or tic-like muscle movements. These movements most frequently involve the tongue, mouth, or face, but they may occur in any muscle group. Tardive dyskinesia occurs in approximately 20% of patients treated with long-term (over 1 year) neuroleptics, but most cases are extremely mild, and only around 5% of patients display severe, obvious movements. Severe cases can, however, be quite debilitating, i.e., affecting walking, talking, breathing, and eating. Predisposing factors may include advanced age, female sex, and high-dose or long-term neuroleptic treatment. Patients with affective or organic disorders may also be more likely to develop tardive dyskinesia. The symptoms disappear with sleep, may wax and wane over time, and generally worsen with withdrawal of neuroleptics. The differential diagnosis when considering tardive dyskinesia includes Huntington disease, Sydenham chorea, spontaneous dyskinesias, tics, and drug-induced dyskinesias (e.g., levodopa, stimulants, etc.) Of note, tardive dyskinesia, which is thought to be due to postsynaptic dopamine receptor supersensitivity due to chronic blockade, may coexist with Parkinson syndrome, which is thought to be due to insufficient dopamnergic activity. Early or mild tardive dyskinesias are easy to miss, and some feel that systematic evaluations, such as the Abnormal Involuntary Movement Scale (AIMS) described below, should be documented every 6 months for patients receiving long-term neuroleptic treatment.

1. **Examination procedure for AIMS.**

a. Either before or after completing the examination procedure, observe the patient unobtrusively, at rest (e.g., in the waiting room). The chair to be used in this examination should be hard, firm, and without arms.

b. Ask patient whether there is anything in his/her mouth (i.e., gum, candy) and, if there is, to remove it.

c. Ask patient about the current condition of his/her teeth. Ask patient if he/she wears dentures. Do teeth or dentures bother patient now?

d. Ask patient whether he/she notices any movements in mouth, face, hands, or feet. If yes, ask to describe and to what extent they currently bother patient or interfere with his/her activities.

e. Have patient sit on a chair with hands on knees, legs slightly apart, and feet flat on floor. (Look at entire body for movements while in this position.)

f. Ask patient to sit with hands hanging, unsupported. If male, between legs; if female and wearing a dress, hanging over knees. (Observe hands and other body areas.)

g. Ask patient to open mouth. (Observe tongue at rest within mouth.) Do this twice.

h. Ask patient to protrude tongue. (Observe abnormalities of tongue movement.) Do this twice.

i. Ask patient to tap thumb, with each finger, as rapidly as possible for 10 to 15 seconds, separately with right hand, and then with left hand. (Observe facial and leg movements.)

j. Ask patient to stand up. (Observe in profile. Observe all body areas again, with hips included.)

k. Ask patient to extend both arms outstretched in front, with both palms down. (Observe trunk, legs, and mouth.)

l. Have patient walk a few paces, turn, and walk back to a chair. (Observe hands and gait.) Do this twice.

2. **AIMS Screen/baseline.** Instructions: Complete examination procedure as described above before making ratings. For movement ratings, rate highest severity observed. Rate movements that occur on activation one less than those observed spontaneously. Rate 1 to 9 as follows: 0 = none or normal, 1 = minimal, 2 = mild, 3 = moderate, and 4 = severe. Rate 10 as follows: 0 = no awareness, 1 = aware and no distress, 2 = aware and mild distress, 3 = aware and moderate distress, and 4 = aware and severe distress. Rate 11 and 12 as follows: 0 = no and 1 = yes. The total score should be recorded and compared over time to note any change that indicates an increase in involuntary movements.

a. Facial and oral movements.

(i) Muscles of facial expression, e.g., movements of forehead, eyebrows, periorbital area, and cheeks; these include frowning, blinking, smiling, and grimacing.

(ii) Lips and perioral area, e.g., puckering, pouting, and smacking.

(iii) Jaw, e.g., biting, clenching, chewing, mouth opening, and lateral movement.

(iv) Tongue, e.g., rate only an increase in movement in and out of mouth but not an inability to sustain movement.

b. Extremity movements.

(i) Upper (arms, wrists, hands, and fingers) include choreic movements (i.e., rapid, objectively purposeless, irregular, and spontaneous) and athetoid movements (i.e., repetitive, regular, and rhythmic).

(ii) Lower (legs, knees, ankles, and toes), e.g., lateral knee movement, foot tapping, heel dropping, and foot squirming; inversion and eversion of foot.

c. Trunk movements.

(i) Neck, shoulders, hips, e.g., rocking, twisting, squirming, pelvic gyrations.

d. Global judgments.

(i) Severity of abnormal movements.

(ii) Incapacitation due to abnormal movements.

(iii) Patient's awareness of abnormal movements (rate only patient's report).

e. Dental status.

(i) Are there current problems with teeth and/or dentures?

(ii) Does patient usually wear dentures?

III. **Treatment of EPS.**

A. General guidelines (please also refer to Table 23–1).

1. Extrapyramidal symptoms can be quite distressing, so many authorities recommend prophylactic treatment. This is particularly important in patients with a history of EPSs, or those patients receiving high-dose potent neuroleptics.

2. The anti-EPS medications have side effects of their own, which may result in poor compliance. The anticholinergics commonly cause dry mouth, blurred vision, memory impairment, constipation, and urinary retention. Amantadine may exacerbate psychotic symptoms. For more complete information, refer to Table 23–1.

3. It is generally recommended that an attempt be made every 6 months to withdraw a patient's anti-EPS medication, watching carefully for a return of symptoms.

B. **ADR.** The anticholinergic medications are the primary form of treatment of ADRs, and pretreatment with one of these drugs usually prevents their occurrence. Common treatment regimens include benztropine (Cogentin), 0.5 to 2 mg twice daily (BID) to three times daily (TID), or trihexyphenidyl (Artane), 2 to 5 mg TID. Benztropine may be more effective than trihexyphenidyl in the treatment of ADRs, and some patients abuse the latter drug for the "buzz" that they get from it. A patient presenting with an acute, severe ADR should be treated rapidly and aggressively. If an intravenous (IV) line is in place, benztropine 1 mg by IV push, may be given. Generally, it is more practical to give diphenhydramine (Benadryl), 50 mg intramuscularly (IM), or if this is not available, use benztropine 2 mg IM. Dramatic remission of the ADR occurs within 5 minutes.

C. **Akathisia.** The treatment of akathisia may be quite difficult, and often, it requires much experimentation. The most commonly used agents are the anticholinergic and amantadine (Symmetrel); these may also be used together. Recent studies suggest that propranolol (Inderal) is very effective, and the benzodiazepines, particularly clonazepam (Klonopin) and lorazepam (Ativan), may also be helpful.

D. **Parkinson syndrome.** The mainstay of treatment for neuroleptic-induced Parkinson syndrome consists of the anticholinergic agents. Amantadine is also frequently used. Levodopa, used in the treatment of idiopathic Parkinson disease, is generally not effective due to its severe side effects.

E. **Tardive dyskinesia.** Prevention, through the judicious use of neuroleptic medication, is the preferred treatment of this syndrome. Once present, involuntary movements may decrease with raising the dose of antipsychotic medication, but this only exacerbates the underlying problem. After the initial worsening, most involuntary movements will disappear, or greatly diminish, after discontinuation of neuroleptic medication, but this may take up to 2 years. The benzo-

TABLE 23–1.
General Guidelines to Treat EPSSs*

Medication PO, mg	Dose Range, mg/Day	Dosing Interval	Mechanism of Action	Indications	Common Side Effects
Benztropine mesylate (Cogentin), 1 and 2	1–8	BID-QID	Antichol, antihistaminic	+++, ++, +++, and 0	Dry mouth, blurred vision, impaired sweating, constipation, memory and concentration impairment, urinary rentention, tachycardia, anticholinergic delirium, contraindication with narrow-angle glaucoma
Biperiden (Akineton), 2	2–10	TID-QID	Antichol	+++, ++, +++, and 0	
Procyclidine hydrochloride (Kemadrin), 5	5–20	TID-QID	Antichol	+++, ++, +++, and 0	
Trihexyphenidyl (Artane), 2 and 5	2–12	QID		+++, ++, +++, and 0	
Diphenhydramine hydrochloride (Benadryl), 25 and 50	25–200	QID	Antichol, antihistaminic	+++, ++, +++, and 0	Also sedation with diphenhydramine hydrochloride may exacerbate psychotic symptoms
Amantadine hydrochloride (Symmetrel), 100	200–300	BID-TID	Dopamine agonist	+++, ++, +++, and 0	
Bromocriptine mesylate (Parlodel), 2.5 and 5	2.5–10	QD-BID	Dopamine agonist	0, 0, +, and 0	Headache, constipation, confusion, nausea
Clonazepam (Klonopin), 0.5, 1, and 2	0.5–8	BID	Sedation? anxiolytic? GABA-ergic?	0, ++, +, and 0/+	Sedation, ataxia

Drug	Dose	Frequency	Mechanism	Effectiveness*	Side effects
Lorazepam (Ativan), 0.5, 1, and 2	1–10	TID-QID	Sedation? anxiolytic? GABA-ergic?	0, ++, 0, and 0/+	Sedation, ataxia
Propranolol hydrochloride (Inderal), 10, 20, 40, 60, and 80	20–120	QID	Beta-blocker	0, ++, 0, and 0/+	Sedation, depression, bradycardia, hypotension
Reserpine (Serpasil), 0.1 and 0.25	0.1–1	QD-BID	Catecholamine depletion, GABA?	0, 0, 0, and 0/+	Sedation, depression, bradycardia
Baclofen (Lioresal), 10	15–60	TID	GABA?	0, 0, 0, and 0/+	Sedation
Methyldopa (Aldomet), 125, 250, and 500	250–2,000	QID	Block catecholamine synthesis	0, 0, 0, and 0/+	Sedation, depression, hypotension

*EPSSs = extrapyramidal symptoms: PO = by mouth; BID = twice daily; QID = four times daily; Antichol = anticholinergic; +++ = very effective, acute dystonic reaction, akathisia, parkinsonism, and tardive dyskinesia; ++ = effective; 0 = not used; TID = three times daily; QD = every day; + = slightly effective; GABA = gamma-aminobutyric acid.

diazepines may decrease involuntary movements in some patients, perhaps through central gamma-aminobutyric acid–ergic mechanisms. Baclofen (Lioresal) and propranolol may also be helpful in some cases. Reserpine (Serpasil) has also described as effective, but depression and hypotension are common side effects. The choline-rich lipid lecithin has been helpful according to some investigators, but its efficacy is controversial. Dosage reduction is generally the best course of action in patients who appear to be developing tardive dyskinesia, but still require treatment. Discontinuing treatment can precipitate a severe decompensation, while treatment at the lowest effective dose can maintain a patient while minimizing risk, but one should be certain to document the need for continued treatment.

IV. Neuroleptic malignant syndrome.

A. Definition and clinical features. Neuroleptic malignant syndrome is a serious disorder that is estimated to occur in between 0.5% and 1% of patients exposed to neuroleptic medication. It may occur at any time during treatment, and in any patient, although young males may be at higher risk. Other predisposing factors include dehydration, physical exhaustion, concurrent organic brain disease, and treatment with long-acting depot neuroleptics. The major symptoms, which usually develop over 24 to 72 hours, include hyperthermia, muscular hypertonicity, delirium, and autonomic instability. Mortality ranges from 20% to 30%, probably even higher with depot neuroleptics, and mortality is generally a result of respiratory failure, cardiovascular collapse, renal failure, or cardiac arrhythmias. Laboratory test may show an elevated creatine phosphokinase level (which may progress to rhabdomyolysis with renal failure), leukocytosis, and elevated liver function test values (aspartate and alanine aminotransferase, lactic dehydrogenase, and alkaline phosphatase levels).

B. Treatment. Early diagnosis is critical to treatment. If a patient receiving neuroleptic medication shows a fluctuating level of consciousness, be sure to check vital signs (particularly temperature) and to check for rigidity. The syndrome lasts approximately 5 to 10 days after discontinuation of oral neuroleptics, but it may last two to three times as long with depot medication. During this period, good supportive care to minimize the fluctuations in vital sign parameters due to the autonomic instability is crucial. Medications that are most often used to treat neuroleptic malignant syndrome include dantrolene sodium and bromocriptine mesylate. The usual initial dosage of dantrolene sodium is 2 to 3 mg/kg of body weight per day given IV in four times daily dosing. The dose may be increased up to 10 mg/kg/day, but above this point, hepatic toxicity is a problem. It may also be given orally, 50 to 200 mg/day. Bromocriptine mesylate is generally given in the dosage range of 2.5 to 10 mg by mouth TID. Amantadine hydrochloride, a dopamine against like bromocriptine, has also been used at the dose of 100 mg by mouth BID.

REFERENCES

1. McEvoy JP: The clinical use of anticholinergic drugs as treatment for extrapyramidal side effects of neuroleptic drugs. *J Clin Psychopharmacol* 1983; 3:288–302.
2. Lipinski JF, Zubenko GS, et al: Propranolol in the treatment of neuroleptic-induced akathisia. *Am J Psychiatry* 1984; 141:412–415.
3. Guze BH, Baxter LR: Neuroleptic malignant syndrome. *N Engl J Med* 1985; 313:163–166.
4. Guy W: *ECDEU Assessment Manual for Psychopharmacology*. Rockville, Md, National Institute of Mental Health Psychopharmacology Branch, 1976.

24

Psychotropic Drug Use and Pregnancy

I. **Introduction.**

A. On occasion, a woman taking psychotropic medication will discover that she has become pregnant. She may turn to her physician for advice concerning the relative risk to her unborn child. The patient's concern may include both the risk from previous exposure and the possible risk to the fetus from continued exposure, if such a course is clinically indicated.

B. When a major mental disorder arises in a pregnant patient, and nonbiologic methods (e.g., individual, couple or family psychotherapy, social casework, and hospitalization) have been exhausted, it is often necessary to consider pharmacologic methods of treatment.

C. If the risks associated with the use of psychotropic drugs are outweighed by the anticipated benefits, and if the risks of inadequately treated disease outweigh the risks associated with a potentially useful medication, then most prudent physicians will opt to treat the disease.

D. No psychotropic drug has been proved to be safe for use during pregnancy, and all drugs carry warnings from the Food and Drug Administration.

II. Lithium

A. Metabolism of lithium during pregnancy.

1. Both the glomerular filtration rate (GFR) and effective renal plasma flow increase during pregnancy to approximately 45% above pregestational levels. During this time, plasma volume increases by about 50%. Renal lithium clearance increases in parallel with the increase in the GFR during pregnancy. Due to this, it may be necessary to increase progressively the intake of lithium to maintain a steady serum lithium level. During the postpartum period, a corresponding reduction in the amount of administered lithium is necessary to avoid possible toxic levels.

2. The dosages to each individual's needs by frequent clinical and laboratory evaluations to maintain therapeutic serum lithium levels should be tailored.

3. To minimize the risk of toxicity to the newborn and the mother, some investigators have advocated discontinuing lithium immediately before delivery. It can be restarted, if indicated, as the mother stabilizes in the postpartum period.

B. Fetal exposure.
The fetus is presumed to be exposed to the same serum concentrations of lithium as are found in maternal blood. There have been reports of lithium toxicity in newborns. Symptoms of neonatal lithium intoxication have included cyanosis, jaundice, hypothermia, lethargy, hypotonia, poor suck reflex, poor respiratory effort, absent Moro reflex, low Apgar scores, and altered thyroid and cardiac function that may take up to 10 days to resolve. Other reports have included nephrogenic diabetes insipidus, functional tricuspid regurgitation, congestive heart failure, and atrial flutter. Symptoms usually remit with supportive care.

C. Breast-feeding.
Breast-feeding is complicated by the fact that the concentration of lithium in breast milk

is about 50% of that in the mother's serum. Lithium ingestion during pregnancy is discouraged because of the concern for the development of toxicity if there are fluid and electrolyte alterations in the infant (e.g., dehydration) that could produce such toxicity and because the effects of ingestions of below therapeutic levels of lithium are unknown on the infant.

D. **Congenital anomalies.** A Lithium Baby Register was established in 1969 to collect information about the effects of lithium on in utero development. Of 217 cases that were reported as having been exposed to lithium during at least the first trimester, 25 infants were born with congenital anomalies. Of those, 18 had cardiovascular malformations, six of of which involved Ebstein anomaly of the tricuspid valve, atrial septum, and right ventricle. Because of this, it has been suggested that lithium may be a cardiovascular teratogen. Even though the absolute incidence of malformations reported in the Register is no higher than what is found in the general population, the Register has suggested that lithium not be used during the first trimester unless it is absolutely essential.

E. **General guidelines for lithium use during pregnancy.** Every attempt should be made to keep the patient off lithium if possible. Whenever possible, lithium should be avoided during the first trimester. If an assessment of the risks vs. benefits and alternative therapies suggests that lithium is indeed indicated, then every attempt should be made to use the lowest serum levels possible that will provide adequate behavioral improvement. The total dose should be spread throughout the day, with each individual dose being as low as possible. Lithium should be discontinued for at least 1 month before attempting pregnancy. If possible, the patient should be maintained free of lithium throughout the pregnancy. Lithium should be reinstated only when the risk of relapse appears to exceed the potential morbidity of drug use. Lithium should be discontinued, if possible, if a patient becomes pregnant while receiving lithium. The mother should be told that many normal infants have been born to mothers who take lithium while they are pregnant. In addition, it is now possible to follow infant development in utero via such imaging modalities as ultrasound to monitor the possible development of anatomic congenital anomalies.

III. **Antidepressants.**

A. **Teratogenicity.** While direct proof of their teratogenicity is lacking, cyclic antidepressants have been assumed by some investigators to cause an increased risk of birth defects. In a study of 19 mothers who took imipramine and 28 mothers who received amitriptyline during the first trimester, there was no evidence of congenital malformations. In a study of 15,000 births, there was no evidence of gross congenital abnormalities in infants born to mothers who received tricyclic antidepressants during the first trimester. The teratogenic potential was estimated to be fairly low, even with exposure during the first trimester, from data contained in a register of 2,784 cases of birth defects matched to an equal number of normal controls.

B. **Postpartum period.** In the immediate postpartum period, the newborn can demonstrate the effects of antidepressants received while in utero. There have been reports of infants, showing signs of respiratory distress, urinary retention, myoclonus, tachycardia, and heart failure. Some of these infants have subsequently demonstrated signs of withdrawal. Some investigators have suggested a period of washout of the antidepressant for the fetus; this washout period has been estimated as about 1 week, due to the half-life of most antidepressants.

C. **Monoamine oxidase inhibitors.** Monoamine oxidase inhibitors have been avoided for several reasons. The possibility of a hypertensive reaction, leading to severe vascular difficulties for both the mother and the fetus, has been a common concern. In addition, phenelzine has been shown to be teratogenic in animals.

IV. **Antipsychotic drugs.**

A. **Teratogenicity.** Most reviews of the effects of neuroleptics have not found a statistically increased incidence of structural birth defects in those infants exposed in utero. For example, a retrospective examination of 100 women given haloperidol while they were pregnant revealed no significant effects on the sex ratio of the offspring, birth weight, intrauterine or neonatal survival, fecundity, or duration of gestation compared with controls. A review of 341 cases of intrauterine exposure to trifluperazine revealed no increased incidence of congenital anomalies compared with the general population. In a study of 19,952 women treated with phenothiazines during their first trimester, there was no significant increase in the incidence of a severe congenital anomaly and perinatal death for the exposed group vs. controls. A prospective study of 12,764 women and their offspring exposed to phenothiazines in the first trimester revealed a statistically significant increase compared with controls in the incidence of major congenital anomalies when exposed to phenothiazines with a three-carbon aliphatic side chain (chlorpromazine, methotrimeprazine, trimeprazine, and oxomemazine). These side effects included malformations of the central nervous, cardiovascular, digestive, musculoskeletal, and genitourinary systems. In addition, there was a very high incidence of microcephaly, ventricular septal defect, cleft lip, hypospadias, polydactyly, and syndactyly. This was not observed with promethazine or the piperidine or the piperazine antipsychotics. Of the drugs suggested to have a deleterious effect by this report, only chlorpromazine is used as an antipsychotic in the United States.

B. **Postpartum period.** There have been reports of toxic side effects observed in newborns. These have included restlessness, abnormal movements, hypertonia, and an extrapyramidal syndrome that includes tremor, hypertonia, weakness, and poor sucking and sluggish primitive reflexes. This syndrome is most likely dose dependent. It has been reported that extrapyramidal symptoms in the newborn may persist for up to 6 months.

C. **Atypical agents.** Nonphenothiazine or nonbutyrophenone antipsychotics, such as thiothixene, molindone, or loxaprine succinate, have not been investigated sufficiently to report accurately the incidence of fetal abnormalities associated with their use during pregnancy.

D. **Precaution.** As a generalization about the use of antipsychotics during pregnancy, some authorities have suggested that it is best to avoid their use during the first trimester and to consider their use during subsequent trimesters only under urgent circumstances.

V. **Benzodiazepines.**

A. **Teratogenicity.** There has been an increasing number of reports of congenital malformations with the use of these agents during pregnancy. Deformities have included a fourfold to sixfold increased incidence in cleft lip or palate from diazepam exposure.

B. **Perinatal period.** When given before delivery, it may result in depression of the neonatal central nervous and respiratory systems. Neonatal withdrawal symptoms include irritability, jittery movements, tremors, diarrhea, vomiting, and a high-pitched cry.

VI. **Conclusion.** The available data on neuroleptics suggest that with proper selection, use, and supervision, most of these drugs can be used during pregnancy. The same cannot be said for lithium, benzodiazepines, or most antidepressants. In general, it is most prudent to avoid all medications, if possible, during the first trimester. However, the decision of how and when to start treatment depends on an assessment of the risks associated, both with the drug and with the untreated illness.

25

Drug Treatments in Child Psychiatry

I. **Introduction.** Psychopharmacology is an established part of child psychiatry; yet, its development generally has lagged behind the notable advances in adult psychopharmacology. Drugs are given to suppress target symptoms rather than to ameliorate well-defined syndromes more often in child psychiatry than in adult psychiatry. It is assumed in this chapter that pediatric psychopharmacology can provide a moderate degree of improvement rather than a cure for some childhood and adolescent psychiatric disorders, and that most treatments are necessarily multimodal. This chapter briefly reviews the indications and side effects of the drug classes widely used in child psychiatry, and provides clinical guidelines for the most frequently used drugs.

II. **Stimulants.** The stimulants are the best-studied class of drugs in child psychiatry. They continue to be the most safe and effective pharmacologic treatment for attention deficit hyperactivity disorder (ADHD). Their use in the treatment of attentional deficits without hyperactivity is not as well established. Whether conduct disorder without ADHD is responsive to stimulants has not been documented adequately. Dextroamphetamine has been reported to increase hyperactivity, irritability, and sterotypic movements in children with pervasive developmental disorder (PDD). But recent reports suggest that methylphenidate may improve hyperactivity and sterotypies in children with PDD. Fenfluramine, a primarily serotonergic stimulant, has been reported to provide symptomatic improvement in some cases of infantile autism.

Side effects from stimulants are generally mild and transient, so that they only occasionally interfere with treatment. Appetite suppression and insomnia sometimes occur initially, but usually subside in 1 to 2 weeks. Other side effects include headaches, abdominal pain, weight loss, dysphoria, irritability, and stereotyped movements. Whether stimulants actually precipitate tics is controversial, but it is clear that stimulants exacerbate tics and Tourette syndrome. The studies of growth velocity in children treated with stimulants for several years have yielded contradictory results. The weight of the evidence seems to be that stimulants have significant effects on growth velocity in childhood. But the growth spurt compensates for these earlier effects, so that eventual height is not compromised.

A. **ADHD.**

1. **General.** Stimulants are indicated in the treatment of ADHD, but not all children with ADHD require medication. Methylphenidate and dextroamphetamine remain the drugs of choice; sustained-release preparations of both drugs are also available. Pemoline has a more delayed onset of action and is thought to be less effective than the other stimulants. Despite much research, there is no reliable method for predicting which children will benefit from medication. Furthermore, an individual patient may respond to one of the stimulants but not to the others. The development of tolerance to stimulants in children is rare, and dependence or abuse has been almost nonexistent. Other medications for ADHD include tricyclic antidepressants (TCAs), monoamine oxidase inhibitors (MAOIs), clonidine, and neuroleptics.

2. **Dosage and monitoring.** Teacher and parent rating scales are necessary to document the pervasiveness and severity of symptoms before starting medication and to measure the response to medication. Methylphenidate and dextroamphetamine are usually started at 5 mg in the morning and at noon. The medication is usually increased every 3 to 7 days, with regular monitoring of pulse rate and blood pressure during the titration. The dosage range for methylphenidate is 0.3 to 1.0 mg/kg per dose, with a maximum dose of 60 mg. The dosage range for amphetamine is 0.15 to 0.5 mg/kg per dose, with a maximum dose of 40 mg. It has been claimed that the optimal dose for clinically significant improvement in social behavior may impair performance in learning and cognition. But numerous recent studies of stimulant effects have not found a dissociation between the effects on behavior and cognition. A lack of improvement after 1 to 2 weeks at a maximum dosage is an indication to change medication. An afternoon dose is occasionally useful for children with significant amounts of homework or with behavior problems at home.

B. **Infantile autism.**

1. **General.** The treatment of infantile autism with fenfluramine has been assessed recently in a multicenter study. It appears that its benefits are more limited than initially hoped, and that it may be effective mainly in verbal, high-functioning autistic children. As a treatment for autism, it is experimental and should not be considered until more standard treatments have been implemented. It suppresses appetite and weight gain more than the other stimulants; its other common side effects include drowsiness, fatigue, irritability, and insomnia. Finally, long-term treatment with low doses has been neurotoxic in rats. Lithium has been reported to be effective in suppressing tantrums and self-mutilation in an autistic child. Propranolol has been reported in open trials to decrease previously intractable aggression in autistic adults.

2. **Dosage.** The initial fenfluramine dosage usually reported in the literature has been 0.75 mg/kg twice each day. Dosage may be adjusted subsequently to yield a total daily dosage range from 20 to 60 mg.

III. **Antidepressants.** Tricyclic antidepressants have been used in the treatment of enuresis, ADHD, major depression, separation anxiety disorder, and bulimia. Desipramine (DMI) is a possible alternative to the neuroleptics and clonidine in the amelioration of Tourette syndrome. Chlomipramine (CMI) is effective in the treatment of obsessive-compulsive disorder, but it has not been approved by the Food and Drug Administration (FDA) for use in the United States. The MAOIs are as effective, if not more effective than the TCAs, in treating ADHD, major depression, and bulimia; however, dietary restrictions limit their use in children and adolescents.

The most common side effects from TCAs are anticholinergic side effects, which include mouth dryness, blurred vision, tachycardia, urinary retention, and constipation. Other TCA side effects include sedation, insomnia, orthostatic hypotension, and dizziness. The MAOIs are essentially free from anticholinergic side effects, but they produce sedation, postural hypotension, and, more seriously, hypertensive crisis following ingestion of tyramine or sympathomimetic drugs.

A. **Enuresis.**

1. **General.** Imipramine (IMI) and the other TCAs usually suppress enuresis within 1 week. However, tolerance often occurs, and the relapse rate after stopping medication is high. Medication is not as effective as conditioning techniques, so that it is indicated only for temporary suppression (e.g., a school outing) or when other interventions have failed.

2. **Dosage.** Imipramine, 0.5 to 1.5 mg/kg at bedtime, is usually sufficient to suppress enuresis. The optimum effect occurs with a total imipramine-desipramine plasma level greater than 60 ng/mL.

B. **Major depression.**

1. **General.** Prepubertal depression appears to be highly responsive to both placebo and TCAs. The treatment of major depression with TCAs may be less effective in adolescents than in adults. Lithium augmentation in adolescent major depression resistant to a TCA is sometimes helpful. Starting a neuroleptic, along with a TCA, is probably mandatory in treating delusional depression.

2. **Dosage and monitoring.** Imipramine and desipramine are usually started at 1.5 mg/kg/day in two or three divided doses. If the patient tolerates the medication, the dose can be increased every 3 days from 1.5 to 3, 4, and 5 mg/kg/day. An electrocardiogram, blood pressure (BP) reading, and side effects should be assessed before each dosage increase. If any of the FDA limits are reached, the dosage should not be increased. These limits are (1) a PR interval greater than 0.21 second, (2) a QRS complex greater than 130% of baseline (or 0.02 second plus baseline), (3) a resting heart rate greater than 130 beats per minute, and (4) a systolic BP greater than 145 mm Hg or a diastolic BP greater than 95 mm Hg. Plasma tricyclic levels should be obtained after a dose has been maintained for a week. When treating with imipramine, the total imipramine-desipramine plasma level should be at least 150 ng/mL. Occasionally, up to 7 mg/kg/day of imipramine is necessary to achieve a therapeutic plasma level and clinical response. When an effective plasma level cannot be reached, switching to a secondary amine or MAOI is indicated.

3. **Duration.** An adequate antidepressant trial should last at least 6 weeks. Some depressed children and adolescents do not respond until after 7 or 8 weeks of treatment. A prepubertal responder should continue to receive medication for at least 3 more months and a postpubertal for 6 more months.

C. **Separation anxiety disorder.**

1. **General.** School phobia secondary to separation anxiety is responsive to imipramine and probably other TCAs. Panic disorder in adolescents and adults is suppressed by TCAs and MAOIs, but this disorder has not been described in prepubertal children. Finally, social phobia in adults is decreased by TCAs and MAOIs, but this has not been studied in the pediatric age range.

2. **Dosage and duration.** The imipramine dosage reported in the literature for children and young adolescents has ranged from 100 to 200 mg/day, divided into two doses. An adequate trial should last 6 weeks.

D. **ADHD.**

1. **General.** The MAOIs appear to be as effective as the stimulants in treating ADHD, but dietary restrictions and side effects make them less practical than the stimulants. The TCAs are less effective, have more side effects, and are more likely to develop tolerance than the stimulants. Yet, they can be useful in treating patients with ADHD who have depression, anxiety, or tics, or who have been unresponsive or intolerant to stimulants.

2. **Dosage.** Effective imipramine dosages reportedly range from 1.0 to 4.0 mg/kg/day in two or three divided doses. Comparative studies of dose, plasma level, and response have not been done.

IV. **Antipsychotics.** Antipsychotics (neuroleptics) are well established in the treatment of adults with schizophrenia, affective and organic psychoses, Tourette syndrome, and intermittent aggression. The limited evidence suggests that antipsychotics are indicated in the temporary treatment of children and adolescents with similar conditions and in the prophylactic treatment of some juveniles with schizophrenia or Tourette syndrome. In addition, they can be a useful adjunct to other treatments for PDDs and ADHD. But their long-term use for these disorders is often unjustified.

Side effects from antipsychotics are numerous and occasionally grave. Oversedation and anticholinergic side effects are common with the low-potency neuroleptics. These side effects appear to impair learning, memory, and cognition—areas often already impaired in those children and adolescents commonly given phenothiazines. Especially with the high-potency neuroleptics, acute dystonic reactions occur occasionally during the first week of treatment and appear to be more common in children than in adults.

A. **Schizophrenia.**

1. **General.** Thioridazine is the most popular and widely used antipsychotic for treating children. In addition to the usual side effects from phenothiazines, pigmentary retinopathy is a serious complication of treatment with high-dose thioridazine. High-potency neuroleptics, such as haloperidol and fluphenazine, are less sedating but more likely to produce extrapyramidal reactions when antiparkinsonian medication is not given.

2. **Dosage and monitoring.** The calculation of dosage should not follow body weight exclusively since there are large individual differences in pharmacokinetics, symptoms, and treatment objectives. Thioridazine and chlorpromazine are usually given in a total daily dosage of 1.0 to 5.0 mg/kg. With haloperidol, control of psychotic symptoms is usually achieved with 0.05 to 0.2 mg/kg/day. Maintenance haloperidol treatment is with lower doses from 0.02 to 0.1 mg/kg/day, usually given as a bedtime dose. School progress, blood pressure, skin, retinas, and movement require regular monitoring. The Abnormal Involuntary Movement Scale is useful for assessing dyskinesias.

B. **Tourette syndrome.**

1. **General.** Several drugs are effective in suppressing the symptoms of Tourette syndrome in the majority of patients. Drugs are not curative, so that

patients may need to continue them for extended periods of time. Haloperidol has been the drug of choice and is effective in about 80% of patients. But, because of side effects, only about 30% of the responders continue the medication for more than a year. In addition to the side effects listed above, patients with Tourette syndrome given haloperidol often experience cognitive dulling, dysphoria, school phobia, and weight gain. Tardive dyskinesia is distinguishable from Tourette syndrome and is a risk with prolonged neuroleptic therapy. Pimozide, clonidine, desipramine, and possibly the calcium-channel blockers are alternatives to haloperidol.

2. **Dosage.** Haloperidol is usually started at 0.25 to 0.5 mg/day and is increased by 0.5 mg/wk until maximum benefit is achieved with minimum side effects. Patients rarely have a favorable response to greater than 5 mg/day. An adequate maintenance dose is likely to be around 0.1 mg/kg/day. The dose may need to be adjusted to compensate for changes in symptom severity.

C. **PDD.**

1. **General.** Antipsychotics have been used to treat patients with PDD, not to cure or relieve the psychosis itself, but to decrease hyperactivity, stereotypies, and aggression and to improve frustration tolerance, mood, sleep, and appetite.

2. **Dosage.** Dose-response curves have not been determined. Relatively low doses, for example, 50 to 100 mg/day of thioridazine, appear to be as effective as higher doses. The dosage and duration of neuroleptic therapy should be limited whenever possible.

D. **ADHD.**

1. **General.** The high-potency neuroleptics appear to have a dissociated dose-response curve for cognitive performance and social behavior. That is, a low dose improves performance on laboratory tests of attention

and short-term memory, whereas a high dose impairs some aspects of cognitive performance. All of the neuroleptics can diminish hyperactivity and other behavior problems. But, if dosage titration is based solely on social responses, cognitive functioning is likely to be compromised. The use of a neuroleptic as the only treatment of ADHD or aggression is unjustified. The addition of a neuroleptic to a stimulant in the treatment of ADHD should be reserved for the most severe and refractory cases. Lithium has been shown to be as effective as a neuroleptic in the treatment of aggressive conduct disorder. Propranolol and carbamazepine also appear to be effective in the treatment of irritability and episodic violence.

2. **Dosage.** Haloperidol, 0.025 mg/kg, may improve attention and short-term memory. Doses above 0.05 mg/kg are likely to impair cognitive functioning.

REFERENCES

1. Elliott G, Ciaranello R: Biological aspects of and drug treatments for selected childhood mental disorders, in Berger P, Brodie H (eds): *American Handbook of Psychiatry: VIII. Biological Psychiatry.* New York, Basic Books, Inc, Publishers, 1986, pp 620–650.
2. Greenhill L: Pediatric psychopharmacology, in Schaffer D, Ehrhardt A, Greenhill L (eds): *The Clinical Guide to Child Psychiatry.* New York, The Free Press, 1985, pp 493–518.
3. Meltzer H (ed): *Psychopharmacology: A Third Generation of Progress.* New York, Raven Press, 1987.
4. Taylor E: Drug treatment, in Rutter M, Herson L (eds): *Child and Adolescent Psychiatry: Modern Approaches,* ed 2. London, Blackwell Scientific Publications, Inc, 1985, pp 780–793.
5. Weiner J (ed): *Diagnosis and Psychopharmacology of Childhood and Adolescent Disorders.* New York, John Wiley & Sons, Inc, 1985.

26
Geriatric Psychopharmacology

I. **Overview.** The psychopharmacologic management of geriatric patients requires special consideration due to the physiologic changes associated with aging, the frequency of medical complications, and the types of disorders that are prevalent in this age group. In general, the elderly are less capable of metabolizing and responding to psychotropic drugs. Therapy should be initiated at lower doses, medications should be increased more gradually, and lower maximum doses should be used. Since side effects are more pronounced, agents with a milder side effect profile are preferred.

A. There are numerous physiologic changes associated with aging that affect response to medication in the elderly. These include a decrease in the volume of distribution, protein binding, hepatic metabolism, and renal clearance. Central nervous system (CNS) neurotransmitters and enzymes are also decreased, with the exception of some of the enzymes that degrade neurotransmitters (e.g., monoamine oxidase [MAO]). These changes result in an increase in drug accumulation, elimination half-life, drug levels, side effects, and toxicity. The CNS changes also predispose the elderly to depression and memory loss. Age-related changes make the elderly more vulnerable both to the effects and side effects of psychotropic drugs. This sensitivity is further complicated by the polypharmacy that is common in this age group.

B. The following are recommended to rule out the more common medical conditions that can cause or contribute to psychiatric presentations.

1. Complete physical examination.

2. Determinations of electrolyte, blood urea nitrogen, creatinine, glucose, total protein, albumin, globulin, calcium, phosphorus, cholesterol, and triglyceride levels; liver function tests; thyroid function tests with thyroid-stimulating hormone; VDRL; complete blood cell count with differential cell count; erythrocyte sedimentation rate; urinalysis; electrocardiogram; and chest x-ray film.

3. For evaluation of dementia, add folate, vitamin B_{12}, and possibly heavy metal (e.g., lead and bromine) determinations.

4. Head computed tomography or magnetic resonance imaging is appropriate for a new onset of depression, psychosis, or memory loss, or a change in mental status of unknown etiology.

5. A lumbar puncture or electroencephalogram may also be indicated (e.g., to exclude suspected CNS infection or seizure focus).

II. **Treatment of affective disorders.**

A. **Unipolar depression.**

1. Cyclic antidepressants are the drugs of choice. Those medications with milder side effects, such as desipramine, doxepin, nortriptyline, and trazodone, are recommended. The selection of a specific drug is based on the same factors considered in younger patients, such as the history of response, depressive subtype, and methylphenidate response. It is even more important in these patients to consider the side effect profile, as this may contraindicate the selection of some agents

(e.g., amitriptyline in patients with prostatic hypertrophy) (see Table 26–1 and Section VII.). All of these drugs, including trazodone, may be prescribed in a single daily dose, although split dosing may help reduce side effects in some patients. It is important to note that cyclic antidepressants block the effect of centrally acting antihypertensive drugs (e.g., clonidine). Also, neuroleptics may potentiate the effects of cyclic antidepressants by decreasing liver metabolism.

2. Monoamine oxidase inhibitors (MAOIs) are effective in the treatment of typical or atypical depression. They have milder anticholinergic and cardiac side effects than the antidepressants. Given the increased CNS MAO that is present in the elderly, they offer a theoretical advantage as well. Patients must be educated about the MAOI diet and particularly about the hazards of over-the-counter preparations, which are used frequently by this population.

The maximum dosages of these agents are highly variable and are best determined on an individual basis by increasing the dose until either desirable effects are achieved or side effects limit further increases. The usual limiting side effects are orthostatic hypotension accompanied by a sensation of light-headedness or anticholinergic effects.

B. **Refractory depression.**

1. Lithium carbonate is the usual first choice to add when a patient has an incomplete response to a cyclic antidepressant. It often has a potentiating effect on other antidepressants when serum levels are in the 0.3- to 0.5-mEq/L range.

2. L-Triiodothyronine (T_3) (25 μg QD) may also be added, but should be discontinued after 4 to 8 weeks. It is relatively contraindicated in patients with cardiovascular disease because it may induce cardiac arrhythmias and hypoxia.

3. Methylphenidate (5 to 10 mg QD-BID) is effective

TABLE 26–1.
Antidepressant Drugs, Doses, and Side Effects*

Drug	Starting Dose, mg/Day	Dosing Interval	Increase	Maximum Daily Dose, mg	Primary Side Effects
Desipramine, doxepin, nortriptyline	25	QD	25 mg every 2–3 days for inpatients; every 5–7 days for outpatients	75–200	Hypotension, anticholinergic, sedation/anxiety
Trazodone	50	QD	50 mg every 2–3 days for inpatients; every 5–7 days for outpatients	100–300	Hypotension, sedation, dietary, priapism in males
Phenelzine	7.5–15	BID-TID	7.5–15 mg every 2–3 days for inpatients; every 5–7 days for outpatients	15–60	Hypotension, hypertension with dietary indiscretion
Tranylcypromine	2.5–5	BID-TID	2.5–5 mg every 2–3 days for inpatients; every 5–7 days for outpatients	5–15	Hypotension, hypertension with dietary indiscretion

*QD = every day; BID = twice daily; and TID = three times daily.

when used alone or to augment cyclic antidepressants. Patients rapidly develop tolerance to its effects.

4. The MAOIs may also be used alone or in combination with cyclic antidepressants.

5. Electroconvulsive therapy (ECT) is effective and possibly safer than drugs. The usual indications are a nonresponse to or intolerance of antidepressants. Some patients with medical problems, such as cardiac disease, may tolerate ECT better than drugs. Although this remains controversial, ECT may cause mild memory deficits, particularly with bilateral lead placement.

C. **Mania.**

1. Lithium carbonate is the agent of choice. The starting doses are usually 150 to 300 mg/day, but one may start as low as 75 mg (one can get 75 mg from elixir and 150 mg by breaking a tablet in half). Initially, a serum level in the 0.3- to 0.7-mEq/L range should be effective for acute mania within 5 to 10 days. Maintenance or prophylaxis can be achieved with doses as low as 150 mg/day, with levels of 0.2 to 0.5 mg/dL. There will be significant side effects at lower doses and lower serum levels than in younger patients. These may include confusion, disorientation, memory deficits, and arrhythmias, although lithium is generally well tolerated in patients with cardiac disease. It is important to warn patients about fluid and sodium intake, as well as diuretics.

2. Neuroleptics are more often used for treatment of an acute episode than for prophylaxis (see Section III.A.). A low dose of a high-potency agent, such as haloperidol, thiothixene, or fluphenazine, is effective and best tolerated, but occasionally, a more sedating agent, such as thioridazine, is necessary.

3. Carbamazepine may be used alone or in combination with lithium. The side effects are more pronounced than in younger patients; the complete blood cell count and liver function test results must be mon-

itored. Carbamazepine may be preferable to lithium in patients with medical problems, such as renal disease, congestive heart failure, or hypertension, particularly when they are receiving high-dose diuretics.

4. Benzodiazepines, such as lorazepam or clonazepam (0.25 mg BID-TID up to a daily maximum of approximately 4 mg), may provide a temporary adjunct to control mania. They can, however, cause excessive sedation and confusion.

5. Electroconvulsive therapy is recommended if the mania remains refractory, or if medical illness contraindicates other treatments (see Section II.B.5.).

III. **Psychosis and agitation.** When elderly patients present with psychosis or agitation, it is important to rule out medical illness and delirium. Whatever the etiology, pharmacologic intervention may be required.

A. Neuroleptics are the usual choice both for psychosis and agitation. It is preferable to use a mildly anticholinergic drug, particularly in patients with medical illness or confusion. One should start with low doses and increase the dose as needed and tolerated, but the increased accumulation and elimination half-life in the elderly (see Section I.A.) may cause sudden overmedication. Extrapyramidal symptoms (EPSs), anticholinergic effects, and hypotension are the usual dose-limiting side effects. The more sedating and anticholinergic neuroleptics may be useful for severe agitation, but these drugs should generally be used for patients who are younger and not for patients who are confused (Table 26–2).

B. Benzodiazepines, such as lorazepam or clonazepam (see Section II.C.4.), may be useful alone or in combination with a neuroleptic. They are relatively contraindicated in patients who are confused, as they may cause increased sedation and confusion.

C. Beta-blocking agents are sometimes effective. Propranolol is the agent most often used for agitation or explosiveness. The starting dose is 10 mg BID-TID, and it is increased 10 mg/day, but may be increased more rapidly. The therapeutic range is usually from 80 to 200 mg/day. The usual side effects are hypotension, bradycardia, and depression.

D. Other agents that have some reported usefulness include lithium, carbamazepine, and trazodone.

IV. **Anxiety.** Anxiety may be the presenting symptom of virtually any psychiatric condition and many medical conditions in the elderly. Depression in this age group is not uncommonly of the anxious or agitated type and may be particularly difficult to distinguish from an anxiety disorder.

A. Cyclic antidepressants, particularly sedating agents, such as doxepin or trazodone in doses as low as 5 mg/day, are the usual first-choice agents for panic or phobic anxiety. They may also function well, if nonspecifically, for generalized anxiety.

B. The MAOIs are also effective for panic or phobic anxiety (use as described in Section II.A.2.).

C. Benzodiazepines are useful for panic, phobic, or generalized anxiety, but because of their habituation potential, they should be used in a time-limited fashion. The elimination half-life of the long-acting agents is prolonged (see Section I.A.), so that shorter-acting agents, such as oxazepam, lorazepam, and alprazolam, are preferred (their metabolism is little affected by aging) (Table 26–3).

D. Neuroleptics are sometimes used for treating severe anxiety, particularly when it is associated with agitation. The more sedating drugs, such as thioridazine, may be the most effective.

E. Buspirone is a new agent, and there is not yet much experience with its use. It appears to be safe and effective in treating the elderly, and its lack of sedation may make it particularly useful in this population. It is

TABLE 26–2.
Neuroleptic and Anticholinergic Drugs, Doses, and Side Effects*

Drugs	Starting Dose, mg/Day	Maximum Daily Dose, mg	Primary Side Effects
Haloperidol, fluphenazine	0.5	8–10	EPSs, mild sedation, mildly anticholinergic
Thiothixene	1	10–20	EPSs, but less than with haloperidol; more sedating than haloperidol; mildly anticholinergic
Perphenazine	2	16–32	EPSs, less than thiothixene; anticholinergic; more sedating than thiothixene
Thioridazine	10–25	100–300	Sedation, hypotension, anticholinergic
Benztropine mesylate/ trihexyphenidyl	0.5–1	4–6	Anticholinergic

*EPSs = extrapyramidal symptoms.

TABLE 26–3.
Anxiolytics: Half-Lives and Doses*

Drug	Half-life, hr	Starting Dose, mg	Maximum Daily Dose, mg
Oxazepam	5–10	15 QD–BID	120
Lorazepam	10–20	0.25 BID	4
Alprazolam	12–15	0.25 BID	2
Buspirone	?	5 TID	40–60 (?)

*QD = every day; BID = twice daily; and TID = three times daily.

not yet known how the dosing may differ in the elderly, so it is best to use the general principle of lower dosing and titrating to symptom relief. It is safe to use, along with other psychotropic drugs, but may cause an increase in serum haloperidol levels.

V. **Insomnia.** Declining function of the "biologic clock" and decreased rapid eye movement sleep are normal changes that occur with aging. Sleep is also affected by medical illness, such as congestive heart failure, chronic obstructive pulmonary disease, pain, "restless legs," caffeine, and nicotine. Therefore, it can be difficult to assess disturbances of sleep that may be due to depression or other causes. Additionally, many elderly persons sleep during the day, leading to decreased sleep at night. It is important to encourage regular exercise and activity, no daytime sleeping, and the use of relaxation techniques. Like anxiolytics, sedatives are habit forming, and they should be used in a time-limited fashion and on an as-needed rather than daily basis.

A. Benzodiazepines, such as triazolam (0.125 to 0.5 mg), temazepam (10 to 20 mg), oxazepam (15 to 30 mg), or alprazolam (0.25 to 1 mg), are typically the drugs of first choice.

B. Chloral hydrate (0.5 to 2 mg) is safe, effective, and less expensive than most other agents.

C. Barbiturates (e.g., amobarbital, 100 to 200 mg) may cause oversedation and confusion and, generally, should be used only in an inpatient setting, as a second-line agent.

D. Neuroleptics (e.g., thioridazine, 25 to 75 mg) should be used only for severe anxiety, psychosis, or agitation that interferes with sleep.

E. Antihistamines (e.g., diphenhydramine, 25 to 50 mg) should be used only for severe anxiety, psychosis, or agitation that interferes with sleep.

F. Cyclic antidepressants should be avoided, except for depression associated with sleep disturbance.

VI. **Dementia.** In patients with dementia, it is important to rule out reversible causes, such as depressive pseudodementia or hypothyroidism. Having determined that the dementia is irreversible, it is still important to make a definitive diagnosis, as this will have implications for treatment. In multi-infarct dementia, for example, one might first focus on prevention of additional ischemic events, whereas in the dementia associated with Parkinson disease, one might focus on maximizing dopaminergic function. It is important to avoid the use of low-potency neuroleptics, benzodiazepines, barbiturates, and antihistamines in these patients. These drugs tend to increase confusion, and those medications with anticholinergic side effects will further impair memory.

The features of primary degenerative dementia of the Alzheimer type, which may respond to drug treatment, fall primarily into two areas: (1) diminished memory and (2) altered behavior, such as agitation. For the latter, see Section III. Treatment of the memory deficit remains marginally effective or experimental.

A. Hydergine (3 to 4.5 mg/day) contains ergot alkaloids, which are thought to improve brain metabolism in mildly demented patients by their effect on cerebral cyclic adenosine monophosphate. The effect is variable, but it may improve behavior and mood within 8 to 12 weeks. If no improvement is noted within 12 weeks, it should be discontinued.

B. Other drugs, such as vasodilators, psychostimulants, naloxone, procaine, adrenocorticotropic hormone, vasopressin, enkephalins, and L-dopa, have, so far, demonstrated inconsistent effects and cannot be recommended. Methods for increasing acetylcholine neurotransmission are promising for theoretical reasons, but, so far, have not yielded consistent and convincing results.

VII. **Special problems.**

A. Heart disease and depression—A screening electrocardiogram is recommended before the use of antidepressants in any patient over 40 years of age. Cyclic antidepressants are contraindicated in patients with a recent myocardial infaction (i.e., within 1 month) or heart block. They are relatively contraindicated with arrhythmias and congestive heart failure. With any significant increase in the PR or QRS interval, or other evidence of abnormal conduction or cardiac instability, an internist should be consulted and therapy started as an inpatient. Cardiac conduction may be further prolonged by the concurrent use of cyclic antidepressants and quinidine or procainamide. The MAOIs or ECT may be particularly useful in treating these patients.

B. Hypotension—This is often the limiting factor in treatment with antidepressants, which can lead to falling, fractures, head injuries, etc. Orthostatic blood pressure and pulse rate should be monitored while increasing the dose. Nortriptyline is the antidepressant least likely to cause hypotension. Fludrocortisone (Florinef) acetate (0.05 to 0.2 mg/day) and/or sodium can be used to maintain adequate blood pressure.

C. Prostatic hypertrophy—This is common in elderly males, and it is a relative contraindication to the use of anticholinergic agents. Trazodone or MAOIs may be used safely for depression, and high-potency neuroleptics may be used for psychosis and agitation.

D. Narrow-angle glaucoma—Anticholinergic agents are contraindicated. There are no contraindications with open-angle glaucoma, the more common variety.

E. Impotence/inhibited orgasm—This is common with antidepressants and neuroleptics in the elderly, and often it is not reported unless inquired about. It may be treated with bethanechol chloride (starting with 10 mg and increasing to 50 mg as needed, 1 to 2 hours before sex). Alternatively, cyproheptadine (4 to 8 mg QD-BID) may be effective.

F. Tardive dyskinesia—The only well-established risk

factors for tardive dyskinesia are drug exposure greater than 3 months, advancing age, and female gender. Suspected risk factors include increasing dose, potency, and duration of exposure over 3 months, affective illness, or brain injury. It is important to be aware of many other possible causes of dyskinesia, such as idiopathic Parkinson disease, cerebrovascular accidents, etc. Spontaneous orofacial dyskinesias appear in up to 16% of elderly persons without neuroleptic exposure. Treatment is the same as for younger patients.

G. Constipation—Decreased bowel motility is a normal part of the aging process and often leads to constipation. This is exacerbated by even mildly anticholinergic medications. It is important to educate patients regarding dietary fiber (i.e., fresh fruit, whole grains, and leafy green vegetables). Psyllium preparations (1 teaspoon to 1 tablespoon QD-TID) are often helpful. If the patient remains constipated, one can add a stool softener, such as ducosate sodium (100 mg BID). If this fails, a laxative may be recommended, but should be used no more often than every 2 to 3 days. Finally, an enema is occasionally required, and while not desirable, it may prevent fecal impaction.

27
Electroconvulsive Therapy

I. **Introduction.** Electroconvulsive therapy (ECT) is a treatment for severe psychiatric illness in which a brief application of electrical current to the head is used to produce a generalized tonic-clonic seizure. Despite its effectiveness, particularly in major depression with melancholia or psychotic features, ECT is typically used as a second line of treatment. At present, it is used in patients in the diagnostic categories listed below (see Section II) when, in addition:

A. They have not responded to adequate trials of pharmacologic agents, or

B. Their medical condition precludes the use of psychotropic agents, or medication side effects have proved to be intolerable for them (e.g., geriatric depressed patients with pre-existing cardiac conduction disturbances, or bipolar depressives in whom antidepressants may precipitate a manic episode), and/or

C. Their condition (because of marked hyperactivity or hypoactivity, sleeplessness, refusal to eat or drink, or suicidal behavior) requires the rapid improvement obtainable with ECT.

In addition, ECT may also be considered in treating patients with severe depression or psychosis during pregnancy, especially the first trimester, as an alternative to psychotropic medication (see Chapter 24).

II. **Indications.**

A. **Depression.** The major indication for ECT is the presence of a *major depressive episode*, particularly with *melancholia* or *psychotic* features. Electroconvulsive therapy is at least as effective as medications in these illnesses (80% to 90% of patients show marked improvement), and it has a more rapid onset of action. Electroconvulsive therapy is usually not effective for treating milder depressions, i.e., dysthymic disorder or adjustment disorder with depressed mood.

B. **Mania.** Electroconvulsive therapy is as effective in treating acute *mania* as lithium, but because of the efficacy of pharmacotherapy, ECT is less frequently prescribed for acute manic episodes.

C. **Other.** Neuroleptics are the first line of treatment for *schizophrenia*, but ECT may be quite efficacious in treating schizophrenics with a shorter duration of illness, a more acute onset, and particularly with *acute affective symptoms*. Electroconvulsive therapy is generally not effective in treating chronic schizophrenia. *Catatonic symptoms*, however, often respond rapidly to ECT.

III. **Contraindications/precautions.** There are few, if any, absolute contraindications to ECT, but certain situations increase the risk of the procedure and must be evaluated with each patient.

A. The patient must be able to tolerate the effects of *brief general anesthesia*. Hence, patients with severe respiratory problems are at greater risk.

B. Patients with a recent *acute myocardial infarction* or other severe myocardial disease are at high risk because of increased cardiovascular demands during ECT. Patients with other cardiac problems generally tolerate ECT very well, but they must be assessed individually for their possible response to drugs used during the procedure (e.g., atropine) and to cardiac responses to the treatment.

C. Electroconvulsive therapy causes a transient increase in intracranial pressure; thus, it is contraindicated in cases with known *increased intracranial pressure*, and relatively contraindicated for space-occupying lesions (tumors, hematomas, evolving strokes, and large aneurysms).

D. Electroconvulsive therapy transiently increases blood pressure, so severe underlying *hypertension* must be brought under control, at least before each treatment.

IV. **Preparation for ECT.**

A. **Informed consent.** Written informed consent must be obtained before treating voluntary patients. The psychiatrist and the patient (and, if possible, close relatives) should discuss:

1. The nature and seriousness of the mental disorder.

2. Its probable course with and without ECT.

3. The nature of the procedure.

4. Its possible risks and benefits (including acknowledgment of post-treatment confusion and memory dysfunction).

5. The alternative treatment options (including the option of no treatment).

This should be done in as simple and empathic a manner as possible. It should be clear to the patient that his/her consent may be rescinded at any time.

B. **Records.** Meticulous records should be kept by the psychiatrist and the hospital or clinic involved in ECT. These should include:

1. The nature and history of the condition, leading to consideration of ECT.

2. The details of previous treatment, including therapeutic response and adverse reactions.

3. The reasons for selecting ECT.

4. The details of all discussions relevant to consent to ECT.

5. The consent form with the signature of the patient and/or relative or guardian when appropriate.

6. Signed opinions of consultants, if these are requested.

Relevant statutes and regulations and the policies of the individual institution must be considered.

C. **Involuntary ECT.** The use of involuntary ECT is rare and is reserved for cases where the patient lacks the capacity to understand or to consent legally to the procedure. In these cases, court proceedings are required in most jurisdictions, except in some instances where there is already a legally appointed guardian with authority to consent on behalf of the patient. In some states, ECT may, in no circumstances, be administered to an involuntarily committed patient.

D. **Pretreatment evaluation.**

1. Electroconvulsive therapy is a procedure that may stress the cardiovascular, respiratory, musculoskeletal, and nervous systems, so a careful pretreatment evaluation is required, as follows:

a. A standard medical history and physical examination (including neurologic examination).

b. Blood and urine tests (as indicated by history and examination, but to include electrolytes and routine urinalysis).

c. An electrocardiogram.

2. In many settings (for instance, the presence of skeletal disease or a history of ECT), thoracolumbar spine x-ray films should be obtained. In cases of suspected cranial or intracranial disease, electroencephalograms (EEGs) and/or head computed tomographic scans are appropriate.

3. Patients should be evaluated before the procedure by an anesthetist or a physician skilled in the use of anesthesia, to evaluate fully the risks of anesthesia and possible drug interactions for each individual.

Patients should be essentially lithium free, as lithium increases the central nervous system sequelae of ECT and prolongs the action of neuromuscular-blocking agents.

Some believe monoamine oxidase (MAO) inhibitors should be discontinued 2 weeks before treatment to avoid anesthetic complications, although more recent evidence suggests that ECT may be given safely in the presence of MAO inhibitors, probably due to the short duration of anesthesia.

Sedative-hypnotics and anticonvulsants may interfere with the ability to induce a seizure, and they should be decreased or discontinued as rapidly as clinically feasible.

Reserpine increases the possibility of hypotensive collapse. It should be discontinued for 1 week before ECT.

A variety of agents influence succinylcholine metabolism, including anticholinesterase ophthalmic solutions, streptomycin, and lithium.

V. **Procedure.**

A. The treatment should be given in an area designated for ECT and equipped for supervised medical recovery, including equipment and medications for cardiopulmonary resuscitation. An electrocardiogram, blood pressure, pulse rate, and respirations should be monitored throughout the procedure.

B. The patient should be given nothing by mouth for 8 to 12 hours before each treatment, and immediately before the procedure, the staff should attempt to have the patient fully empty his/her bladder and rectum.

C. To prevent potential treatment-related bradycardia

and to minimize secretions, an anticholinergic agent (0.6 to 1.2 mg of atropine or 0.2 to 0.4 mg of glycopyrrolate) is often administered intramuscularly or subcutaneously approximately 30 minutes before treatment, or intravenously at the time of treatment.

D. Peripheral venous access should be started and maintained until the patient is fully recovered. Teeth should be examined just before starting treatment, to remove dental appliances or to note chipped or loose teeth.

E. Light anesthesia minimizes both adverse effects of anesthesia and the tendency of the usual agents employed to elevate the seizure threshold (and thus to require higher intensity electrical stimulation). The usual anesthetics used are methohexital (0.5 to 1.0 mg/kg) or thiopental (3 mg/kg). Occasionally, etomidate (0.15 to 0.30 mg/kg) or intramuscular ketamine (6–10 mg/kg) is used instead. The patient should be ventilated by mask with 100% oxygen from the onset of anesthesia to the resumption of adequate spontaneous respiration.

F. Following the onset of anesthetic effect, the muscle relaxant succinylcholine (0.5 to 1.5 mg/kg) is given. The goal is enough relaxation to stop most but not all ictal body movements, except in some cases of musculoskeletal or cardiac disease where total muscle relaxation may be required.

The action of succinylcholine, a depolarizing blocker, is marked by muscle fasciculations that move rostrocaudally. When these disappear, maximal relaxation has occurred. Relaxation should also be assessed by stroking the patient's foot in the manner used to elicit the Babinski sign. With maximal muscle relaxation, no plantar response should take place. A nerve stimulator may be used as an alternative method of testing for muscle relaxation.

Succinylcholine-induced apnea usually does not last longer than the effects of anesthesia. Pseudocholinesterase deficiency (inborn or acquired) or drug interactions that prolong the effect of succinylcholine may produce prolonged apnea. If apnea is greatly prolonged after the treatment, endotracheal intubation should be considered.

G. Seizure monitoring may be accomplished by an EEG and/or by the "cuff" technique. With this, a blood pressure cuff is placed on an arm or leg of the patient and inflated to a pressure greater than systolic before injection of succinylcholine. This allows unmodified convulsive movements of that extremity to occur and to be timed. With unilateral ECT, the cuff should be on the same side as the electrodes, to ensure that a bilateral seizure has occurred.

H. **Electrode placement.** Many alternatives for electrode placement exist. Leads should be applied with conductive gel, onto a clean scalp. In bilateral ECT, the two electrodes may be placed bifrontotemporally, with each one approximately 2 in. above the midpoint of a line drawn from the external auditory meatus to the lateral angle of the eye. In unilateral ECT, both electrodes are placed over the nondominant hemisphere. One is placed over the frontotemporal area, as for bilateral ECT, while the other is usually placed on the nondominant centroparietal scalp, just lateral to the midline vertex. The distance between the midpoint of the two electrodes is approximately 4.5 in. Right-handedness is highly correlated with left hemispheric dominance.

Controversy exists about the relative efficacy of lead placements and their contribution to memory deficits. Many believe that bilateral ECT is more uniformly effective; unilateral nondominant ECT, however, has been shown to be associated with less confusion and fewer memory deficits. For most patients, it is now recommended that treatment be initiated with unilateral electrode placement, switching to bilateral placement if there is little or no response after four or five unilateral treatments.

I. **The electrical stimulus and the seizure.** Seizure thresholds and durations vary greatly among patients and may be difficult to determine. The goal is to achieve a seizure between 25 and 60 seconds by using the lowest amount of electrical energy. Some ECT devices allow determination of actual stimulus energy, and this value should be kept as low as possible. Seizures of greater than 60 seconds often indicate that the stimulus is suprathreshold and should be diminished at a subsequent treatment session. If no seizure occurs, stimulation should be followed immediately by a repeated stimulation at a higher stimulus intensity. With seizures lasting less than 25 seconds, the stimulus should be repeated once. If this also produces a short seizure, the stimulus intensity should be increased, and a third stimulus should be given. If three stimulations fail to elicit an adequate seizure, the treatment session should be terminated. Because of the refractoriness to further seizures that follows a seizure, an interval of 60 to 90 seconds should be allowed to elapse before repeating the stimulation, during which time the patient should be ventilated with oxygen. Waiting too long may allow the effects of anesthesia or of the muscle relaxant to wear off. The maintenance of adequate muscle relaxation should be assured before each stimulation. Seizure thresholds increase with anesthetic dose, age, number of treatments in the current ECT course, and a number of medications, especially anticonvulsants, sedative-hypnotics, and lidocaine.

J. **Number and spacing of ECT treatments.** The number of treatments in a course varies and should be determined on the basis of clinical response. The decision to stop the ECT course is usually based on the achievement of a maximal response or the lack of substantial improvement after a fixed number of treatments. Six to 12 treatments are usually effective, although some patients may require up to 20 to 25 treatments.

The usual frequency of treatments is three times weekly. Some believe that because of lower central nervous system side effects, unilateral ECT can be given four to five times weekly. On occasion, with a severely ill patient, the first few treatments may be given on a daily basis even with bilateral ECT. In all cases, if the patient begins to show a severe and lengthening confusional state after treatments, the frequency of the treatments should be decreased.

Records of the specifics of each treatment should be kept, including date, electrode placement, drugs administered, characteristics of the electrical stimulus, seizure duration, and any complications.

VI. **Adverse effects.** The mortality rate for a complete series of ECT is roughly the same as that associated with brief general anesthesia (approximately 1/10,000), while for a single treatment session it is less than 5/100,000. It is usually on the basis of cardiovascular complications and is more likely to occur in patients whose cardiac status is compromised.

A. **Systemic.** Occasional, usually benign, transient cardiac arrhythmias occur. These are often secondary to the postictal bradycardia caused by central vagal stimulation and thus may be prevented by anticholinergic premedication. Some short-lived arrhythmias occur due to the sinus tachycardia and sympathetic hyperactivity that follow the seizure-induced bradycardia. There is also a marked transient increase in blood pressure that may be worse in patients with pre-existing hypertension. Prophylactic beta-blockers, calcium-channel blockers, or other antihypertensive agents can be useful.

B. **Central nervous system.** Immediately after the treatment, patients commonly experience short-term confusion, transient memory loss, headache, and sometimes nausea. The severity of the confusion is greatest after bilateral ECT. It is also increased by the following:

1. Longer seizure duration.

2. Closer spacing of the treatments.

3. Increasing dose of electrical stimulation.

4. Each additional treatment.

5. The age of the patient.

Gentle reorientation and close observation are generally all that is required. Headaches may be treated with acetaminophen, and if they recur with each treatment, pretreatment before each session with an acetaminophen suppository is often helpful.

Patients receiving ECT have a retrograde amnesia for events just before each treatment, as well as an anterograde amnesia, i.e., an impaired ability to learn and retain new information. After a series of treatments, the patient's retrograde amnesia extends to more remote events, although the effect is always greatest for more recent memory. The ability to learn returns to normal several weeks after the termination of treatment. Memory and other forms of cognitive function return at least to baseline by 1 to 6 months after ECT, as assessed by neuropsychologic testing. Persistent mild spotty memory losses, particularly for the period surrounding ECT treatment, are described by some individuals. Other patients complain of more severe and lasting impairment of memory, although there is little objective evidence for this. The same factors that increase the severity of the acute confusional state increase the severity of post-ECT memory deficits.

VII. **Maintenance treatment.** Electroconvulsive therapy produces a remission but does not, in itself, prevent relapse. In most cases, patients should continue to receive antidepressant medication or lithium to reduce the likelihood of relapse. A role for periodic maintenance ECT to prevent recurrent illness remains to be clarified.

In summary, as with all treatments, the choice of ECT is based on the assessment of risks and benefits of all available forms of treatment for a given condition, and it depends as well on the particular constellation of symptoms and risks present in each individual case. Even the pharmacotherapeutic agents have significant morbidity, however, so that in addition to being effective, ECT may represent the safest form of treatment for some patients.

REFERENCES

1. American Psychiatric Association: *Electroconvulsive Therapy*, task force report 14. Washington, DC, American Psychiatric Association, 1978.
2. *Consensus Development Conference Statement: Electroconvulsive Therapy 5 (No. 1)*. Washington, DC, US Dept of Health and Human Services, 1985.
3. Fink M: *Convulsive Therapy: Theory and Practice*. New York, Raven Press, 1979.
4. Fink M: Convulsive therapy: A manual of practice, in (Hales RE, Frances AJ (eds): *Annual Review of Psychiatry*, vol 6. Washington, DC, American Psychiatric Press, Inc, 1988, pp 482–497.
5. Glenn MD, Weiner RD: *Electroconvulsive Therapy: A Programmed Text*. Washington, DC, American Psychiatric Press, Inc, 1985.

28 | Interactions Between Psychotropic and Other Drugs

The following Tables 28–1 through 28–6 are provided to assist the clinician who is treating a patient who is taking more than one psychotropic drug or a combination of medical and psychiatric drugs at one time. (All tables in this chapter are reproduced with permission from Glassman R, Salzman C: Psychopharmacology: Interactions between psychotropic and other drugs: An update. *Hosp Community Psychiatry* 1987; 38:236–242.)

TABLE 28-1.

Drug Interactions With Neuroleptics*

Drug Interacting With Neuroleptic	Clinical Effect of Interaction
Anticholinergics	Delayed onset of neuroleptic effect in acute oral dose; may alter neuroleptic blood levels; increased anticholinergic effect (delirium, disorientation); possible increased risk of hyperthermia
Lithium	May reduce plasma chlorpromazine levels and clinical effect, may increase CNS toxicity
Narcotics	Increased sedation, analgesia augmented, hypotension augmented, respiratory depression augmented, anticholinergic effects augmented by meperidine
Benzodiazepines	Increased CNS sedation, decreased akathisia
Cyclic antidepressants	Increased sedation, increased hypotension, increased anticholinergic effect, may increase clinical effect

	of neuroleptic, possible increased risk of seizures
Levodopa	May exacerbate psychosis, decreased antiparkinsonian effect of levodopa
Amphetamines	May exacerbate psychosis by counteracting effects of neuroleptics
Barbiturates, nonbarbiturate hypnotics	Increased sedation, decreased clinical effect of neuroleptic
Iproniazid	Hepatic toxicity and encephalopathy, decreased neuroleptic effect
Epinephrine	Hypotension augmented
Enflurane, isoflurane anesthetics	Profound hypotension with phenothiazines
Indomethacin	May cause severe drowsiness with haloperidol

*CNS = central nervous system.

TABLE 28-2.

Drug Interactions With Cyclic Antidepressants

Drug Interacting With Cyclic Antidepressant	Clinical Effect of Interaction
Cimetidine	Inhibits metabolism, increasing blood levels and toxicity of antidepressants
Guanethidine, debrisoquin, bethanidine	Decreased antihypertensive effect, decreased antidepressant effect
Quinidine, procainamide	Cardiac conduction prolonged
Coumarin anticoagulants	Increased bleeding
Phenytoin	Induces hepatic metabolism, decreasing clinical effect of antidepressants
Anticholinergic drugs	Increased anticholinergic toxicity
Triiodothyronine, lithium	Possible potentiation of antidepressant effect
Activated charcoal, kaolin	Helpful in overdose by decreasing absorption
Epinephrine, local anesthetic dissolved in epinephrine	Hypotension augmented, increased bleeding in nasal surgery
Alcohol	Increased sedation

TABLE 28-3.

Drug Interactions With MAO Inhibitors*

Drug Interacting With MAO Inhibitors	Clinical Effect of Interaction
Amphetamines, ephedrine, metaraminol, levarterenol, methylphenidate, phenylephrine, pseudoephedrine, levodopa, dopamine, mephentermine, chlorpheniramine, procaine hydrochloride (Novacain) (dissolved in epinephrine)	Increased blood pressure
Cyclic antidepressants	May have enhanced clinical effect; conflicting reports on toxicity—hyperpyrexia, excitability, muscle rigidity, convulsions, coma; use with caution; weight gain
Meperidine, dextromethorphan	Excitation, sweating, hypotension; use other narcotics; can be life threatening
Alcohol	Decreased MAO inhibition, CNS depression

*MAO = monoamine oxidase; CNS = central nervous system.

TABLE 28–4.

Drug Interactions With Lithium*

Drug Interacting With Lithium	Clinical Effect of Interaction
Indomethacin, piroxicam, sulindac, ibuprofen	Increased lithium effect and toxicity due to decreased renal lithium clearance
Phenylbutazone, naproxen, zomepirac	Increased lithium effect and toxicity due to decreased renal lithium clearance
Thiazide diuretics, phenylbutazone, spironolactone, triamterene, amiloride	Increased lithium effect and toxicity due to decreased renal lithium clearance
Neuroleptics	Decreased neuroleptic blood levels, decreased nausea and vomiting from lithium, increased neurotoxicity (may be severe)
Theophylline, acetazolamide, aminophylline	Increased renal excretion of lithium, decreasing its effect
Succinylcholine, pancuronium, decamethonium	Prolonged apnea with ECT
Sodium bicarbonate, sodium chloride, urea, mannitol	Increased renal excretion of lithium, decreasing its effect
Tetracycline, spectinomycin	Increased lithium effect and toxicity due to decreased renal lithium clearance
Carbamazepine	Increased neurotoxicity of both drugs; increased polyuria, ataxia, and dizziness due to antidiuretic

	property of carbamazepine; enhanced antidepressant effect
Cyclic antidepressants	May increase lithium neurotoxicity; may increase lithium tremor; enhanced antidepressant effect
Ketamine	Increased lithium toxicity, resulting from sodium depletion
Furosemide	Increased lithium toxicity, resulting from sodium depletion

ECT = electroconvulsive therapy.

TABLE 28–5.

Drug Interactions With Benzodiazepines*

Drug Interacting With Benzodiazepine	Clinical Effect of Interaction
Cimetidine	Increased toxicity of diazepam and chlordiazepoxide due to inhibition of metabolism
Alcohol, neuroleptics, narcotics, antihistamines, sedative-hypnotics	Increased CNS sedation
Cyclic antidepressants	Increased CNS sedation, increased amitriptyline levels
Levodopa	Possible decreased effect of levodopa

CNS = central nervous system.

TABLE 28–6.

Drug Interactions With Carbamazepine

Drug Interacting With Carbamazepine	Clinical Effect of Interaction
Lithium	Inhibits diuresis and polyuria associated with lithium; in combination, may increase ataxia, feelings of unreality, dizziness; neurotoxicity with normal levels of both
Cimetidine, erythromycin, isoniazid	Increased carbamazepine levels; may produce somnolence, lethargy, nystagmus, dizziness, nausea, vomiting in combination
Propoxyphene	Increased carbamazepine levels; may produce headache, dizziness, nausea, ataxia

IV
Psychotherapies

29 Choosing the Appropriate Psychotherapy

I. **Introduction.** This section reviews the process of going from the psychiatric assessment and diagnosis to the selection of the appropriate therapeutic intervention. The section begins with an overview of psychotherapy and the process of how to choose the appropriate type of psychotherapy for a given patient.

Psychotherapy is an effective tool in helping distressed individuals to increase their sense of flexibility, independence, and pleasure in life. Psychotherapy helps people become more competent problem solvers and more adaptive.

II. **Establishing a therapeutic alliance.**

A. **Psychiatric evaluation and the therapeutic relationship.** Psychiatric intervention can be divided into a *first stage* of *assessment* and *diagnosis* and a *second stage of psychiatric therapy*. The distinction between evaluation and therapy emphasizes the need to obtain a data base and to develop a formulation of "what is going on" with the patient before choosing "what can be done."

The *choice of therapy* is based on establishing what the patient is seeking help for and what type of interventions would be effective to meet these goals. Every form of therapy involves two areas: (1) the establishment of a *therapeutic relationship* and (2) the choice of *therapeutic techniques*. Although the evaluation period may appear to be a separate, information-gathering phase, it is the beginning of the therapeutic alliance between the patient and mental health professional.

Patients may present for psychiatric evaluation and/or treatment for a variety of reasons (see Lazare, 1976). The evaluator's goal is to understand what the patient's experiences have been and what brings them to attention *at this time*. This is establishing an "intimate relationship" that may reach to the "core" of the patient's sense of self. If done with warmth, empathy, and sensitivity, the patient may find a sense of connection and relief in being listened to and understood. Thus, "making contact" in the beginning can be therapeutic. Respect for this privileged connection is warranted and can set the stage for being able and willing to reach out for help during the "therapeutic phase" following evaluation.

Involvement of the patient's support system (family, friends) may be helpful. How others view the patient at the present time can be crucial in understanding what brings the patient in for help. This information can also be essential in determining which form of psychotherapy (e.g., individual vs. family) will be most helpful. Family members or close friends should not be brought into the evaluation process if it is requested by the patient or at the hesitancy of the evaluator for fear of breaking confidentiality. Interviewing these individuals should be seen as supportive of the effort to understand and help the patient. In this way, involving others should not pose a threat to the development of the emerging therapeutic alliance during the assessment period.

B. **Therapeutic inquiry.** Psychiatric history taking can be an extensive process that is felt by some patients to be awkward and intrusive. To help the patient feel more comfortable in giving information and to align ourselves with them in a therapeutic way, empathic statements of various kinds can be made (Sullivan, 1954; Havens, 1986). Simple statements that reflect the patient's ideas, phrases that reveal the evaluator's sense of the nature and magnitude of the difficulty being described, and open-ended questions can be helpful (e.g., "That must have been a very difficult time . . . how did you cope with all of that?").

A general rule of thumb for the psychiatric evaluation interview is to have the first part with open-ended questions (e.g., "What brings you to the clinic today?" or "What was that like for you?"), followed by more directive questions aimed at specific information required (e.g., "Were you ever hospitalized?" or "Did your mother or father ever receive psychiatric help?"). Once a general formulation is being considered, then even more specific information that elaborates these hypotheses can be pursued. A final portion is to allow the patient to ask any questions and to share how he/she feels after revealing personal information. It can be helpful to acknowledge the potential stressfulness of the interview and give the patient the chance to express his/her concerns about what the evaluation experience has been like and what the results will mean to him/her.

C. **Communicating the diagnosis and treatment recommendations.** Some psychiatric diagnoses require a careful and accurate history or longitudinal observations and, thus, cannot be made definitively in the short-term setting. The acknowledgment of the limitations in this situation can be frustrating but important to patients and their relatives. When an assessment and a diagnostic formulation can be made, clinical judgment is warranted to determine who should be informed of the findings. Involvement of the family can be crucial in cases of gravely disabled individuals. The assessment summation should be tailored to the needs of the patient. Done with sensitivity, the process of explaining the psychiatric view of what is troubling the patient can be a relieving experience. This stage, carried out with warmth and compassion, can further help to develop the therapeutic relationship.

The decision of which treatment modality to recommend is a process which should involve collaboration with the patient. This involves them actively in the therapeutic process. Certain patients may resist treatment recommendations.

D. **Some "Do's" and "Don'ts" in the establishment of the therapeutic alliance during the psychiatric evaluation.**

1. Do:

a. Show concern, empathy, warmth, acceptance, and genuineness.

b. Explain to the patient the limits and nature of your involvement (i.e., the evaluation session is only for a certain amount of time at the end of which you will be discussing together what will be most helpful).

c. Ask the patient what his/her view is of what is troubling him/her and what would be most helpful.

2. Don't:

a. Offer the patient premature conclusions about the nature of his/her illness.

b. Imply that you will personally see the patient as his/her therapist unless this will definitely occur.

c. Forget to respect the psychiatric encounter as a stressful experience that will be reviewing the intimate, subjective world of the patient.

III. **Choosing appropriate psychotherapy.**

A. **Introduction.** Choosing the appropriate therapy is *not* based solely on the diagnosis. There is no simple "cookbook" method for placing an individual with a specific diagnosis into a corresponding treatment modality. Several factors, in addition to the diagnosis, need to be carefully considered. The patient's "problems" need to be viewed in a context of his/her possible biologically based mental illness and his/her intrapsychic world, personality style, behavioral difficulties, and sociocultural factors. Thus, two individuals with the same categories on all five *DSM III-R* axes may be quite different people and require different therapeutic interventions.

All psychotherapies are based on a relationship between therapist and patient and specific technical procedures. The relative emphasis between these two areas and the emphasis on particular techniques are what distinguishes one school of therapy from another. Research has attempted to correlate the effects of these "nonspecific" and "specific" interventions with a positive outcome (see Karasu, 1984). For example, a simple, conditioned avoidance response may respond best to systematic desensitization, while prevention of relapse in chronic schizophrenia is best attained with a combination of neuroleptic medications and family psychoeducational interventions.

Jules Masserman (in Karasu, 1984) has written, "Comprehensive treatment must be exquisitely individualized as to age, physical state, education, intellectual level, familial and economic status, cultural and religious orientations, special talents and potentialities, treatment objectives, and many other factors and contingencies. How each therapist, acting as clinician, social ombudsman, and philosophic mentor, combines elements of various parameters of influence constitutes his or her unique therapeutic craft. Analysis of the interrelated vectors of physical, psychosocial, and metapsychologic influences can then lead to a more comprehensive rationale for, and more specific and effective applications of, various modalities of psychiatric therapy."

B. **Conceptualizing the "issues."** The evaluator must have a thorough view of the different levels of realities that effect the patient. It may be helpful to refer to the following "checklist," making a diagnostic formulation and treatment plan.

Conceptual Hypotheses Checklist

Biologic	Includes organic mental states, affective illness, psychosis, substance abuse
Psychodynamic	Includes psychologic meaning of a precipitating event and its effect on a rigid or malfunctioning defensive style, post-traumatic sequelae, unresolved grief, developmental crises
Cognitive/behavioral	Includes stressful event-induced and -reinforced dysfunctional behaviors, thoughts, emotional responses
Systems/sociocultural	Includes difficulties with social support systems, social/cultural meaning of symptoms, family issues

C. **The presenting "problem."** Patients may present with a number of chief complaints. Lazare (1976) noted several as follows: administrative request, advice clarification, community triage, confession, control, limit setting, medical or psychologic expertise, psychotherapy, social intervention, reality contact, succorance, ventilation, or nothing. Table 29–1 (below) shows one way in which to conceptualize the presenting problem.

D. **Patient characteristics.** Personality characteristics are relevant to what form of therapy is indicated. An understanding of these features helps to clarify the patient's present difficulties and what resources are available to alleviate these problems. Table 29–2 (below) lists some of these characteristics adapted from Lazare (1976).

E. **How to decide which therapeutic interventions to use.** Psychotherapy is a relationship plus a *combination* of techniques from psychodynamic to psychopharmacologic interventions. As psychotherapists from different schools of therapy become more experienced, what they actually do in therapy becomes more and more similar. Combinations of therapies may be more effective than strict adherence to one school or another.

Masserman (see Karasu, 1984) has described seven basic "parameters of influence" that comprise the common elements in all types of psychotherapies. These include the societal role ("prestige") of the psychotherapist, rapport (therapeutic alliance), right, retrospection, re-education, rehabilitation, resocialization, and recapitulation.

Psychotherapeutic elements can be chosen for each patient initially and modified as therapy continues. These features may be changed as the therapeutic goals, mental state, and patient needs change. Psychotherapy is characterized by goals, setting, format, timing, techniques, and concomitant use of other therapeutic modalities. These variables can be outlined as follows:

PSYCHOTHERAPY CHARACTERISTICS

Psychotherapy Goals

Acute care (crisis intervention and stabilization)

Rehabilitation (improving severe behavioral impairments)

Maintenance (long-term prevention of deterioration)

Restructuring (promoting a lasting change in the patient)

TABLE 29–1.
Conceptualization of Presenting Problem and Initial Therapeutic Implications

Presenting Problem Features	Therapeutic Implications
Acute crisis:	Generally shorter duration
Precipitant?	Brief therapy, exploratory therapy
Life stage issue?	Brief therapy, exploratory therapy
Internally driven?	Longer term Tx
Chronic disturbance:	Generally longer duration
Periodic episodes?	May require long-term therapy
Chronic personality traits?	May require long-term therapy
Anniversary reaction?	Exploratory therapy
Pathologic grief	Exploratory therapy
Post-traumatic syndrome	Exploratory therapy
Premorbid functioning	
Good	Shorter duration
Poor	Longer duration
Behavioral manifestations	
Addictions, compulsions?	Directive therapy; homogeneous group (e.g., AA)
Eating disorder?	
Thought disorder	
Acute or chronic	Supportive therapy and psychotropic medication

Mood disturbance
  Reactive?
  Autonomous?
	Various therapies: exploratory directive, and psychotropic medication

Post-traumatic sequelae
  Acute or chronic?
  Dissociative symptoms?
	Crisis therapy initially; exploratory therapy with directive techniques

Interpersonal deterioration:
  Progressive withdrawal?
  Sudden?
	Long-term therapy
	
	Crisis therapy

Complexity of symptoms:
  Highly complex
  Relatively "simple"
	
	Longer-term therapy
	Shorter-term therapy

Severity of symptoms:
  Markedly incapacitating
 	
  Mildly distressing
	
	Increased frequency of therapy
	Generally less frequent therapy

TABLE 29-2.
Patient Characteristics and Therapy Implications

Patient Characteristics	Implications for Therapy
Motivation for change	Receptive to therapeutic influence
Belief systems and therapeutic expectations	Convergence of therapist and patient expectations important (especially regarding duration, format, and orientation)
(Patient's sense of) Locus of control	
Internal (self)	Insight/exploratory therapy
External (fate, others)	Supportive or directive therapy
Ego strengths	
Object relatedness good	Insight/exploratory
Impulse control (ability to delay gratification)	
High	Insight
Low	Directive
Cognitive style (Horwitz, 1974)	
Obsessive	Affect experiencing via experiential, insight
Hysterical	Cognitive understanding of emotions via insight, directive
Interpersonal relatedness	
Low	May suggest need for group therapy

High	May tolerate dyadic setting or group
Verbal ability/intelligence	Possible ability to use insight/exploratory (watch for rigid intellectual defenses)
Ability to introspect "psychologic mindedness"	Exploratory/insight
Social support system difficulties (e.g., scapegoating, interpersonal conflicts)	May require marital or family therapy

Notes: The goals depend on the present "state" (relatively short-lived mental status features) and "traits" (more enduring characteristics of the patient's personality) that need to be changed to benefit the patient. Acute care generally focuses on stabilizing a deteriorated state of functioning; the other goals tend to focus on traits. The goals determine how the therapy features are chosen and combined.

Psychotherapy Setting

Hospital

Partial hospitalization (day-hospital)

Outpatient

Notes: An increased acuity, severity of impairment with an inability to care for self, and dangerousness to self or others are generally associated with the hospital setting. Hospital settings may be required for diagnostic evaluations. Partial hospitalization may be useful as an intermediate step between inpatient and outpatient status. Outpatient care is the least costly and most easily integrated, with the patient functioning in the society as a whole.

Psychotherapy Format

Individual

Family/marital

Group (homogeneous or heterogeneous)

Notes: This format may be used in various combinations at different phases of therapy. One therapist may see a given patient in various formats, or different therapists may be seen. Selection criteria for the various formats are reviewed in detail later in this chapter and in subsequent chapters.

Psychotherapy Timing

Session frequency

Session duration

Treatment duration

Notes: Frequency may vary from one to several times per week for most forms of psychotherapy. Maintenance goals with supportive techniques may be less frequent (once a month to every 2 or 3 months). Frequency may be increased during acute episodes as indicated.

Session duration varies, depending on the goals and techniques of the therapy and the patient's attention span and tolerance during the session. Session duration generally varies from 20 to 30 minutes, 45 to 50 minutes, and 75 to 90 minutes per session. These durations generally correspond to individual supportive, individual restructuring, and group or family/marital therapy, respectively.

Treatment duration also varies, depending on the goals that are set and the techniques that are chosen. Limited, specific goals and directive techniques are associated with shorter lengths of therapy. Therapy may be "preset" as time limited or open ended. Time-limited therapies include ultrabrief (up to six sessions) and brief therapy (ten to 20 sessions or 3 to 6 months). Open-ended therapies may range from several visits to several years of therapy. Ideally, maintenance therapy would be the only therapeutic goal that requires a lifelong duration.

Psychotherapy Techniques

Exploratory (includes psychodynamically oriented therapy, psychoanalysis, hypnoanalysis, and guided imagery)

Directive (includes cognitive and rational-emotive biofeedback, desensitization, and reality therapy)

Experiential (includes existential, client-centered, gestalt, and Zen therapy, psychodrama, and art therapy)

Supportive (includes procedures of advice, praise, reassurance, lending ego, and limit setting)

Notes: Please see this chapter's section on selection of therapeutic techniques.

Concomitant Use of Other Therapeutic Modalities

Somatic therapies (includes psychotropic medications, electroconvulsive shock therapy, sleep deprivation, and exercise)

"Bibliotherapy" (includes assignments to keep a personal journal, daily symptom log, and reading of appropriate relevant literature)

Rehabilitation (includes social skills training and occupational therapy and may include some self-help groups)

F. **Is psychotherapy for everyone?**

1. **"No treatment" as a disposition.** Certain patients who are seen for evaluation will, for a variety of reasons, either not benefit from treatment at the present time or will have a probable negative response to intervention. In these cases, psychiatric assessment will result in the recommendation that no treatment be initiated. It is important to state that psychotherapy is *not* appropriate for all patients who are seen for psychiatric evaluation. Some general features relevant to this issue include a past response to well-conducted therapy, dependency issues and personality traits, fostering unnecessary and unhealthy forms of regression in certain patients, legal suits, and psychiatric compensation cases. There are exceptions to every attempt to categorize "no indicated treatment" patients; therefore, no more specific guidelines will be offered.

It is probably best to provide an extended evaluation before stating that therapy is not indicated or that the patient is not suitable for any form of therapy.

Some patients may be appropriate for therapy but opposed to accepting treatment. If they are legally not holdable and are opposed to psychotherapy, then these patients should be offered the appropriate treatment and their refusal carefully documented in the chart.

2. **Psychotherapy and the "medication patient."** The "medication patient" may require working through the loss of reliability of his/her own mind if he/she has had an acute episode and then an ongoing supportive therapeutic relationship during his/her long-term maintenance on psychotropic medications. In addition, medications are more likely to be appropriately taken in the context of an ongoing supportive relationship with the psychiatrist as therapist rather than merely as a dispenser of drugs.

Caution should be used in carefully assessing the ego strength of an individual who has a history of psychosis before entering into potentially stressful exploratory therapy.

G. **Selection criteria for treatment format.** The following is adapted from Frances et al., 1984.

1. **Individual.**

a. **Relative indications.** (1) The patient's symptoms or character is based on a firmly structured intrapsychic conflict that causes repetitive life patterns that more or less transcend the particulars of the current interpersonal situation (e.g., family, job relationships). (2) An adolescent, young adult who is striving for autonomy. (3) Psychiatric problems that are of such a private and/or embarrassing matter that they need the privacy of individual treatment, at least for the beginning phase.

b. **Enabling factors.** (1) A patient who is comfortable in a dyadic situation and able to handle the potential intimacy of the individual treatment setting. (2) Financial and temporal resources that are needed for individual treatment.

c. **Relative contraindications.** (1) A family (systems) problem. (2) Patient regresses (in a nontherapeutically advantageous manner) in individual therapy relationships.

2. **Family/marital.**

a. **Relative indications.**

(1) Family/marital problems are presented as such, without either spouse or any family member designated as the identified patient; symptoms are predominantly within the marital relationship.

(2) Family presents with difficulties in intrafamilial relationships, with each person contributing collusively or openly to the problem.

(3) Family has fixed and severe deficits in perception and communication.

(4) Adolescent behavioral disturbances, including drug abuse, delinquency, promiscuity, or vandalism.

(5) Another format of treatment is stalemated or has failed, e.g., individual therapy has focused only on family problems.

(6) One family member's improvement has led to deterioration in another.

(7) Limited resources and the need for treatment of more than one family member make this format desirable.

b. **Enabling factors.**

(1) Motivation is strongest to be seen as a couple or family, or an individual patient will accept no other format.

(2) No family member has a psychopathologic condition of such proportions that family therapy would be prevented.

(3) Crucial members of a defined functional social system are available for family treatment.

c. **Relative contraindications.**

(1) The presenting problem of the individual does not have a significant cause in or effect on the family system.

(2) Marital problems, if present, are chronic and ego-syntonic.

(3) Defensive misuse of family therapy to deny individual responsibility for major personality or character illness.

(4) A massive but minimally relevant or unworkable parental pathologic condition that indicates a symptomatic child or adolescent should be treated alone.

(5) Individuation of one or more family members requires that they have their own and separate treatment.

(6) Family treatment has stalemated or failed and has resolved what crises it can, and one or more individual members require additional sessions to establish trust.

(7) There is a need for another modality of treatment before family therapy, e.g., detoxification, medication, individual sessions to establish trust.

(8) Motivation is to be seen alone, e.g., adolescents who state emphatically that they have personal problems for which they want individual help.

3. **Group.**

a. **Relative indications.**

(1) A patient's most pressing problems occur in current interpersonal relationships, both outside and inside family situations, such as (a) loneliness, social and work inhibitions, excessive embarrassment with others, shyness, and feelings of being unlovable; (b) inability to share, needs excessive admiration from others, and has difficulty understanding or caring about the

needs of others; (c) being excessively argumentative, unable to cooperate, and oppositional, and having authority problems; and (d) being excessively dependent, timid, unable to separate from family, and unable to be properly assertive.

(2) The patient presents with problems that are significantly attributable to a specific disorder (e.g., alcoholism) for which a specialized ("homogeneous") group is available.

(3) The patient has problems that are not predominantly interpersonal, but group indicated because (a) other modalities of treatment have been unsuccessful or have reached maximum returns and further treatment is needed; (b) the patient has a tendency to actualize the transference and to become excessively involved with and persistently distort the relationship with an individual therapist; and (c) the patient cannot tolerate a dyadic intimacy and is not motivated or ready to change this characteristic.

b. **Enabling factors.**

(1) The patient is capable of participation in group treatment as evidenced by characteristics, such as an openness to influence from other patients and a willingness to listen to others and to participate in and maintain a group process.

(2) Motivation for group treatment is at least adequate.

(3) Availability or cost of treatment makes group referral desirable.

C. **Relative contraindications.**

(1) There is an acute psychiatric emergency or crisis that requires more urgent, intense, specialized, and individualized attention (e.g., acute depression, suicidal ideation, psychosis, mania, etc.).

(2) The patient is likely to respond to brief therapy.

(3) The patient refuses group treatment, and his/her resistances are unmovable.

(4) The patient manifests a condition that makes interpersonal relatedness disorganizing, impossible, or possibly harmful to the individual, group, or both. Examples would include patients with severe organic brain syndrome and/or severe impairment in reality testing, and patients who are so dishonest, manipulative, suspicious, or explosive that it is impossible to form a therapeutic group alliance.

(5) Group participation would be an avoidance of another form of treatment that is more indicated.

H. **Selection criteria for treatment techniques.** The selection of treatment techniques is based on the therapeutic goals and the patient's personality characteristics, including ego strengths, motivation for change, and belief systems. An overview of the various psychotherapy approaches or schools is given at the end of the chapter.

1. **Exploratory.**

a. **Relative indications.**

(1) The patient's problem can be understood as a manifestation of an intrapsychic conflict.

(2) The goals of treatment increase flexibility of defensive structure, uncovering and working through traumatic past experiences (as opposed to simply symptom reduction).

b. **Enabling factors.**

(1) Motivation to change behavior and to understand oneself better vs. merely attaining symptom relief.

(2) The patient is willing to make sacrifices (in time, money) to be involved in therapy.

(3) The patient is attempting to be honest and open about personal motivations and self.

(4) The patient has psychologic mindedness and is eager to study his/her own behaviors and feelings, including those that occur in response to the therapist.

(5) The patient has the potential ability to experience, express, tolerate, and discuss painful affects.

(6) The patient has relatively high ego strengths (as evidenced in interpersonal relations, educational and work performance, and the ability to accept responsibility).

(7) The patient is intelligent and able to communicate verbally thoughts, feelings, fantasies, and perceptions.

c. **Relative contraindications.**

(1) Discussing unconscious conflicts and examining mechanisms of defense have led to psychotic fragmentation, destructive regression, and/or actualized transference in previous treatments or these are likely to occur based on the evaluation of present ego weaknesses.

(2) The use of exploratory techniques should not preempt the use of more expedient, directive techniques when specific symptoms (e.g., phobia, depression, sexual dysfunction) that demand immediate attention dominate the presenting picture. After the specific dysfunction is being addressed, exploratory techniques may be helpful.

2. **Directive.**

a. **Relative indications.**

(1) The goal is to change maladaptive behaviors and/or symptom reduction (e.g., simple phobias, compulsions, psychophysiologic response patterns, and covert behavior, such as depressive thinking).

(2) The goal is to increase or learn more adaptive behaviors (e.g., problem solving, assertiveness, social skills).

b. **Enabling factors.**

(1) Willingness to take direction from others.

(2) Motivation to do homework assignments.

(3) Willingness to expose oneself to anxiety-provoking situations.

(4) Willingness to accept the focused and limited goals.

c. **Relative contraindications.**

(1) The patient feels the goals are too limited, and techniques are too concrete.

(2) The patient requires a more exploratory process to uncover traumatic memories and emotionally work through their sequelae. Here, it is important that directive techniques do not predominate the therapy when more expressive strategies are indicated.

3. **Experiential.**

a. **Relative indications.**

(1) Intense feelings of existential angst, emptiness, lack of identity, and alienation from self and others.

(2) Difficulty in expressing and/or experiencing an inner emotional world, including responses to others.

(3) Difficulty in perceiving interpersonal cues, including others' emotional responses and social communication.

b. **Enabling factors.**

(1) An ability to be emotionally involved with the therapist or other patients while also accepting the limits of the therapeutic relationship.

(2) The motivation to become more aware of one's own and others' emotions and forms of communication.

c. **Relative contraindications.**

(1) The presence of specific problems that are more amenable to change by more specific techniques.

(2) The tendency to avoid experiencing life by restricting experiential goals to the therapy session.

4. **Supportive.**

a. **Relative indications.**

(1) Patients present ego strengths that require help in adapting to reality and developing coping skills.

(2) The patient's sense of self is deficient and requires the benefit of the therapist's provision of encouragement, reassurance, and nurturing beyond that supplied by the supportive therapeutic relationship.

b. **Enabling factors.**

(1) A willingness to accept praise from a therapist as not being condescending or infantilizing.

(2) An ability to accept encouragement and use this support to a patient's benefit outside of therapy.

c. **Relative contraindications.**

(1) The excessive use of supportive techniques, especially in predominantly exploratory therapies, can inhibit working through transference issues and foster an unnecessarily prolonged dependency on the therapist.

(2) The patient's sense of self does not require support beyond that of the supportive therapeutic relationship, and the provision of such overt encouragement may actually slow the development of the patient's internal resources.

IV. **An overview of the major psychotherapies.** This section will review the major "schools" of psychotherapy and offers one way of conceptualizing and categorizing the different orientations and their specific techniques and proponents. The reader is encouraged to turn to some of the references in the bibliography for a more in-depth understanding of the theoretical and clinical applications of these therapeutic techniques. An excellent source for both a practical and historical perspective on the diverse "vocabulary" of the psychotherapies can be found in Walrond-Skinner's *Dictionary of Psychotherapy* (1986).

The psychotherapies differ in their relative emphasis on the therapeutic relationship vs. therapeutic technique. Techniques differ significantly, i.e., from a markedly passive role of the therapist that allows development of transference and free associations (e.g., psychoanalytic therapy) to very active and directive techniques that urge the patient to think in certain ways and stop behaving in other ways (e.g., rational-emotive therapy). In "pure psychotherapy schools," one technique is felt to be contraindicated in that it will theoretically contaminate the therapeutic endeavor.

More often, the "eclectic" therapist may find it most efficacious to utilize various techniques at different phases in psychotherapy. An example would be the use of experiential techniques to aid an overintellectualized patient to experience emotions in a nonthreatening setting, followed by the use of more uncovering strategies that might involve transference issues. An understanding of the principles of more directive techniques to analyze maladaptive-thinking patterns might also be applied judiciously to increase the flexibility of this patient's rigid intellectual defensive structure. Thus, a given patient may require that the therapist be able to utilize *various* techniques, depending on the primary clinical/therapeutic aim at a particular time.

The following outline may be applied primarily to the individual format, with some general features applicable to the group and family/marital setting. It is adapted from the work of Frances et al. (1984), Karasu (1977 and 1984), and Winston et al. (1986). The reader is encouraged to refer to these works for a more detailed discussion of these therapeutic techniques.

A. **Exploratory psychotherapy.**

   1. **Purpose/goal.**

   a. Reduce rigidity of defensive style and personality structure.

   b. Improve ability to integrate intellectual understanding with emotional insight.

   c. Uncover and "work through" painful past traumatic experiences.

   2. **Clinical data.**

   a. Family of origin information.

   b. Unconscious material brought into awareness, including free association, dreams, and fantasies.

   c. Transference and resistances.

   3. **Role of therapist.**

   a. Neutral; "blank-screen" to foster transference issues.

   b. Anonymous; empathic.

   4. Techniques.

   a. Mirroring (empathic reflection).

   b. Reframing; clarifying; interpreting.

   c. Reconstructing (connecting previously isolated clinical data, especially pertaining to developmental history in the family of origin).

   5. **Specific "schools" and their proponents.**

   a. Classic psychoanalysis (Freud).

   b. Psychoanalytically oriented psychotherapy (Lange).

   c. Individual psychology (Adler).

   d. Interpersonal psychiatry (Sullivan).

   e. Ego analysis (Klein).

Choosing the Appropriate Psychotherapy **499**

   f. Focal therapy (Sifneos).

   g. Time-oriented therapy (Mann).

   h. Character analysis (Horney).

   i. Analytical psychology (Jung).

   j. Intensive psychotherapy (Fromm-Reichman).

   k. Hypnoanalysis (Wolberg).

   l. Guided imagery (Fuller).

B. **Directive psychotherapy.**

   1. **Purpose/goal.**

   a. Change maladaptive behaviors and/or symptom reduction.

   b. Enhance or learn more adaptive behavioral options.

   2. **Clinical data.**

   a. Analysis of symptom-based history and daily log.

   b. Patterns of repeated behavioral sequences.

   c. Analysis of thought patterns and their related behavioral and emotional correlates.

   3. **Role of therapist.**

   4. **Techniques**

   a. Consultant; teacher; advisor.

   4. **Techniques**

   a. Confronting; reassuring; suggestion; desensitization.

   b. Systematic exposure; flooding; modeling; relaxation training.

   c. Self-hypnosis training; paradoxical homework assignments.

   d. Strategic maneuvers; positive reinforcement and contingency contracting.

5. **Specific "schools" and their proponents.**

a. Cognitive therapy (Beck).

b. Reciprocal inhibition therapy (Wolpe).

c. Learning theory therapy (Dollard).

d. Strategic psychotherapy (Haley).

e. Rational-emotive therapy (Ellis).

f. Hypnotherapy (Spiegel).

g. Reality therapy (Glasser).

h. Sex therapy (Kaplan).

i. Direct decision therapy (Greenwald).

j. Biofeedback training (Green).

k. Assertion-structured therapy (Phillips).

l. Interpersonal therapy (Weissman).

C. **Experiential psychotherapy.**

1. **Purpose/goal.**

a. Enhance awareness of inner experience.

b. Improve ability to express emotions.

c. Enhance sense of being understood by another human being.

2. **Clinical data.**

a. "Process" information of the "here and now" experience.

b. Atheoretical/ahistorical.

c. Therapist's inner experience/empathic awareness of patient.

3. **Role of therapist.**

a. Nonauthoritarian; partner or "fellow human being."

4. Techniques.

a. Empathy; "getting" or "being" with the patient; permission for abreaction; imitation; confrontation.

5. Specific "schools" and their proponents.

a. Client-centered therapy (Rogers).

b. Gestalt therapy (Perls).

c. Existential therapy (Yalom).

d. Logotherapy (Frankl).

e. Corrective emotional experience (Alexander).

f. Primal scream therapy (Janov).

g. Zen psychotherapy (Watts).

h. Psychodrama (Moreno).

i. Dance therapy (Barnieff).

j. Art therapy (Naumberg).

D. Supportive psychotherapy.

1. Purpose/goal.

a. Enhance reality testing.

b. Help develop coping skills and reality-adapting behaviors.

c. Provide encouragement and nurturing.

2. Clinical data.

a. Patient's description of daily activities.

b. Interpersonal relatedness to therapist and others.

c. Decision-making abilities.

3. Role of therapist.

a. Parental surrogate; friendly mentor; supportive teacher.

4. **Techniques.**

a. Respectful statement; praise; reassurance; advice.

b. Lending ego functions; education.

5. **Specific "schools" and their proponents.**

a. Various applications of supportive techniques as written by Werman (1984), Kernberg (1984), and Winston et al. (1986).

REFERENCES AND SUGGESTED READING

1. Butheil TG: The psychology of psychopharmacology. *Bull Menninger Clin* 1982; 46:321–330.
2. Frances A, Clarkin JF, Perry S: *Differential Therapeutics in Psychiatry: The Art and Science of Treatment Selection.* New York, Brunner/Mazel, Inc, 1984.
3. Frank J: *Persuasion and Healing.* Baltimore, The Johns Hopkins Press, 1961.
4. Havens L: *Making Contact—Use of Language in Psychotherapy.* Cambridge, Mass, Harvard University Press, 1986.
5. Horowitz M: Stress response syndromes. *Arch Gen Psychiatry* 1974; 31:768–781.
6. Karasu TB (ed): *American Psychiatric Association Commission on Psychotherapies.* Washington, DC, 1984. American Psychiatric Association, 1984.
7. Karasu TB: Psychotherapies: An overview. *Am J Psychiatry*, 1977; 134:8.
8. Lazare A: The psychiatric examination in the walk-in clinic. *Arch Gen Psychiatry* 1976; 33:96–102.
9. Perry S, Cooper AM, Michels R: The psychodynamic formulation: Its purpose, structure and clinical application. *Am J Psychiatry* 1987; 144:543–550.
10. Sullivan HS: *The Psychiatric Interview.* New York, WW Norton & Co, Inc, 1954.

11. Walrond-Skinner S: *A Dictionary of Psychotherapy*. London, Routledge & Kegan Paul, 1986.
12. Werman DS: *The Practice of Supportive Psychotherapy*. New York, Brunner/Mazel, Inc, 1984.
13. Winston A, Pinsker H, McCullough L: A review of supportive psychotherapy. *J Hosp Community Psychiatry* 1986; 37:1105–1114.

30
Psychodynamic Psychotherapies

I. **Introduction.** Psychotherapies can be divided into three major categories: behavioral/directive, experiential, and psychodynamic. These categories refer to the different theoretical constructs that form the foundation for most of the hundreds of kinds of psychotherapies in existence today. These three major theoretical frameworks are found in practice in all types of psychotherapy settings, including individual, group, and family (see Chapters 29, 32, 33, and 36 under those headings). While there are technically pure forms of these theoretical approaches, in practice, a mixture of approaches is usually employed. This chapter will focus on some of the basic concepts in psychodynamic psychotherapy. It is important to mention that during residency training, the patients who are treated by residents are often severely disturbed and require a combination of approaches, with more emphasis usually on behavioral techniques. This is in direct contrast to the experience a resident might be having in his/her own therapy, when a more technically pure psychodynamic approach is warranted. Aside from the practice of psychotherapy, psychodynamic principles are critical to grasp as they are often the preferred method for understanding the personality and development of the individual in psychiatric evaluation.

II. Definitions.

A. **Countertransference.** It is useful to define countertransference as the total emotional response of a therapist to a patient. This reflects the belief, clarified by Otto Kernberg, that the total response includes conscious and unconscious elements and that these elements are reactions to the patient's real and transferential needs. This response, in turn, reflects the therapist's real and transferential needs. It is critical to delineate countertransference, especially when it is negative. The reactions may be subtle and usually impede a patient's progress and a therapist's capacity to work when they are not made conscious.

B. **Defense mechanisms.** These reactions are generated in the unconscious and deflect consciousness from elements that would generate anxiety. Defense mechanisms are normal protective intrapsychic phenomena. Some are considered to be indicative of more mature developmental stages, while others are representative of earlier stages.

1. **Blocking.** This is an inhibition of affect, thinking, or impulse.

2. **Denial.** This involves seeing reality, but refusing to acknowledge it, i.e., negating what is heard, seen, or perceived.

3. **Displacement.** This is an unconscious process that shifts the focus of attention from one subject to another object, usually one less threatening to allow emotional expression in relative safety.

4. **Dissociation.** This is a temporary but drastic modification of character, sense of personal identity, or awareness to avoid emotional distress. It exists on a continuum that ranges from normal dissociative states (brief, nondisruptive) to severe dissociation, resulting in the development of discrete, separate personalities (see Chapter 12 on multiple personality disorder).

5. **Intellectualization.** This is the control of affects and impulses by thinking about them instead of experiencing them. A systematic excess of thinking is used to defend against anxiety that is created by unacceptable impulses or feelings.

6. **Isolation.** This involves intrapsychic splitting or separation of one's affect from content, which results in the repression of either an idea or an affect. It could also result in displacement.

7. **Projection.** This is the perception of one's own feelings in another and the acting on that perception. It is the attribution of one's own unacknowledged feelings to others, e.g., prejudice, suspiciousness.

8. **Projective identification.** This term refers to a process similar to projection. Projection, as a term, has its historical basis in drive theory; projective identification has its roots in object relations theory. Thus, projection has one dimension, subject-object; the process of projective identification adds one more dimension, subject-object-subject (via internal objects in the subject). This process reflects a dynamic structure with internalized objects (internal representations of people and relationships to those people) that are disavowed, split off, and then projected out and into someone else. This process also can elicit behaviors in the object that reflect this disavowed aspect of the subject.

9. **Reaction formation.** This is the management of unacceptable impulses by permitting expression of the impulse in its antithetical form.

10. **Regression.** This is a return to a previous state of psychologic development to avoid anxieties or hostilities experienced in later stages.

11. **Repression.** This refers to expelling and withholding from the conscious state of awareness an idea or a feeling. This exclusionary process is often accompanied by symbolic behavior that may reveal whatever is repressed.

12. **Somatization.** This involves the defensive conversion of emotions, impulses, psychologic conflicts, and feelings into bodily symptoms.

13. **Splitting.** This is a developmentally early mechanism that occurs because ambivalence cannot be tolerated by the developing ego (it is too complex). Experience is understood in all-or-none terms. A person is considered either all good or all bad. Splitting is a common defense in some personality disorders. It is thought to represent arrested development and leads to the consistent impairment in a person's ability to integrate experiences.

14. **Sublimation.** This refers to the indirect or attenuated expression of emotions or instincts without adverse consequences or loss of pleasure. This defense is a late developmental response that allows for the expression of intense emotions in work, art, sports, and other productive outlets. In this process, impulses and affects are transformed into other modes of expression.

C. **Free association.** This is a technique that was used in psychodynamic therapy and originally developed by Freud. A patient should be encouraged to talk as freely as possible, saying whatever comes to mind and not censoring any material. The relationship should be as trusting as possible to facilitate this process. It is, however, true that it is very difficult for anyone to speak uncensored, but the process is encouraged while the difficulty is recognized.

D. **Insight.** This is the intrapsychic process of understanding a psychologic truth. It involves the simultaneous experiencing and observing of affects and/or cognitions. The development of insight is accompanied by feelings and behaviors that then demonstrate enhanced self-understanding. Essentially, there are two types of insight: intellectual and emotional. Intellectual insight is primarily a cognitive process, while emotional insight usually includes both cognitive and affective components. Both types of insight lead to a useful change in the process of therapy. Emotional insight, however, usually yields the most profound realization and acceptance.

E. **Interpretation.** This is the technique used in psychodynamic psychotherapy that connects elements, such as events, affects, and perceptions, into a pattern that patients can then better understand in terms of dominant themes in their lives. It is essentially a formulation or an explanation of behavior or feelings that is placed into a context rather than viewed as isolated. Interpretations are usually based both on an understanding of the patient's life and on a theoretical framework. Interpretations can be made by the therapist or by the patient. It is often true that the interpretations made by the patient are the most enduring.

F. **Psychoanalytic.** This refers to a psychotherapeutic treatment approach that is provided by a therapist who has been trained by one of the psychoanalytic institutes. The course usually involves at least 6 years of training and is not necessarily limited to psychiatrists. This training involves the trainee's own analysis. Patients are usually seen four to five times per week. The therapist, in addition, adheres to technical principles that are common to psychoanalytic therapy: (1) free association, (2) interpretation, (3) dynamic understanding of behavior and emotions, and (4) avoidance of reassurance and guidance with a focus on empathic understanding to allow for the full development of transference.

G. **Psychodynamic.** The original concept refers to the observation that internal forces are in various states of disequilibrium or equilibrium within the psyche. These mental events are the result of the interaction between life experiences and psychobiologic development. This term reflects the complex, changing nature of these forces as unconscious and preconscious elements drive conscious thought, behavior, and affects.

H. **Resistance.** This term refers to a concept that the

mind often works to keep painful, disturbing thoughts and affects outside of awareness. Resistance refers to this phenomenon in the course of psychodynamic psychotherapy. Such resistance may sometimes be adaptive for the individual, since awareness of painful self-truths may lead to overwhelming anxiety.

I. **Transference.** This term has several levels of definition. The classic definition originated with Freud who noted that patients, at times, would react to him as if he were someone else. He concluded that patients were transferring attitudes to him from other significant relationships in their lives because of unresolved conflicts. A broader definition of transference is often most helpful in the process of psychotherapy whereby all subsequent relationships are considered to be interspersed with "transferred" elements. Thus, all of a patient's fears, affects, and patterns of relating, in part, reflect his/her past relationships. The broader concept implies that the patient's dominant life themes (e.g., abandonment, the search for an idealized parent, etc.) are thus recapitulated and can be observed directly in the relationship to the therapist. Interestingly, it is often the seemingly trivial details (e.g., lateness to therapy sessions) that provide the richest source of transference information that can be of crucial benefit for the therapeutic process.

J. **Unconscious.** This term refers to information, memories, thoughts, or feelings that lay outside of awareness. Between the unconscious and conscious is the preconscious that includes elements that can be retrieved relatively easily but that are not immediately available to the conscious mind.

III. **The process of therapy.**

A. **Goals.**

1. To allow a constructive mutually satisfactory relationship to develop.

2. To identify current conflicts and their early developmental antecedents.

3. To elucidate unconscious wishes and fears.

4. To help the patient to develop insight into aspects of the self that may be sabotaging adaptation, personal development, and contentment.

5. To enhance the patient's ability to relate to the self, to others, and to work.

B. **Technical considerations.**

1. **The process of therapy.** A patient's free associations, feelings, and behavior are studied. Special attention is focused on the relationship between the therapist and the patient (the transference relationship), from which critical information is gleaned that allows the patient's maladaptive emotional and behavioral patterns to be revealed. When unconscious conflicts are made conscious and resolved, the typical maladaptive patterns may abate and then may become less destructive in the patient's life. There is also a search during therapy for traumatic events, unresolved issues, such as losses, grief, unexpressed resentments, and unidentified buried affects. Each of these areas is explored as to the meaning to the patient and worked through, with special attention to related thoughts, affects, and behaviors. Dreams also present important sources of data for understanding the psyche. There are several *phases* during this process as follows:

a. **Beginning.** It is important initially to establish rapport and begin building trust with the patient. It is also helpful at this time to establish the formal structure of therapy (see helpful hints section further): the *guidelines*. The patient should be educated as much as possible as to what to expect, what to do, what the theory is, and also as to what therapy is not. Interpretations should be minimal in this phase.

b. **Middle.** This phase involves furthering the therapeutic relationship and elaboration of the basic process of therapy as mentioned above.

c. **Termination.** This phase focuses on separation

issues and reclarification of earlier identified psychodynamic issues.

2. Additional mention must be made of the process of termination that is often the critical focus during residency training. When the therapist and the patient feel satisfactory progress has been made and consolidated, a process of termination should be set in motion. At times, termination can lead to an increase in symptoms sufficient to require the resumption of therapy. The termination phase can often be a difficult time, especially if separation issues were critical in the patient's early development.

C. **Helpful hints in preparing the patient for therapy.**

1. Make appointments as consistently as possible, both in terms of time and place.

2. Explain as much of the process as possible. Include such concepts as free association and transference. Let the patient know that there may be times, such as termination, when a worsening of symptoms may occur as part of the therapeutic process. It is also important to stress the long-term nature of the treatment and to identify any unreasonable expectations early in the phase of treatment.

3. Have a clear vacation and emergency coverage policy with telephone numbers available to the patient.

4. Have a clear policy about missed sessions and about telephone contact with the therapist.

5. Discuss the possibilities, when appropriate, of medication, hospitalization, or alternative forms of treatment.

6. Discuss any potential change in treatment as far in advance as possible to assure the patient that you will assist in any transitions and in finding the appropriate modes of therapy.

7. Do not abandon a patient. Always refer to several alternative types of therapeutic situations. Keep a clear

documentation of your recommendations and transactions.

8. In cases of dangerousness, keep good communication with the patient's whole support system to protect both the patient and/or any potential victims. It is also essential to get good legal supervision on cases when dangerous behavior might occur.

D. **Criteria that favor the use of psychodynamic psychotherapies.**

1. A history of forming lasting relationships.

2. Verbal ability.

3. Ability to think abstractly.

4. Psychotherapy is consistent with the patient's cultural values.

5. The patient is capable of committing reliably to a long-term relationship.

6. The patient is motivated to change. If the patient is willing to make a change only in a specific behavior but does not want a broader approach, then he/she may be referred for behavioral/directive therapy. (See Chapter 31.)

7. The patient is able to tolerate another's point of view.

8. The patient is able to delay gratification.

9. This type of therapy is usually not the appropriate primary mode of treatment for a patient who is suffering from acute psychosis, organic brain syndrome, antisocial personality disorder, or major depressive disorder.

CONTRIBUTORS TO THE FIELD OF PSYCHODYNAMIC THEORY AND PRACTICE

Sigmund Freud was one of the first and most significant contributors to the field of psychodynamic thinking; an incomplete list of additional important authors includes:

Adler, G.	Klein, M.
Bailant, M.	Kohut, H.
Bettelheim, B.	Laing, R. D.
Bion, W. R.	Langs, R.
Erickson, E.	Mahler, M.
Fairbairn, W. R. D.	Rosenfeld, H.
Freud, A.	Searles, H.
Greenson, R.	Sullivan, H. S.
Jung, C.	Winnicott, D. W.
Kernberg, O.	

REFERENCES

1. Baker HS, Baker MN: Heinz Kohut's self psychology: An overview. *Am J Psychiatry* 1987; 144:1–9.
2. Brenner C: *An Elementary Textbook of Psychoanalysis,* revised edition. New York, International University Press, Inc, 1973.
3. Freud S: *Interpretation of Dreams.* New York, Avon Books, 1965.
4. Karasu TB: Psychotherapies: An overview. *Am J Psychiatry* 1977; 134:8.
5. Grotstein JG, Malin A: Projective identification in the therapeutic process. *Int J Psychoanal* 1966; 47:26.
6. Kernberg O: *Borderline Conditions and Pathological Narcissism.* New York, Jason Aronson, Inc, 1975.
7. Kohut H: *The Restoration of the Self.* New York, International University Press, Inc, 1977.
8. Lansky MR: On blame. *Int J Psychoanal Psychotherapy* 1980; 8:429–456.
9. Mason A: *Notes on Melanie Klein,* unpublished lecture, 1984.

31 Behavioral and Cognitive Therapies

I. **Introduction.** It has been argued that insight alone is neither sufficient nor necessary to evoke change. While insight-oriented therapies provide an unstructured and permissive environment in which to examine thoughts and behavior, the actual change is left up to the patient. Most behavioral and cognitive therapies are considered directive therapies, and the therapeutic situation is actively structured by the therapist. In fact, the directive therapist "does not hesitate to use any of the familiar forms of persuasion including exhortation, advice, instruction, and providing a good example" (Frank, 1974). In contrast to insight-oriented therapies, the focus is on conscious problems labeled "symptoms," the therapy is often time limited, and any transference is used more to gain leverage over the patient to help achieve the set goals, than to promote self-understanding.

Generally, behavioral therapies are those that focus on changing observable behaviors, while cognitive therapies are those that focus on changing thoughts.

A clear distinction between the two therapies often cannot be made, and many therapies that contain components of each are aptly termed cognitive-behavioral therapy.

II. **Behavioral therapy.** Formally defined, behavioral therapy is "the use of experimentally established principles and paradigms of learning to overcome unadaptive habits" (Wolpe, 1982). In practice, what is common to all behavioral therapies is the emphasis on behavior, the use of a methodology, and the use of a behavioral analysis to test systematically the hypotheses on which the therapy is based.

The origins of behavioral therapy date back to the 1950s and 1960s, were rooted in the work of experimental psychologists and derived from learning theory, and represented a radical departure from the psychoanalytic view predominant at the time. It was hoped that successful psychotherapeutic methods based on scientific principles could be established. Behavioral therapy developed on several different fronts independently and simultaneously. First, Joseph Wolpe, in 1958, used classical, pavlovian techniques to produce neuroses experimentally in cats. He then developed a method to cure the neuroses. This method became the prototype of systematic desensitization, a technique with wide applicability in psychiatry for eliminating maladaptive anxiety. Second, B. F. Skinner used operant conditioning principles established in animals, and he applied them to humans, making famous the practice of reinforcers to alter behavior. Finally, H. J. Eyesenck and M. B. Shapiro used modern learning theory and stressed the importance of using an experimental approach to the individual patient, thus devising single-case paradigms.

A. **Definitions.** Classical conditioning: This is based on the work of Ivan Pavlov, a Russian physiologist. When a neutral stimulus, such as a bell, is paired with an unconditioned stimulus (one that automatically elicits a response), such as the sight of meat, an animal will learn to respond (i.e., salivate) to the neutral stimulus, that is, the bell, alone. The bell becomes the conditioned stimulus.

Operant conditioning: This is also termed instrumental conditioning and was first demonstrated with animals by R. L. Thorndike, then made famous by B. F. Skinner. The frequency of a response, such as a hungry rat pressing a bar, is determined by the stimulus consequence, such as receiving food, that follows the response. The animal "operates" on environment, and what the animal does is thus instrumental to the outcome.

Reinforcers: These terms are used in operant conditioning. A positive reinforcer is a consequence that increases the likelihood of the associated response occurring, e.g., presenting food in response to lever pressing increases the frequency of lever pressing. A negative reinforcer is a consequence that increases the likelihood that the associated response will occur where the response results in the removal of a negative stimulus. For example, allowing a rat to escape from a shock by pressing the lever increases the frequency of lever pressing.

Extinction: In classical conditioning, when the conditioned stimulus, such as the bell, is repeatedly presented without the unconditioned stimulus, such as the meat, the conditioned response (salivating to the bell alone) gradually disappears. In operant conditioning, a learned response is extinguished by withholding the reinforcer.

Partial reinforcement: Many behaviors are learned by partial reinforcement. For example, temper tantrums may be learned this way in that they are sometimes successful i.e., reinforced, and sometimes not. Behaviors learned by partial reinforcement are very difficult to extinguish.

Spontaneous recovery: Once it appears that a behavior has been extinguished, if the animal is removed from the situation for a matter of days and then returned, the rat will spontaneously resume the behavior that had appeared to be extinguished (i.e., if a rat is cured of running a maze for food, taken out of the maze a few days, and then replaced, the rat will begin running again even though there is no food). The phenomenon of spontaneous recovery and the difficulty of extinguishing behavior learned by partial reinforcement account, in part, for why some habits are so hard to break.

Counterconditioning: Since it is often nearly impossible to extinguish a behavior totally, counterconditioning, the technique whereby one habit is replaced by another, is often useful. It is most effective when the substitute or replacement behavior is incompatible with the undesired behavior.

Positive counterconditioning: When a pleasant stimulus of sufficient strength (such as intense relaxation) is paired with an unpleasant emotion (such as severe anxiety), the unpleasant emotion is over-ridden or neutralized. Systematic desensitization is based on the use of positive counterconditioning.

Negative counterconditioning: When an aversive stimulus of sufficient strength, such as an electric shock, is paired with a pleasant but undesirable response, such as sexual excitement at the sight of a fetish, the sexual excitement will be reduced. Aversive therapy, used for many disorders (sex offenders, alcoholics, and obese persons), is based on negative counterconditioning.

Premack principle: If two behaviors differ in their frequency of occurrence, the frequency of the less likely event can be increased by using the more frequent event as a positive reinforcer. For example, the frequency of a student doing his/her homework may be increased by reinforcing that behavior with a higher frequency behavior, such as watching television.

B. **Specific behavioral therapy techniques.**

1. **Systematic desensitization.** Systematic desensitization is a technique discovered by Joseph Wolpe

and used to reduce maladaptive anxiety. It is based on the principle of reciprocal inhibition that states that anxiety will be extinguished if, at the same time, a psychophysiologic response incompatible with the anxiety (such as intense relaxation) is elicited. The three components of systematic desensitization are the construction of a hierarchy (of the situations provoking anxiety), relaxation training, and the desensitization proper.

a. **Hierarchy construction.** For a given anxiety, the patient is asked to assign a subjective unit of anxiety or "sud" score to different situations that elicit the anxiety. The situations are then arranged according to the sud score in a hierarchy from the situation that elicited the least to the most anxiety. A score of 0 is assigned to a situation in which the patient is completely calm, and a score of 100 to the worst anxiety imaginable. For a polysymptomatic patient, a separate hierarchy is constructed for each problem. Note the sample hierarchy (below) to follow that was constructed by Wolpe (1982) for a 24-year-old woman to be successfully treated for a test anxiety. The sud scores are in parentheses.

Hierarchy: Test Anxiety

1. On the way to the university on the day of an examination. (95)
2. In the process of answering an examination paper. (90)
3. Standing before the unopened doors of the examination room. (80)
4. Awaiting the distribution of examination papers. (70)
5. The examination paper lies face down before her. (60)
6. The night before an examination. (50)
7. One day before an examination. (40)
8. Two days before an examination. (30)
9. Three days before an examination. (20)

10. Four days before an examination. (15)
11. A week before an examination. (10)
12. Two weeks before an examination. (5)

---

b. **Relaxation training.** The patient is taught some method of profound muscular relaxation, usually the progressive relaxation method of Jacobson. This method focuses on tensing and then relaxing all muscle groups in a systematic order. Other methods of relaxation, such as hypnosis or audiotapes, may be used. Wolpe devotes a full six sessions to teach the relaxation.

c. **Desensitization proper.** The patient is first helped to achieve a state of deep relaxation. Once deeply relaxed, he/she is asked to imagine vividly the scene lowest on the hierarchy. The patient is asked to signal the therapist by raising a finger if any anxiety is experienced. The therapist proceeds up the hierarchy, but it is essential that the patient can imagine the scene without anxiety before the next scene is attempted. This may require repeating a scene or even proceeding down the hierarchy. The process is continued until all scenes, including the one that elicits the most anxiety, are able to be imagined vividly without eliciting anxiety.

The expectation is that when the patient can imagine the most anxiety-provoking scene without anxiety, little anxiety will be experienced in the real-life situation. The carryover process into real life should be facilitated by having the patient, between sessions, enter real-life hierarchy scenes that have been successfully imagined in the relaxed state without producing anxiety. It is very important that the patient not be sent prematurely into the situation that previously provoked anxiety, lest the patient become anxious, flee, and reinforce the avoidance behavior. Supportive and enthusiastic reinforcement from the therapist as the patient proceeds up the hierarchy is very powerful.

d. Clinical application. Indications include any anxiety where the stimulus that triggers the anxiety can be identified. Treatable disorders include phobias, such as claustrophobia, agoraphobia, and snake phobia, a host of anxieties, including test anxiety, fear of disapproval, and social anxiety, and some cases of obsessive-compulsive disorders. Limitations include some obsessive-compulsive disorders, situations in which the phobic behavior is strongly reinforced (such as an agoraphobic whose behavior is strongly reinforced by family members, in which case behavioral family therapy may be needed as well), and spontaneous panic attacks in which there is no identifiable stimulus for the anxiety. Spontaneous panic attacks may precede the development of anticipatory anxiety, and in such cases, medication (tricyclic antidepressants or monoamine oxidase inhibitors) alone or in addition to systmatic desensitization is indicated. The average duration of treatment based on Wolpe's (1982) successful treatment of 68 patients was 11 sessions/fear.

2. Treatment of sexual dysfunction. The behavioral therapist approach to the treatment of sexual dysfunction is based on the assumption that sexual dysfunction is a learned maladaptive behavior. Specifically, anxiety has become a conditioned response to some stimulus associated with sexual functioning, and it has come to inhibit the natural response of intense arousal and pleasure. Therapy consists of using the pleasurable response produced by arousal to overcome and inhibit the anxiety response with which it is incompatible; thus, it is very similar to systematic desensitization in that a relaxed and pleasurable state is used to overcome anxiety. A difference is that the treatment of sexual dysfunction is carried out in the real-life situation. The first step is to define the exact point at which the anxiety begins. The patient is then trained to proceed in a stepwise manner up a hierarchy, such that, at each step, the pleasure from arousal is sufficient to inhibit the anxiety previously associated with that step. This is continued until the patient is able to achieve orgasm or intercourse without anxiety.

a. **Clinical application.** Indications include inadequate penile erections and premature ejaculation in men, inability to achieve orgasm in women, general inhibition of arousal, and situational frigidity. Limitations include cases where there is an underlying physical cause for the dysfunction (e.g., diabetes mellitus causing erectile dysfunction in men) or a pharmacologic agent causing sexual dysfunction (e.g., many tricyclic antidepressants, neuroleptics, antihypertensives, etc). Regarding duration, in a study by Wolpe (1982), 78% of a group of men with an inhibited sexual response were successfully treated with an average of 11 sessions. In addition to the general treatment outlined, partner participation and assertiveness training to help the patient openly discuss his/her desires may be employed.

3. **Token economies: positive reinforcement and extinction.** The token economy is based on the principle of operant conditioning, i.e., the frequency of a certain behavior will be increased if it is followed by a positive consequence. The development of the token economy is credited to Ayllon and Azrin (1968) who began a program for "hopeless" long-term institutionalized psychotic patients in a state hospital. The patients were given the opportunity to take on "jobs" that consisted of self-care activities, such as grooming, making their own beds, etc. They were rewarded with tokens that could be exchanged for desirable items (candy, cigarettes, etc.). In addition to the positive reinforcement, negative behaviors, such as head banging and delusional speech, were ignored on the principle that many such behaviors were being inadvertently reinforced by the staff, and that they could therefore be extinguished by discontinuing the reinforcement. A study by Paul and Lentz (1977) that compared patient treatment on a "token economy" ward, compared with

a "milieu therapy" ward, demonstrated a 89% improvement in the former compared with a 46% improvement in the latter. In addition to patient improvement, the staff morale was raised, and the ward became cleaner. Verbal reinforcement for appropriate behaviors is also very effective. A schizophrenic patient who continues to burn himself/herself with a cigarette can be examined and praised at intervals when found free of burns, until his/her habit is extinguished.

4. **Aversive therapy.** Aversive therapies are based on the principle that many behaviors are performed to avoid unpleasant consequences. There are three main types: (1) classical conditioning in which a noxious stimulus, such as a shock, is paired with the stimulus leading to the unwanted behavior, such as the sight of alcohol; (2) punishment in which the problem behavior, such as drinking alcohol, is followed by a noxious stimulus, such as a shock; and (3) avoidance training in which a noxious stimulus can be avoided by avoiding the problem behavior, such as a patient receiving disulfiram (Antabuse) can avoid vomiting by avoiding alcohol.

a. **Clinical application.** Regarding indications, aversive procedures are most useful in two general cases: (1) situations where the problem behavior is naturally reinforcing to the patient, such as alcohol and drug abuse, smoking, sexual offenders, and overeating; and (2) cases where the behavior is self-destructive and must be immediately controlled. A variety of techniques are available for each problem behavior, and the aversive techniques are most effective when used in conjunction with other forms of treatment that help reinforce the desired behavior. It has been established that aversive therapy carried out in the imagination alone (imagining taking a drink and then vomiting all over oneself) is also effective (Cautela, 1971). Lovaas and Simmons (1969) demonstrated the effectiveness of aversive therapy for self-destructive behavior in a 16-year-old retarded girl. The girl had bitten her hands (one finger required amputation), banged her head, and ripped out her nails. Following such behaviors, five 1-second shocks were delivered, and her behavior was eliminated.

Sexual offenders have been successfully treated with aversive therapy. Men convicted of repeated rapes are required to watch videos of sexual offenses while their penile tumescence is monitored. An electric shock is delivered once they become sexually aroused. Limitations include unmotivated patients (in which there is little carryover into the real-life situation), patients unable to give consent, and patients particularly sensitive to any painful procedure used. The duration is highly variable and depends on the behavior involved.

5. **Flooding and implosive therapy.** Flooding and implosive therapy are examples of exposure therapies and are used to treat classically conditioned fears, as is systematic desensitization. While the latter technique is based on pairing imagined anxiety-provoking scenes with a state of relaxation, the exposure therapies are based on prolonged exposure to the actual feared stimulus. The assumption is that if a person is exposed to the feared situation (placing an acrophobic on the roof of a 20-story building) long enough, and the fear is not reinforced (nothing bad happens), then the fear will be extinguished. It is essential that the exposure be continued until there is a reduction in the anxiety. Flooding is carried out by in vivo exposure to the feared stimulus, whereas implosive therapy is carried out in the imagination. An acrophobic would be treated by flooding by taking him/her to the top of a tall building and forcing him/her to stay there until the fear began to diminish. This usually takes 5 to 25 minutes the first time but less time when repeated in 1 to 2 days. Additional sessions are held regularly until there is no or little anxiety. Additional sessions are then held at increasing intervals to prevent spontaneous recovery. It is very important that the patient not withdraw from treatment until it is completed, as withdrawal may reinforce the fear and the phobic behavior.

a. **Clinical application.** Indications include agoraphobia, simple phobias, obsessive-compulsive disorders (especially those that involve fears of contamination), post-traumatic stress disorders, and some types of sexual dysfunction. Limitations include certain disorders that may require, in addition, the use of medication (agoraphobia, obsessive-compulsive disorders) and cases where the anxiety evoked by direct exposure could be physically damaging (taking a post-MI patient to the top of a tall building). In addition, there are cases where the fear is nonextinguishable by repeated exposure (some cases of acrophobics), and the stronger the emotional arousal, the more difficult to extinguish. In such cases, graded exposure may be useful in which the full exposure is built up to in small steps. The duration and frequency of exposure depend on the particular problem.

6. **Modeling.** Modeling or observational learning has been shown by Albert Bandura to be a faster and more effective way of learning than learning by reinforcement in many cases. Modeling is usually carried out in a stepwise fashion as, e.g., in the treatment of a child with a dog phobia, and it may either be accomplished symbolically (watching a film of the modeled behavior) or by live modeling with graded participation. The latter has been shown to be more effective. In the treatment of a child with a dog phobia, modeling might begin by watching the model see the dog in the distance; then, the model should begin to approach the dog, stand next to the dog, and finally pet the dog. The model would, in addition, help the child participate until he/she was able to do so without fear.

7. **Treatment of eating disorders.** Behavioral therapy techniques exist for the treatment of anorexia nervosa, bulimia, and obesity and are based primarily on the principles of operant conditioning, namely, the use of rewards and punishment. Most behavioral programs for anorexia nervosa and bulimia take place within the hospital. Anorectic patients are given a goal weight and

rewarded for weight gains by being granted visiting passes and more freedom in the hospital, and they are allowed to exercise. They may be punished by a restriction of these privileges and tube feeding when indicated. Similarly, bulimic patients are rewarded for maintaining a normal weight and for not binging, purging, or using laxatives. A contract is often drawn up defining clearly the goals and desired behavior, as well as the consequences of the actual behavior in terms of the rewards and punishments. In the treatment of anorectic patients, it is important that the emphasis be on the actual weight (which should be gradual, i.e., approximately 0.25 lb/day) rather than on eating disorders, to minimize strife between staff and patient. Regarding the frequency of the reinforcement, the treatment of obesity is more often done on an outpatient basis and includes teaching the patient to identify the antecedent stimulus associated with overeating, teaching relaxation techniques as competing responses to eating, and teaching how to use rewards and punishments effectively.

a. **Clinical applications.** Indications include anorexia nervosa, bulimia, and obesity. Regarding limitations, behavioral therapy for the treatment of anorexia is most effective in the severe stage of the illness, requiring medical management and nutritional support. However, several studies show that when compared with other treatments carried out in the hospital, there is no advantage, especially in the long run to behavior therapy (Eckert et al., 1979; Pertschuk, 1977; and Garfinkel et al., 1977). The treatment of bulimia by behavioral therapy has been more successful, especially when combined with cognitive therapy (Fairburn, 1981). The use of tricyclic antidepressants and monoamine oxidase inhibitors has also shown some benefit in the treatment of bulimia (Pope and Hudson, 1984). Behavioral therapy for weight loss has been shown to be superior to social pressure and insight-oriented groups (Wollersheim, 1970).

8. **Behavioral medicine.** Behavioral therapy techniques have many applications to the treatment and prevention of medical disorders. Many of the problem behaviors, as well as the techniques, have already been mentioned. Relaxation training may be useful in the treatment of essential hypertension: (1) to change from a type A behavior pattern to type B to reduce the risk of cardiovascular heart disease, and (2) to help avoid unwanted behaviors that may occur more while under stress, such as overeating, substance abuse, and smoking. Many of these disorders, referred to as disorders of self-control, may be changed by using a reward-and-punishment system. Other applications include using reinforcement to help with noncompliance to medications, as, e.g., with an insulin-dependent diabetic patient who refuses to take insulin.

9. **Assertion training.** Assertion training is a type of social skills training that is based on the assumption that people have a right to express their attitudes, beliefs, and desires, and it supplies patients with an increased behavioral repertoire. It includes the following basic strategies: instruction (teaching the patient to speak clearly and make eye contact); feedback by the instructor on a given behavior, modeling by the instructor, of the desired behavior, behavior rehearsal (role-playing of difficult situations); and social reinforcement by the instructor and other participants (this would include shaping, which is the reinforcement of behaviors that approach the desired behavior); and homework assignments (practicing the skills in real life, recording successes, etc.) (Bellack and Herson, 1977).

a. **Clinical application.** Regarding indications, training is useful for patients with interpersonal difficulties, particularly those who are overly polite, unable to say no, unable to express positive or negative emotions, and unable to ask for what they want. Many types of assertion training employ the principle of cognitive therapy to help the patient deal with negative self-statements and self-defeating beliefs that may underlie the unassertive behaviors. The duration is often eight to 12 weekly sessions. For further details and a good resource for patients, the reader is referred to *Your Perfect Right: A Guide to Assertive Behavior* by Alberti and Emmons (1982).

III. **Cognitive therapy.** "Men are disturbed not by events, but by the views which they take of them."

The central tenet of cognitive therapy is that the way in which individuals think will determine how they feel and behave. When a young boy sees a dog and thinks, "this is dangerous," he may feel afraid and run. When the same boy sees a dog and thinks, "this is safe," he may feel safe and approach the dog. The goal of cognitive therapy is to identify and correct any thoughts that lead to undesirable feelings and behaviors.

The theoretical underpinnings of cognitive therapy are rich, diverse, and date back at least to the Greek stoic philosophers. The principles on which cognitive therapy are based are ones that are widely used and not unique to cognitive therapy: e.g., psychoanalysis places a strong emphasis on examining one's internal dialogues that underlie beliefs and the effect that these have on behavior.

Cognitive therapy generally refers to that developed by Aaron Beck et al. (1976 and 1979), and rational-emotive therapy (RET) is that developed independently by Albert Ellis (1962, 1973, and 1977). Both therapies are usually time limited, directive, and structured, and they focus on the alleviation of symptoms caused by the dysfunction thoughts. The relationship between the patient and therapist is one of collaboration, and although great importance is assigned to understanding the patient's internal dialogue, no mention is made of unconscious processes. Indications for these therapies include the treatment of depression, anxiety, phobias, pain, and psychosomatic illnesses.

Important and more recent contributions to the cognitive-behavior therapies that will not be discussed here include the multimodal therapy of Arnold Lazarus (1976 and 1981), the cognitive-behavior modification of Donald Meichenbaum (1977), and the rational behavior therapy of Maxie Maultsby (1984).

A. Beck's cognitive therapy. Aaron Beck, a psychoanalytically trained psychiatrist, is credited with the development of cognitive therapy. Cognitive therapy is best known for its application to the treatment of depression, but it has also been extensively developed for the treatment of anxiety and phobias. For a discussion of the latter two applications, the reader is referred elsewhere (Beck and Emery, 1984). Cognitive therapy is best explained by examining its three component parts: (1) the cognitive triad, (2) the cognitive distortions, and (3) the underlying assumptions.

1. **The cognitive triad.** Depression can be explained as the activation of a set of three cognitive patterns: People become depressed when they begin to view themselves negatively, the world negatively, and the future negatively.

a. Negative view of the self: "I'm ugly, stupid, a failure, etc."

b. Negative view of the world: "This shouldn't happen, life isn't fair, etc."

c. Negative view of the future: "I'll always feel bad and have this problem."

2. **Cognitive distortions.** The thinking of depressed individuals actually becomes distorted and different than when they are not depressed. Examples of cognitive distortions that are characteristic of depressed people follow. A depressed person may use any combination. For a practical guide to identifying and correcting cognitive distortions, the reader (and patient) is referred to *Feeling Good: The New Mood Therapy* by Burns (1980).

a. **All-or-nothing thinking.** This refers to evaluating one's performance in black-and-white categories and feeling like you failed if you got less than 100% on the examination.

b. **Overgeneralization.** Because one person turns you down, you think "no girl will ever go out with me."

c. **Arbitrary inference or jumping to conclusions.** You know your friend is thinking something bad about you by the way he/she cleared his/her throat.

d. **Catastrophizing.** A shy person thinks something horrible will happen if someone notices he/she looks uneasy at a party.

e. **Magnification and minimization.** A depressed person magnifies his/her own shortcomings and the positive qualities of others while minimizing his/her own positive qualities and the shortcomings of others.

f. **Disqualifying the positive.** You get the highest score of the anatomy final and say, "It doesn't mean anything, I had anatomy in college."

g. **Selective abstraction.** A small detail is focused on negatively and colors all of reality. You get a haircut that you don't like.

h. **Labeling/mislabeling.** You negatively label yourself on the basis of some behavior, and you believe the label adequately describes you. After going off your diet and eating ice cream you say, "I am a pig with no self-control."

i. **Personalization.** You take responsibility and blame yourself for things for which you are not responsible.

j. **"Should" Statements: "Masturbatory" Thinking According to Ellis.** Although you are depressed, you think, "I should always be happy, I should have more energy, I should be confident, etc."

3. **Underlying assumptions.** Every person has a set of beliefs or rules about how he/she should behave that developed out of the religious, social, cultural, fam-

ily, and legal background in which the person was raised. These underlying assumptions about how one should behave can give rise to cognitive distortions and undesirable behaviors and feelings. It is the job of the cognitive therapist to not stop at identifying the cognitive distortions but to examine the underlying assumptions. The patient is then given the opportunity to change the beliefs or assumptions that may be causing undesirable feelings and behaviors.

4. **Daily log of dysfunctional beliefs.** To teach the patient how thoughts lead to feelings, and particularly how maladaptive or dysfunctional thoughts lead to unpleasant emotions, homework, such as the following daily log, is assigned. Of utmost importance in cognitive therapy is the ability to catch and identify "automatic thoughts." Such thoughts, which occur so quickly and automatically that they are often not even noticed, are often the cause of the unpleasant reaction to a situation. Once identified, automatic thought may be replaced by a more rational thought and result in a more positive outcome.

The following (Table 31–1) is structured after the log presented by Beck et al. (1979) in *Cognitive Therapy of Depression*.

5. **A clinical example.** A young college student presents for the treatment of depression. She learns to identify and correct many cognitive distortions. In attempting to determine what dysfunctional assumptions underlie her distortions, it is found that as a child she was praised for bringing home all As but ignored and berated for bringing home anything less. She is currently left depressed when she is unable to perform perfectly, and she is operating under the belief "to be valued, I must perform perfectly." Once identified, given the opportunity to change this to a more adaptive belief, such as "I am still valuable when I don't perform perfectly," the latter belief will result in a much more positive, less depressed state than the former.

TABLE 31–1.
Daily Log

Date	Situation	Emotion	Automatic Thought	Rational Response	Outcome
1/1	Friend does not acknowledge you on the street	Rejection	"She doesn't like me anymore"	"I don't know if she saw me"	Relief
1/2	Received a "C" on an examination	Anxious/angry	"I'll never be a success"	"One examination does not determine my success"	Hopeful

6. **Clinical application.** The indications of cognitive therapy have been mentioned (depression, anxiety, phobias, and psychosomatic illnesses). Limitations include psychotic depressions and some depressions that require hospitalization (especially those with melancholia and those that require electroconvulsive therapy). Most studies that have demonstrated the efficacy of cognitive therapy have been conducted on nonpsychotic outpatients, and they have shown cognitive therapy to be as effective as pharmacotherapy in this group. Furthermore, one study of moderately to severely depressed outpatients, most of whom were suicidal and had been depressed intermittently or continuously for 8 years, showed that those patients who were treated with cognitive therapy alone had a greater recovery rate, a lesser dropout rate, and more rapid improvement than those patients who were treated with antidepressants alone (Rush et al., 1977). A recent systematic analysis of all controlled studies between 1974 and 1984 on outpatients with unipolar depression has demonstrated that the combined treatment of pharmacotherapy plus cognitive therapy is slightly superior to pharmacotherapy or cognitive therapy alone. The group treated with pharmacotherapy had the greatest relapse rate at 6 months. The relapse rate in the group treated with pharmacotherapy was even greater when hospitalized patients were studied, raising the question of the prophylactic value of cognitive therapy in hospitalized patients (Blackburn et al., 1986).

B. **Rational emotive therapy.** Rational-emotive therapy was first called rational therapy to emphasize the cognitive and philosophic (RET) aspects of it, including Ellis' belief that if one holds a sane view of life, emotional disturbance would rarely occur. The word emotive was added to stress the strong evocative and behavioral components (including in vivo desensitization, homework assignments, and direct confrontation) and to distinguish this therapy from others that were more passive (such as classical analysis and rogerian client-centered therapy).

1. **The philosophy of RET.** The goal of RET is "to help people live longer, minimize their emotional disturbances and self-defeating behaviors, and actualize themselves so that they live a more fulfilling, happier existence" (Ellis and Bernard, 1985). This is accomplished by helping people think more rationally (i.e., flexibly, clearly, and scientifically) and feel more appropriately. Ellis states that inappropriate feelings result from absolutistic or "masturbatory" thinking (the use of musts, shoulds, and oughts): If a husband is left by his wife and thinks, "I absolutely must get her back," he is likely to feel depressed and worthless if this does not happen (inappropriate feelings); however, if he treats this as a preference and says, "I want her to come back but I can survive if she doesn't, he is likely to feel appropriate feelings of sorrow, regret, and disappointment if she does not come back, but not depression and worthlessness.

Rational-emotive therapy holds that the scientific method is the best way to determine which methods are most effective for helping people accomplish these goals. It states that people are born with the capacity for both straight and crooked thinking, but that if one is to change, it requires a concerted effort and practice. Without this, behavior will not change. In contrast to many other therapies, there is no emphasis on attempting to raise one's self-esteem. Rather, the focus is on self-acceptance and on rating behaviors or performance but not one's self or essence. Rational-emotive therapy may go beyond treatment of symptoms and profoundly affect one's personal philosophy. Although RET attempts to be "scientific," it does not claim to be without values. The following is a list of "rational attitudes" that Ellis and Bernard (1985) stated would be beneficial for a person to strive to internalize:

a. Self-interests.

b. Social interests.

c. Self-direction.

d. High frustration tolerance.
e. Flexibility.
f. Acceptance of uncertainty.
g. Commitment to creative pursuits.
h. Scientific thinking.
i. Self-acceptance.
j. Risk taking.
k. Long-range hedonism.
l. Nonutopianism.
m. Self-responsibility.

2. **The ABCs of RET.** Rational-emotive therapy is best known for the ABC's of irrational thinking and emotional disturbance. *A* stands for the activating event (a situation, behavior, and/or thought), *B* stands for the intervening belief (cognition, attitude, self-statement, and/or image), and *C* stands for the consequence (emotional state, behavior, and/or thought). The basic tenet of RET is that when an event occurs (you get fired), it is not the event itself that causes the consequence (your depressed feeling), but rather it is the intervening belief(s) ("I'm a failure. I'll never get another job. My life is ruined.") that causes the feeling. The irrationally held belief may be disputed, *D*, and replaced with a more rational statement ("Even though I lost this job, I will be able to get another one. Losing a job doesn't make me a failure"). The effect, *E*, of disputing the belief is a change in the consequence or feeling (you now feel regret that you lost the job, but hopeful about the future and not depressed).

3. **Clinical application and techniques used in RET.** Indications and useful applications of RET include the treatment of depression, anxiety, phobias, personality disorders, psychotic disorders, sexual and relational problems, and social skills training. The duration is often a few months.

The primary cognitive technique used in disrupting irrational beliefs has been demonstrated above (see the ABCs). The therapist may actively argue the irrational belief with the patient, may assign homework instructing the patient to come up with a list of alternate rational responses, and may instruct the patient to test out the accuracy of the belief in vivo. For example, a shy teenage boy who believes, "No girls will go out with me" may be instructed to go to the local park, ask out 50 girls, and then report back on whether or not his belief, that no girl would go out with him, was correct. Although in vivo techniques are often preferred, rational-emotive imagery is also used. Attention is paid to self-talk, particularly to minimize thinking in absolutistic terms, such as should, must, and ought, and to upgrade such demands to preferences.

BIBLIOGRAPHY

1. Ayllon T, Azrin N: *The Token Economy: A Motivation System for Therapy and Rehabilitation.* East Norwalk, Conn, Appleton-Century-Crofts, 1968.
2. Alberti RE, Emmons ML: *Your Perfect Right: A Guide to Assertive Behavior,* ed. 4. San Luis Obispo, Calif, Impact Publishers, 1982.
3. Bandura A, Blanchard ED, Ritter B: Relative efficacy of desensitization and modeling approaches for inducing behavioral, affective and attitudinal changes. *J Pers Soc Psychol* 1969; 13:173.
4. Beck A: *Cognitive Therapy and Emotional Disorders.* New York, International University Press, Inc, 1976.
5. Beck AT, Emery G: *Anxiety and Phobias: A Cognitive Approach.* New York, Basic Book Inc Publishers, 1984.

6. Beck AT, Rush AF, Emery G: *Cognitive Therapy of Depression*. New York, Guilford Press, 1979.
7. Bellack AS, Herson M: *Behavior Modification: An Introduction Textbook*. Baltimore, Williams & Wilkins, 1977.
8. Blackburn, IM, Eunson KM, Bishop S: A two-year naturalistic follow-up of depressed patients treated with cognitive therapy and a combination of both. *J Affective Disord* 1986; 10:67–75.
9. Burns DD: *Feeling Good: The New Mood Therapy*. New York, Signet—New American Library, Inc, 1980.
10. Conte HR, Plutchik R, Wild KV, et al: Combined psychotherapy and pharmacotherapy for depression: A systematic analysis of the evidence. *Arch Gen Psychiatry* 1986; 43:471–479.
11. Cautela JR: Covert conditioning, in Jacobs A, Sachs LB (eds): *The Psychology of Private Events*. Orlando Fla, Academic Press, Inc, 1971, pp 109–131.
12. Eckert ED, Goldberg SC, Halmi KA, et al: Behavior therapy in anorexia nervosa. *Br J Psychiatry* 1979; 134:55–59.
13. Ellis A: *Reason and Emotion in Psychotherapy*. Secaucus, NJ, Lyle Stuart, Inc, 1962.
14. Ellis A: *Humanistic Psychotherapy:* The Rational-Emotive Approach. New York, Julian Press, 1973.
15. Ellis A, Gieger R (eds): *The Handbook of Rational-Emotive Therapy*. New York, Springer-Verlag NY, Inc, 1977.
16. Ellis A, Bernard ME: Clinical applications of rational-emotive therapy, in *What is Rational-Emotive Therapy?* New York, Plenum Press, 1985, p 5.
17. Fairburn CG: A cognitive behavioral approach to the management of bulimia. *Psychol Med* 1981; 11:707–711.
18. Garfinkel PE, Moldofsky H, Garner DM: The outcome of anorexia nervosa: Significance of clincial features, body image, and behavior

modifications, in Vigersky RA (ed): *Anorexia Nervosa*. New York, Raven Press, 1971, pp 315–329.
19. Frank JD: *Persuasion and Healing*. New York, Schocken Books, Inc, 1974, p 235.
20. Lazarus A: *Multimodal Behavioral Therapy*. New York, Springer-Verlag NY, Inc, 1976.
21. Lazarus A: *The Practice of Multimodal Therapy*. New York, McGraw-Hill International Book Co, 1981.
22. Lovaas, OI, Simmons JQ: Manipulation of self-destruction in three retarded children. *J Appl Behav Anal* 1969; 2:143.
23. Masters WH, Johnson VE: *Human Sexual Inadequacy*. Boston, Little Brown & Co, Inc, 1970.
24. Maultsby MC: *Rational Behavioral Therapy*. Englewood Cliffs, NJ, Prentice-Hall International, Inc, 1984.
25. Meichenbaum D: *Cognitive-Behavior Modification: An Integrative Approach*. New York, Plenum Press, 1977.
26. Paul GL, Lentz RJ: *Psychosocial Treatment of Chronic Mental Patients*. Cambridge, Mass, Harvard University Press, 1977.
27. Pertschuk MJ: Behavior therapy: Extended follow-up, in Vigersky RA (ed): *Anorexia Nervosa*. New York, Raven Press, 1977.
28. Pope HG, Hudson JI: *New Hope for Binge Eaters*. New York, Harper & Row Publishers, Inc, 1984.
29. Rush AJ, Beck AT, Kovacs M, et al: Comparative efficacy of cognitive therapy and pharmacotherapy in the treatment of depressed outpatients. *Cognitive Ther Res* 1977; 1:17–38.
30. Wollersheim JP: Effectiveness of group therapy based upon learning principles in the treatment of overweight women. *J Abnorm Psychol* 1970; 176:462–474.
31. Wolpe J: *The Practice of Behavior Therapy*, ed 3. Elmsford, NY, Pergamon Press, Inc, 1982, p 152.

32
Family Therapy

I. **Family assessment.** Before considering whether family therapy is indicated and should be started, an initial family meeting and assessment are required. Many investigators believe that a family evaluation should be done on every patient, but family therapy should not. A thorough family evaluation may provide additional insight and perspective on work with individual cases even when family therapy is not involved. The ways an individual relates to, perceives, and thinks about his/her environment are influenced by his/her family of origin and his/her current family situation. Utilizing a family assessment and the principles of family systems can lead to a more accurate diagnosis, appropriate treatment, improved compliance, and attempts for prevention.

A. **Practical considerations in family assessment.** As with individual therapy, in family therapy, there are many theoretical orientations that may influence the way a therapist will assess a family. This guide integrates a variety of approaches.

1. **Preinterview task: preparation.** From the initial contact or referral, the therapist should obtain basic information on the family structure and the nature of the presenting problem. At this stage, one may begin

to develop tentative hypotheses to test in the interview. Of note, families pass through various stages as they form, expand, and contract. The sequence of characteristic stages that families go through has been labeled the *family life cycle*. With a knowledge of the family life cycle, one may be able to predict the problems and tasks expected at that stage. One may develop a strategy in preparation for the family meeting, including specific questions.

2. **Greet and join the family.** The therapist should introduce himself/herself, welcome and identify the family members, and invite the family members to sit where they wish (this may give additional information about the family). The seating can always be changed later. Establishing rapport is very crucial, and its importance cannot be understated. The therapist should increase contact with each family member, be aware of the mood of the family and how the members interact with the therapist, and observe the verbal and nonverbal relationship between family members and family subgroups (siblings, parents-children, and the marital couple).

3. **Identify the stated problem.** The therapist should explore each family member's view of the problem, what solutions have been tried, and what is the desired outcome of the current effort for change.

4. **Assess the current functioning of the family.**

a. Observe interactions between family members.

b. Ask questions that bear on the relationships between the members (consider specific behaviors) and study the family's verbal and nonverbal responses.

c. Develop some hypotheses about the family system; tentatively accept these hypotheses to provide a basis for further investigation, from which a verification or refutation can be made.

d. Look for "triangles," i.e., two people in conflict tend to involve a third person in the conflict.

e. Maintain an empathic and neutral position.

f. Recognize the strengths in the family and individual members.

g. Focus on the relationship patterns and habitual ways of interacting.

5. **Review the family's history and construct a genogram.**

a. These assessments are helpful when time permits.

b. For more detail, see Section B.

6. **Develop a diagnostic formulation.**

a. This is done in preparation for providing the family feedback, defining goals, and making recommendations.

b. Consider what you have learned about the family structure and dynamics.

c. Following the interview, a complete family assessment and formulation can be synthesized. A complete diagnostic formulation will be described later.

7. **Family feedback and recommendations.**

a. These can be the start of therapy (if indicated).

b. Give family members more options and alternatives to consider with regard to family dynamics.

c. Arrange whatever further interviews or referrals that you recommend.

B. **The genogram (Fig 32–1).**

1. This gives a concise, graphic summary of a family's current composition.

2. This is a structural representation of the family structure and includes the extended family network, the ages of family members, and the dates of any marriages, divorces, or separations. It also shows who is the identified patient.

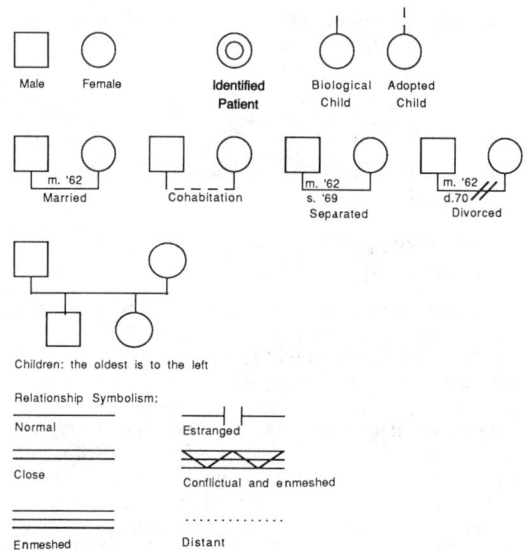

FIG 32–1.
Genogram symbolism. m. = married; s. = separated; d. = divorced.

3. Any information may be included, e.g., details on the health, behavior, strengths, or weaknesses.

4. You may actively involve all family members in making the genogram. This may improve rapport, and get the family to share information and express feelings about the people and events that are discussed.

C. **The family life cycle.** Families pass through various stages as they form, expand, and contract. Each family has a beginning and an end, and is changing over time. Also, the family operates in a changing cultural system. The sequence of characteristic stages has been characterized by several theorists and comprises the following six stages (Haley, 1973):

1. The courtship period.
2. Marriage and its consequences.
3. Childbirth and dealing with the young.
4. Middle marriage.
5. Weaning parents from children.
6. Retirement and old age.

The family has phase-specific developmental tasks in each stage. Presenting problems may be "normal" difficulties for a family in that specific stage, or the problems may represent a maladaptive response to specific stresses of a given stage. Also, chronic problems from a previous stage may still be unresolved. Failure to complete early stages leads to difficulties with later stages. Problems can occur either in a specific stage, or as a family is trying to make a transition to the next stage.

D. **Diagnostic formulation.** Through a formulation, one describes and explains the family's problems and situation. The formulation can be then used as a basis for developing a therapeutic plan. To assess families, it is often necessary to have a theoretical model of how families function and of the ways the functioning becomes dysfunctional. The major models or school of family therapy can be grouped into the structural, strategic, transgenerational, experiential, and behavioral models. These models will be described in more detail later; however, several techniques are available for assessment of families as follows.

1. **Practice.** This is a family assessment tool. The acronym PRACTICE is a tool based on a systems approach and can serve as a guide and a record for a

family interview. The components of the schema are as follows:

Presenting problem or reason for interview.

Roles and structure, including hierarchical organization, boundaries, and individuation, cohesion (from disengagement to enmeshment), and control (from chaos to rigidity).

Affect (emotional expression), i.e., family emotional tone (warmth, sadness, anger, and humor).

Communication (verbal and nonverbal).

Time in the family life cycle. The dynamics of developmental stages are experienced differently by each family and may influence the occurrence and response to illness.

Illness in the family, past and present. A presenting problem may mask dysfunction in the family. Past experiences will influence current problems.

Coping with stress (adaptability, family strengths and resources, and coping in past and present).

Ecology and culture (interaction of the family with the environment). Social, cultural, religious, economic, educational, and medical resources (SCREEM).

2. **Integrated family therapy.** Various authors have emphasized a distinction between the "surface action" of a family (that which is observed) and the underpinning explanatory mechanisms. The therapist must be able to identify "dysfunctional transactional processes," which are defined as maladaptive processes that are directed toward reducing anxiety in the family (see part 6 below).

In this approach, the therapist must ask three questions: First, how is the family's surface action linked to dysfunctional transactional processes in the family? Second, how are the surface action and dysfunctional transactional processes linked with past events, states, and relationships that have been particularly stressful or traumatic for the family? Third, what immediate precipitant, if any, has affected or threatened family homeostasis and resulted in the family's presenting now? The construction of a formulation has four main components.

a. Regarding surface action, this group uses the McMaster dimensions of family functioning as a framework.

b. Dysfunctional transactional processes that may underpin and derive this surface action are identified. Authorities have labeled eight maladaptive processes that are directed toward reducing anxiety: *displacement* (family may avoid a threatening one), *scapegoating, triangulation, family beliefs and family myths, projective identification, persistent dysfunctional communication, manic defenses against depression, and defenses against schizoid anxieties*.

c. The McMaster model of family functioning considers six aspects of family functioning: problem solving, communication, roles, affective responsiveness, affective involvement, and behavioral control (see Table 32–1).

d. **The circumplex model.** Family behavior is grouped into three dimensions: *cohesion*, i.e., a measure of the emotional bonding between family members (enmeshment, expressed emotion); *adaptability*, i.e., a measure of how flexible the family is and how much change is permitted; and *communication*, i.e., a facilitating dimension that allows members to express their needs as they relate on the other two dimensions.

3. **Group for the Advancement of Psychiatry (GAP).** The GAP published a report on family assessment that suggested considering eight dimensions.

TABLE 32–1.
Six Main Dimensions of Family Functioning

Problem Solving	Roles
2 types of problems:	2 areas of family function:
Instrumental and affective	Instrumental and affective
7 stages to the process:	5 stages to the process
1, identification of the problem	1, systems management and maintenance
2, communication of the problem to the appropriate person(s)/resources	2, provision of resources
3, development of alternative action	3, nurturance and support
4, decision on one alternative action	4, sexual gratification of parent or parental figures
5, action	5, life skills development
6, monitoring the action	
7, evaluation of success of action	
Postulated (prescriptive)	Postulated (prescriptive): most effective when all necessary family functions have clear allocation to appropriate individuals and accountability built in

a. The nature of the family as a unit (stable, cohesive, divisive, close, and/or distant).

b. The family capacity for cooperation with treatment plans.

c. The psychologic mindedness of members of the family.

d. The capacity for communication among family members.

e. The degree of mental health or ill health of the family as a unit or in terms of the individual members.

f. The role of the child's disorder in the psychic economy of the family (secondary gain or family misuse of the child's disorder).

g. The relationship of the family to the community (distant, isolated, and/or involved).

h. The subcultural values dominant in the family.

4. **Fischer's schema.** There are many instruments used by different theorists in assessing patients. Fischer evaluated many of these different assessment tools and developed a composite of five dimensions necessary to assess families as follows:

a. **Structural descriptors** (e.g., roles, alliances, scapegoating, boundaries, and/or communication patterns).

b. **Controls and sanctions** (e.g., power and leadership, flexibility, dependence vs. independence, and/or fusion vs. differentiation).

c. **Emotions and needs** (e.g., rules of affective expression, need satisfaction, and/or affective themes).

d. **Cultural aspects** (e.g., social position, cultural heritage, and/or cultural views).

e. **Developmental aspects** (e.g., appropriateness of the above dimensions of the family to the developmental stage in the family life cycle).

TABLE 32–2.
Major Models of Family Therapy: Normally, Dysfunctional, and Therapeutic Goals

Model of Family Therapy	View of Normal Family Functioning	View of Dysfunction/ Symptoms	Goals of Therapy
Structural (Minuchin, Montalvo, and Aponte)	Boundaries clear and firm; hierarchy with strong subsystem; and flexibility of system for autonomy and interdependence, individual growth and system maintenance, continuity and adaptive restructuring in response to changing internal (developmental) and external (environmental) demands	Symptoms result from current family structural imbalance, i.e., malfunctioning hierarchical arrangement and boundaries; maladaptive reaction to changing requirements (developmental and environmental)	Reorganize family structure: shift members' relative positions to disrupt malfunctioning pattern and strengthen parental hierarchy; create clear, flexible boundaries; and mobilize more adaptive alternative patterns

(Continued.)

TABLE 32–2 (cont.)
Major Models of Family Therapy: Normally, Dysfunctional, and Therapeutic Goals

Model of Family Therapy	View of Normal Family Functioning	View of Dysfunction/Symptoms	Goals of Therapy
Strategic (Haley, Milan team, and Palo Alto group)	Flexibility; large behavioral repertoire for large behavioral and lifecycle passage; and clear rules governing (Haley)	Multiple origins of problems; symptoms maintained by family's unsuccessful problem-solving attempts, inability to adjust to lifecycle transitions (Haley), and malfunctioning hierarchy: tricoalition or coalition across hierarchy; and symptom is a communicative act embedded in interaction pattern	Resolve presenting problem only: specific behaviorally defined objectives; interrupt rigid feedback cycle: change symptom-maintaining sequence to new outcome; and define clearer hierarchy (Haley)

Behavioral-social exchange	Maladaptive behavior is not forced; adaptive behavior is rewarded; exchange of benefits outweighs long-term reciprocity	Maladaptive, symptomatic behavior reinforced by family attention and reward; deficient reward exchanges (e.g.,); and communication deficit	Concrete, observable behavioral goals; change contingencies of reinforcement (interpersonal consequences of behavior): rewards for adaptive behavior and no rewards for maladaptive behavior
Psychodynamic (Ackerman, Boszormenyi-Nagy, Framo, Lidz, Meissner, Paul, and	Parental personalities and relationships well differentiated; relationship perceptions based on current realities, not projections	Symptoms due to family projection process stemming from unresolved conflicts and losses in family of origin	Insight and resolution of family of origin conflict and losses, family projection processes, relationship reconstruction and reunion,

(Continued.)

TABLE 32–2 (cont).
Major Models of Family Therapy: Normally, Dysfunctional, and Therapeutic Goals

Model of Family Therapy	View of Normal Family Functioning	View of Dysfunction/Symptoms	Goals of Therapy
Stierlin	from past; Boszormenyi-Nagy: relational equitability; and Lidz: family task requisites (parental coalition, generation boundaries, and sex-linked parental roles)		and individual and family growth
Family systems therapy (Bowen)	Differentiation of self, intellectual/emotional balance	Functioning impaired by relationships with family of origin: poor differentiation, anxiety (reactivity), family projection process, and triangulation	Insight and resolution of family, cognitive functioning, emotional reactivity, modification of relationships in family system: detriangulation and repair cutoffs

Experiential (Satir and Whitaker)	Satir: Self-worth (high) communication (clear, specific, and honest), and family rules (flexible and appropriate); linkage to society (open and hopeful); and Whitaker: multiple aspects of family structure and shared experience	Symptoms are nonverbal messages in reaction to current communication dysfunction in system	Direct, clear communication; individual and family growth through immediate shared experience

33

Group Therapy

I. **Introduction.** The term *group therapy* covers a broad range of activities, which differ as widely as the therapeutic approaches that can be found in individual psychotherapy. In the most general sense, group therapy includes any gathering of people who generally meet regularly, usually with a trained leader, to work on their psychologic problems or personal growth.

II. **Various forms of group therapy.**

A. **Leadership style.** Therapy groups can be differentiated along a variety of parameters, one of which is leadership style. Some groups are *leader centered* in which the leader is very active, directive, and involved in most of the interactions in the group. In such a group, the leader may attend successively and individually to different members, interacting with them as he/she would in conducting individual therapy. A contrasting role would be the leader who functions as a removed consultant to the group, in which most of the interactions and initiatives are located in the group membership *(group centered)*. A group may have one leader, or possibly two cotherapists. While most therapy groups have professional leaders, others might not. There are a variety of self-help groups that function without a designated leader or where leadership is provided by the more experienced members. Self-help groups are generally organized around a common problem that all the members face (substance abuse, bereavement, a medical illness, and/or an ill family member). The variety of types of self-help groups that can be formed is vast. Up to 14 million Americans participate in such groups. Alcoholics Anonymous is one well-known such group that, with its 12-step program for recovery, has been a paradigm for other addictive disorder groups.

B. **Focus and goals.** Groups can differ in their main focus and goals. There can be groups whose focus is mainly *educational*. These may be time limited with specific information to convey, such as information about a particular psychologic disorder. Similarly, there may be groups whose purpose is to *teach certain skills*, such as assertion training or social skills building, often by means of role-playing. There can be groups whose function is to facilitate communication or to act as a *supportive therapy* for chronically impaired patients or their families. In inpatient settings, there may be "community meetings" where the main focus is to attend to issues related to creating a therapeutic milieu.

Those forms of group therapy that emphasize and facilitate the *interactions between group members* take advantage of what is unique in group work. Here, the interactions among the members are used as a source of learning and are of therapeutic import. In their interactions, the members may again experience the problems for which they are seeking help. The group then provides an in vivo experience in which to learn more about the problems, and it also provides a safe place where persons can try new behaviors to practice the changes that they desire.

In a *group-centered* approach, the therapist's major goal would be to shape the group slowly into being able to conduct its own therapeutic process. This involves getting the members to listen to each other, to make relevant observations and interpretations, to note contradictions, and to challenge each other appropriately. This also requires a group culture in which there is an underlying concern for all the members and their betterment. This culture is fostered when all members feel that they will be heard and respected and when communications are direct and interactions are completed. Initially, the therapist has to take a major role in creating this culture and in providing a safe environment. Creating safety may involve the leader holding people responsible for their behavior, making sure everyone gets heard, and possibly stepping in to limit excessively aggressive or destructive behaviors.

C. **Group membership.** Groups can differ in the nature and severity of the *psychologic illness* of the members. Therapy groups can be created that are *homogeneous* for the main problem or symptom of its members (e.g., for eating disorders or agoraphobia). Most therapy groups, in practice, are *heterogeneous* in the nature of the members' problems and in the demographic mix of the members. The heterogeneity provides the group with a collection of people with varied resources and experiences from which to draw. Sensitivity groups, encounter groups, and groups originating from the human potential movement are examples of groups that emphasize *personal growth* rather than therapy for an "illness." There are also group experiences that emphasize learning about group dynamics ("group process"). Here, the emphasis is to learn more about one's own behavior in groups and about organizational behavior to learn to function better in the work setting. These types of groups include human relations training groups, T-groups (T stands for training), "process" groups, and Tavistock groups.

D. **Group structure.** Groups can differ in their *organizational parameters*. The *frequency* of meeting can vary. Some groups may meet several times a week. There can be groups that are limited to one extended session, possibly a weekend. Marathon groups are meant to go continuously for many hours, with the cumulative fatigue intended to facilitate lowering of resistances. Groups can be *open* or *closed*. In a closed group, the membership is restricted for a certain time period. In an open group, the membership may change from session to session, as might happen for inpatient groups. Groups can differ widely in *size*. For most ongoing therapy groups, an optimum size is between seven and ten members. In multiple family therapy groups, the gathering can be quite large.

E. **Theoretical orientation.** Groups can also vary in terms of the theoretical orientation of the leader and how much this influences the group. Some of the more common theoretical orientations include the existential orientation of gestalt therapy, the interpersonal interactional emphasis of transactional analysis, the psychoanalytic orientation of groups run by psychoanalysts, and the catharsis and role-playing of psychodrama groups. Sometimes, behavior therapy techniques or cognitive therapy are conducted in a group format.

III. **Conceptualizing group therapy and group processes.** One way to conceptualize the experience in a group is to realize that three *levels of phenomena* are getting expressed at any time. First, there are the *intrapsychic* dynamics that are going on in each individual who is present. Second, there are the *dyadic interactions* and dynamics between individual group members. Third, there are *group level phenomena*. These are dynamics that are present in all groups. While there is much theory about group dynamics, unconscious group phenomena, and the development of groups, as with individual therapy, there is no one perspective that is definitive. Group level phenomena (which can only be mentioned in passing here) include the following dynamics: issues of inclusion (who is really regarded as a group member and is anyone excluded); boundary issues (where does the "group" stop, in terms of people, time, location, and confidentiality); issues of subgrouping, special pairings, and intimacy; issues of implicit or explicit norms of behavior; members taking on certain roles; competition and struggles over decision making and leadership; dynamics involving denial and "flight" from dealing with issues; and issues of dependency on the leader.

The group therapist, at any time, may focus the attention of the group to a phenomenon on any of these three levels. While only one level can be directly addressed at any time, the challenge is to attempt to be aware of what is going on at these levels for the different group members. Another distinction is between the *content* of what is being discussed in the group at any time and the *process* of the group (the dynamics of the interactions between the members). The therapist also implicitly has to decide whether to focus the group's attention on the content or the process issues of the group.

Groups have been observed to go through *developmental phases*. There are a variety of different theoretical descriptions of these stages. Initially, when a new group starts, there is no sense of unity or belonging, but this usually quickly develops. The members all enter the group with feelings of insecurity and a preoccupation with their own situation in the group. Often, first meetings may be filled with long silences. Individual members bring up topics that don't connect or relate to each other. Only with time do people become less anxious, start to listen to what others are saying, and take an interest in the other people. Implicitly, issues of belonging, inclusion, and psychologic membership in the group predominate initially. Later, issues of power, roles, alliances, and autonomy typically arise. One such struggle is whether people can retain their differences and individuality without jeopardizing their place in the group. Only later in the life of a group are issues of intimacy and mutuality likely to emerge spontaneously.

IV. **The therapeutic impact of groups.** Irvin Yalom (1985), in his authoritative writing on group therapy, has described 11 factors that he feels are implicated in the therapeutic effect of groups.

A. *Universality* refers to the patient coming to realize that he/she is not alone in having problems, and that his/her struggles are shared by or at least understandable to others.

B. *Instillation of hope* is mediated, in part, by meeting others who have made progress with their problems, and by the emotional support that can be provided by the group.

C. *Imparting information* can range from providing information about the person's disorder to direct feedback about the person's behavior and effect on other group members.

D. *Altruism* can be experienced as members give support to each other and contribute their ideas, not just receiving these from others.

E. There can be a *corrective recapitulation of the primary family*, which for many patients may have been problematic. Both the therapist and the other members can be the recipient of transference reactions that can then be addressed.

F. Further *development of social skills* and the ability to relate to others is possible. The patient can get feedback and have an opportunity to learn and practice new ways of interacting.

G. *Identification, imitative behavior, and modeling* may result from therapists or other members providing good role models.

H. *Interpersonal experiences* involve learning the importance of interpersonal relationships, how to have better relationships, and having the corrective experience of good relationships.

I. *Group cohesiveness* and belonging can be powerful forces in a person's life. If the therapy group comes to develop a sense of togetherness and unity, this may give more influence to the group experience as something that will have impact and provide a sense of belonging and acceptance.

J. *Catharsis* and the sharing of strong emotions may not only help relieve personal emotional tension, but enhance the sense of intimacy in the group.

K. *Existential* factors, for Yalom, subsumes a variety of issues that are intrinsic to personal growth, having to do with acknowledging one's limitations, the limitations of others, responsibility for oneself, and issues of loneliness and death.

To add to this list, there are also the benefits of additional *reality testing* that follows from the interactions and feedback that the group provides. The group may also directly encourage, prompt, and *reinforce* desired behavioral change.

V. **A special precaution.** Groups can be very powerful, and their influence needs to be respected. One of the most destructive group phenomena that a therapist needs to monitor is that of *scapegoating*, which the therapist can be drawn into if not attentive. In scapegoating, one person is singled out for exclusion, attack, or criticism. The emotional force usually has to do with group issues that get projected onto that individual.

VI. **Indications for group therapy.** The following comments are intended as guidelines for a "typical" outpatient psychotherapy group composed of members of heterogeneous characteristics.

Group therapy can be the treatment of choice for people whose problems are *primarily interpersonal* and who do not have major psychiatric impairments. Similarly, groups are good for people who just need an arena in which to try new behaviors and practice new social skills. A group may also be better than individual therapy for a person at risk of forming a strong fixed transference reaction or too great a dependency on an individual therapist. Because individual and group therapies have different benefits, the best solution may be to have the person involved in both. From a certain perspective, individual therapy can be seen as a preparation for group therapy, in that in a group, the person has the opportunity to apply more directly what he/she has learned in his/her individual therapy. Individual therapy may bring the person to the point where he/she can relate well enough to engage in a group and have a psychologic mindedness so that person can start to learn from his/her own experiences.

Groups can be particularly helpful with adolescents where peer pressure to be involved can often engage adolescents who would otherwise be silent or resistant.

VII. **Contraindications for group therapy.** People who are inappropriate for a group are those who cannot learn from their experience, who cannot be influenced by others, and who would be disruptive to the group. This can include people with psychosis, mania or hypomania, organic brain disease, severe depression, or severe character disorders. While groups are typically good for people with neurotic problems or mild character disorders, people with severe disorders may prove too intransigent or difficult for a group. This would include patients with paranoia or somatization. Antisocial personalities may prove too disruptive, domineering, or destructive of group trust. People who cannot control violent impulses are contraindicated. Severely schizoid or withdrawn persons may not be able to become sufficiently engaged. Severely narcissistic people are usually difficult as group members.

One additional consideration is the overall composition of a group. It is not advisable to include a member who will be very different from the others, i.e., on any relevant dimension, such as severity of impairment, race, sex, etc. In general, a balance in the group is desirable, particularly for sex. "Minorities of one" (of any kind) are best avoided.

VIII. Guidelines for the beginning group therapist.

Consider that your main goal is to facilitate interactions and the learning from them. You should attend closely to what is said and try to *get people to respond to each other* around the issues that come up. Having people share the similarities and differences in their experiences can be very helpful. You can redirect indirect communications and have them be made more explicit by encouraging people to express more directly what they are feeling. By attending to the interactions in the group, you may notice how *problems get re-enacted* for different members. You can now encourage them to try different behaviors and to work through their interactions more completely. One important thing is to monitor that people do not feel cut off or unheard; this a major phenomenon in new groups. Particularly when a person is starting to open up and share something of importance, if the group ignores them, this can induce negative reactions and greater guardedness. The position of the therapist is not to do the group's work but to teach them to become more therapeutic for each other.

SUGGESTED READING

Yalom ID: *The Theory and Practice of Group Psychotherapy*, ed 3. New York, Basic Books Inc Publishers, 1985.

Grotjahn M, Kline FM, Friedman CTH: *Handbook of Group Therapy*. New York, Van Nostrand Reinhold Co, 1983.

Kadis AL, Krasner JD, Weiner MF, et al: *Practicum of Group Psychotherapy*. New York, Harper & Row Inc, 1963.

Naar R: *A Primer of Group Psychotherapy*. New York, Basic Books Inc Publishers, 1983.

Yalom ID: *Inpatient Group Psychotherapy*. New York, Basic Books Inc Publishers, 1983.

34 | Relaxation Training, Biofeedback, and Hypnosis

I. **Relaxation training.**

A. **Definition.** Many varieties of relaxation training and stress reduction exist. In general, their goal is to reduce physiologic arousal and tension and thereby reduce anxiety. Along with the reduction in physiologic parameters, such as heart rate, respiratory rate, and muscle tension, a concurrent lowering of psychologic stress is achieved.

B. **Types.**

1. Progressive relaxation.
2. Controlled breathing.
3. Visualization.
4. Meditation.
5. Biofeedback.
6. Hypnosis.

C. **Theory and methods.** The theory behind relaxation training is based on the assumption, described by Edmund Jacobsen in the 1920s, that lowering physiologic arousal lowers the subjective experience of anxiety. Also important is the idea that responses learned in the training situation can be generalized to real-life situations. Learning theory, which, in simple terms, may be thought of as the idea that behavior and responses may be learned, has allowed relaxation training to serve as a foundation for several conditioning techniques as follows: (1) counterconditioning (reciprocal inhibition) where a response inhibitory to anxiety is used when a subject is confronted with anxiety-provoking stimuli, thereby weakening the anxiety response; (2) covert conditioning, which is based on the idea that covert (imagined) and overt psychologic events obey the same laws; and (3) flooding, where patients are exposed to phobic stimuli, real or imagined, for as long as they can tolerate.

1. In progressive relaxation, a subject is taught to lessen muscular tension by progressively tensing and relaxing major muscle groups. A simple procedure for teaching the method is as follows.

a. Have the subject assume a comfortable, relaxed position.

b. Instruct the subject to clench one of his/her fists tightly and note the tremendous tension as compared with the opposite hand and forearm.

c. After 5 to 7 seconds, have the subject relax and note the sensations associated with relaxation as contrasted with tension.

d. Repeat the procedure.

e. Repeat the procedure, with the subject tensing both fists at once, and on relaxing have them again, note the contrasting feelings of relaxation.

f. Repeat the procedure, this time with the subject tensing the forearms and biceps of both arms.

g. Using the same procedure, have the subject alternately tense and relax the muscles of the face, jaw, neck, and shoulders. Then, move on to the legs if desired.

h. Areas of particular tension can be repeated several times.

2. In controlled breathing, the subject is taught to relax via slow, deep diaphragmatic breathing. A simple example of one procedure that can be used for teaching the technique is as follows. (This can be extremely useful for very anxious patients, even in emergency room settings.)

a. Have the subject assume a comfortable position, either sitting or lying, with one hand over his/her stomach.

b. Instruct the subject to breathe in slowly and deeply through his/her nose over a count of five. With the breath, the subject should be breathing into the abdomen, trying to push the hand on his/her abdomen gently away.

c. Instruct the subject to hold the breath for a count of five.

d. In many of the meditation techniques, the mind is given a relatively simple and repetitive task to concentrate on, while slipping into a relaxed state.

e. Biofeedback; see Section II.

f. Hypnosis; see Section III.

g. The various relaxation-training techniques described above may be used alone or in combination.

D. **Applications.**

1. Relaxation training may be used purely to induce a more pleasant, relaxed state of mind.

2. Many psychosomatic disorders respond well to relaxation techniques (see also section II./D.); ones that have been reported to respond especially well include Raynaud disease, irritable bowel syndrome, chronic pain syndrome, and nausea.

3. Sleep disorders also frequently respond well to relaxation techniques.

4. Anxiety disorders, phobias, and even panic attacks may be controlled or lessened (see also Section I./C./2.).

E. **Summary.** The relaxation-training and stress-reduction techniques are usually simple, may be taught in very few sessions, and require little, if any, equipment. They may provide great relief to patients with a wide variety of stress-induced or exacerbated conditions, and they are easily used as an adjunct to other forms of therapy. For general relaxation, they have been found to be as effective as biofeedback and hypnosis.

II. Biofeedback.

A. **Definition.** Biofeedback is a process in which physiologic responses, normally not discernible, are amplified and displayed to the patient through auditory or visual feedback. Commonly measured parameters include heart rate, muscle tension (electromyography), blood pressure, skin temperature, and skin conductance (galvanic skin response).

B. **Types.**

1. The patient is provided feedback about the actual physiologic parameter that he/she wishes to learn to control.

2. The physiologic parameter or symptom itself in which change is desired is not measured, but in using feedback from another parameter, the patient learns a general relaxation response that produces the desired effect.

C. **Theory and methods.**

1. Normally obscure physiologic processes and changes are made evident to both subject and therapist, providing informational feedback that enables the subject to effect change in the desired direction. Biofeedback is generally used in conjunction with other relaxation-training techniques (see Section I). It provides, in addition, an objective measurement of effec-

tiveness, thus giving the subject direct feedback and reinforcement.

2. Biofeedback is based on the concept that the somatoform and psychosomatic disorders develop or worsen when the body's normal homeostatic mechanisms are affected by stress, social isolation, or unconscious conflict.

3. Examples include using biofeedback to minimize heart rate or maximize skin temperature, as indirect ways of lessening sympathetic tone and increasing parasympathetic tone, thereby restoring balance.

D. **Applications.**

1. General stress reduction, as well as control of anxiety disorders, panic attacks, and phobias, are possible using a wide variety of biofeedback modalities.

2. Neuromuscular rehabilitation, including peripheral nerve damage, spasms, cerebral palsy, and upper motor neuron damage may all be aided by biofeedback, especially electromyographic feedback.

3. Fecal incontinence and enuresis may both respond to direct (e.g., sphincter tone monitoring) and indirect techniques.

4. Headaches, both of the tension and migraine type, may be reduced or even averted.

5. Hypertension and orthostatic hypotension may both respond to either direct blood pressure feedback or monitoring another modality, such as the galvanic skin response.

6. Asthmatic symptoms may be lessened, both by an increased airflow and a by a decreased panic associated with an attack using airway resistance feedback and frontalis electromyographic feedback.

7. Musculoskeletal pain can be greatly reduced, along with the need for narcotics or other analgesics, particularly through the use of electromyographic feedback.

8. Epileptic seizures may be suppressed in some patients through the use of electroencephalographic feedback.

E. **Summary.** The equipment needed varies greatly, from a simple handheld thermometer to sophisticated electroencephalographs or sphincter tone monitors. The equipment is, however, becoming increasingly available in many settings. Biofeedback techniques can generally be learned in around six to eight sessions, after which the subject may practice on his/her own. Biofeedback may be an effective adjunct to many other therapies used in the treatment of physical, psychosomatic, and psychiatric disorders. It must be cautioned that these technqiues are still experimental and have not yet been proved to be of substantial clinical value in physical illnesses, such as hypertension.

III. **Hypnosis.**

A. **Definition.** Hypnosis is the induction of a state of focal concentration with a diminution of peripheral awareness, generally, but not exclusively, brought about through the use of suggestion. While in hypnosis, a subject's perceptions may be altered, he/she may become more responsive to suggestion, and he/she may continue to respond to suggestions given during hypnosis after hypnosis has ended (posthypnotic suggestion.) After hypnosis, the subject may be amnestic for all or part of the experience. Hypnotic-like states occur frequently in everyday life. Examples include becoming briefly visually transfixed on an object, or going into reverie while engaging in a repetitive movement during physical exercise.

B. **History.**

1. Hypnotic phenomena have been described far back in history, particularly as trances associated with religious ceremonies.

2. Franz Anton Mesmer, in the 18th century, was the first to attempt a scientific description of states pro-

moted by "healers." The term "mesmerized" refers to his early work with hypnotic states.

3. Freud studied hypnosis under Charcot in France, and he initially used it as his primary method of treating hysterical patients.

4. This century has seen a tremendous increase in the research and clinical application of hypnotic techniques.

C. **Theory and methods.**

1. Approximately 70% to 80% of the psychiatric patient population are hypnotizable.

2. Various scales exist to measure a subject's hypnotizability, such as the Stanford Hypnotic Susceptibility Scales. The susceptibility and depth of hypnosis are generally assessed by gauging the response to a number of suggestions, including altered perception, imagery, dissociation, passive movement or paralysis, age regression, and posthypnotic suggestion.

3. Hypnosis may be induced by a variety of techniques, generally using suggestions and imagery. Suggestions may be quite directive, such as telling the subject, "your eyelids are becoming heavy," or more subtle and permissive, such as "you may or may not notice feelings in your eyelids as you think about how heavy they have been when you tried to read a dull book late at night." Ericksonian techniques use extremely subtle, often confusing and paradoxical, or nonverbal suggestions to induce hypnosis. Please refer to the references listed at the end of this chapter for complete hypnotic induction scripts.

D. **Applications.**

1. Hypnosis is frequently used in the treatment of a specific, well-circumscribed symptom, or to suggest physiologic and emotional changes, but it may also be used in a wide variety of other circumstances, including as an adjunct to psychotherapy.

2. Acute and chronic pain may be treated very effectively with hypnosis. Major surgery has been performed with hypnosis as the sole anesthetic.

3. A wide variety of psychosomatic disorders respond well to hypnosis. These include gastrointestinal disorders, asthma, hypertension, seizure disorders, headaches, and dermatologic disorders.

4. Physical rehabilitation may be aided by hypnotic suggestions.

5. Unwanted habits, such as smoking, nail biting, and even some of the eating disorders, may be successfully treated with hypnosis.

6. Anxiety disorders and phobias may be controlled with hypnosis. Subjects can learn to induce hypnosis when faced with overwhelming anxiety, as in fear of flying or taking an important examination. Panic attacks may be averted or aborted, and anticipatory anxiety associated with medical or surgical procedures also responds well.

7. Nausea, even that associated with cancer chemotherapy, may be markedly diminished with hypnosis.

8. In psychotherapy, hypnosis may assist in a variety of ways, such as memory enhancement, age regression, guided imagery, dream induction, and exploration, and it also allows the patient to relax and share more in the therapy.

9. Sexual dysfunctions have been reported to respond to hypnotic intervention.

10. Hypnotic techniques may be used in group situations, for most of the applications listed above. Similarly, family therapy may be aided by hypnosis.

11. The use of hypnosis in law is an extremely controversial subject, particularly in the area of memory enhancement for witnesses. The veracity of material recalled under hypnosis cannot be guaranteed, although material gathered may be useful for further in-

vestigation. Caution must be exercised before using hypnosis, as witnesses who have been hypnotized sometimes are not permitted to offer testimony.

E. **Summary.** Hypnotic techniques are relatively easy to learn, require no specialized equipment, and are applicable to the majority of psychiatric patients. In addition, a patient may be referred to a qualified hypnotist for a brief period of time to learn hypnotic techniques, without interfering with other treatment modalities.

REFERENCES

1. Wester WC, Smith AH: (eds): *Clinical Hypnosis: A Multidisciplinary Approach.* Philadelphia, JB Lippincott, 1984.
2. Davis M, McKay M, Eshelman ER: *The Relaxation and Stress Workbook,* ed 2. Oakland, Calif, New Harbinger Public, 1982.
3. Kihlstrom JF: Hypnosis. *Annu Rev Psychol* 1985; 36:385–418.
4. Turner JA, Chapman CR: Psychological interventions for chronic pain: A critical review: I. Relaxation training and biofeedback. *Pain* 1982; 12:1–21.
5. Turner JA, Chapman CR: Psychological interventions for chronic pain: A critical review: II. Operant conditioning, hypnosis, and cognitive-behavioral therapy. *Pain* 1982; 12:23–46.
6. Holroyd J: How hypnosis may potentiate psychotherapy. *Am J Clin Hypn* 1987; 29:194–200.
7. Goldberg RJ: Anxiety reduction by self regulation: Theory, practice, and evaluation. *Ann Intern Med* 1982; 96:483–487.
8. Agras WS: Behavioral medicine: An overview. *Annu Rev Am Psychiatr Assoc* 1986; 5:526–539.
9. Braun BG: Introduction: The uses of hypnosis in psychiatry. *Psychiatr Ann* 1986; 16:75–77.
10. Braun BG, Horevitz RP: Hypnosis and psy-

chotherapy. *Psychiatr Ann* 1986; 16:2:81–86.
11. Frischholz EJ, Spiegel D: Adjunctive uses of hypnosis in the treatment of smoking. *Psychiatr Ann* 1986; 16:87–90.
12. Tuite PA, Braun BG, Frischholz EJ: Hypnosis and eyewitness testimony. *Psychiatr Ann* 1986; 16:91–95.
13. Kluft RP: Hypnosis in the treatment of phobias. *Psychiatr Ann* 1986; 16:96–101.
14. Araoz DL: Uses of hypnosis in the treatment of psychogenic sexual dysfunctions. *Psychiatr Ann* 1986; 16:102–105.
15. Wain HJ: Pain control with hypnosis in consultation and liaison psychiatry. *Psychiatr Ann* 1986; 16:106–109.
16. Sachs BC: Stress and self-hypnosis and mental set on major surgery and burns. *Psychiatr Ann* 1986; 16:115–118.

35
Acute Crisis and Intervention

I. **Introduction.** This chapter discusses the various methods by which suicidal, grieving, and traumatized patients may best be managed in the setting of the emergency room. Such patients find themselves in the midst of a stressful situation that represents a major threat to their physical and/or psychologic integrity. This review will focus on the *immediate* management of patients in crisis and on decision making regarding their subsequent care ("crisis intervention"). In Chapter 36, there is a discussion of short-term psychotherapeutic interventions.

II. **Suicidality.** At least 15% of psychiatric visits to a general hospital emergency room involve patients with suicidal ideation and/or a recent suicidal gesture and attempt. The evaluating physician must be able to assess the risk of suicide first and then to implement a feasible plan for disposition and management.

A. Demographic data.

1. There are 22,000 suicides per year in the United States (US). This is probably underestimated. Many true suicides not recorded. Many are labeled as "accidents."

2. US: 11 suicides per 100,000 population. The US is in the middle of the scale of Western countries with respect to rate of suicide. Japan and Sweden are near the top.

3. The association between suicide and gender: Men lead women in completed suicides 3:1; however, women lead men in attempted suicides 3:1.

4. The association between age and suicide: The risk of suicide increases with advancing age, reaching a plateau in the sixth and seventh decades. At highest risk are men in middle and old age.

5. The association between race and suicide: Overall, suicide risk is greater among whites than nonwhites, except for American Indians and Eskimos. However, in cities, black rates approximate white rates.

6. The association between living situation and suicide: Suicides *per 100,000 US population:* married, 11; widowed, 24; and divorced, 40 (divorced men: 69/100,000, divorced women: 18/100,000). Note also that the single, never-married, suicide rate is almost twice that for the married national average.

B. **Risk factors for suicide.** Risk factors can be categorized according to epidemiology, historical data, physical condition of a patient, psychopathologic condition, and suicidal behavior. These risk factors should be recognized, assessed, and utilized in conjunction with careful clinical assessment in deciding the suicidality of a patient. The following clinical indicators of high suicide risk are according to Hanke (*Handbook of Emergency Psychiatry*, 1984).

1. Epidemiologic risk factors.

a. Separated, divorced, widow>single>married.

b. Over 45 years old.

c. Male>female.

d. White>nonwhite.

e. Recent losses (loved one, health, money, job).

f. Protestant>Catholic or Jew.

g. Spring, fall>summer, winter.

2. Historical data.

a. Family history of suicidal behavior.

b. Previous suicide attempts or behavior.

3. Concurrent medical conditions.

a. Chronic or terminal illness.

b. Chronic pain.

c. Severe, persistent insomnia.

d. Hypochondriasis.

4. Current psychopathologic condition.

a. Poor impulse control.

b. Poor reality testing.

c. Psychosis or organicity.

d. Depression.

e. Drug or alcohol abuse.

f. Personality disorders (borderline, paranoid).

5. Suicidal behavior.

a. Lethal method and means.

b. Serious persistent *intent*.

c. Will or suicide note written.

d. High-risk context (lives alone, no social support).

C. Who needs to be evaluated for suicidality?

1. The patient who has recently attempted suicide.

2. The patient who presents with suicidal ideation.

3. The patient who reveals suicidal ideation only when asked.

4. The patient who denies suicidal ideation, but whose behavior indicates possible suicidality (e.g., has recently given away cherished items, carefully cleared up debts, calls friends to vaguely say "good-bye," etc.).

5. The patient with a history of assaultive behavior. Violent patients often turn their violence against themselves.

D. The general approach to an interview of a patient who appears to be suicidal: Empathy is especially important. As long as the interviewer maintains a gentle and reassuring empathic approach, careful questioning usually elicits the information needed to evaluate the risk of suicide. In the final analysis, despite many attempts to devise scales to measure the risk of suicide scientifically, only careful examination coupled with clinical judgment provides each interviewer with the ability to assess the risk of suicide. While the epidemiologic data should be used in the assessment, it is the *clinical* assessment that should assume over-riding importance in each individual evaluation.

E. The interview itself.

1. **Chief complaint.** Is the patient stating that he/she is suicidal? Is the patient indicating ambivalence with regard to suicidal intention? Is the patient complaining of emptiness and a severely and morbidly low mood? Is the patient so paranoid that he/she might commit suicide to escape from intolerable paranoia? Is the patient hearing voices that suggest or order that he/she commit suicide (command hallucinations)?

2. **Complete history of the present illness.** Be sure to include careful but empathic questioning regarding preoccupation with death, suicidal ideation, and intent.

3. Obtain demographic data.

4. Obtain family history. Is there a history of suicide in the family? Is there a family history of unipolar or bipolar affective disorder?

5. Any previous suicide attempts? Inquire about lethality of attempts and whether patient intended to be successful.

6. **Alcohol and drug abuse.** Substance abuse is often associated with depression. An individual under the influence of mind-altering substances often have impaired impulse control and/or reality testing, increasing his/her suicide risk.

7. Have there been any recent losses? This includes death or illness of a significant other, as well as unresolved grief over the loss of a loved one, perhaps precipitated by the anniversary of the loss.

8. Is the patient physically ill? Physical illness is often similar in experience to loss of a significant other, for it involves the loss of health and, therefore, often results in a sense of loss of control or independence. Also, is there a history of violence to others? A significant number of suicides are carried out by people who would be diagnosed primarily as personality disorders (rather than major depression).

F. A synthesis of information is needed to decide on management. The examiner must take into account the presence or absence of a viable support system. The presence of a reliable significant other lessens the risk of suicidality.

All of the data obtained from the patient and available family and friends is then combined with a subjective assessment of the patient's demeanor and ability to relate to the examiner.

An important point to remember is that the assessment of suicidal risk is never foolproof. For this reason, it's best to err on the side of safety in deciding among the several disposition options.

G. *The Suicidal Gesture.* A suicidal gesture that involves nonlethal means of self-harm also deserves attention. Often, the gesture is carried out in front of another person, or immediately reported to a significant other. There is frequently an acute precipitant with secondary gain as an immediate result. Nevertheless, the gesture should be taken seriously, both as an indicator of severe psychologic distress and also because a significant percentage of such gestures are thought to result inadvertently in completed suicide or severe self-harm.

H. Disposition options.

1. Send the patient home, providing appropriate follow-up care. This decision may be made if:

a. The risk of suicide is assessed to be nonexistent or low.

b. The precipitating crisis has been resolved.

c. The patient is not psychotic and has resumed what appears to be good impulse control.

d. There is a good support system in the patient's environment.

e. A follow-up treatment plan has been organized and discussed with the patient, who is in agreement.

2. **Admittance to a general hospital ward.** This decision is made in the case of a suicide attempt where there is medical instability. Consultation psychiatry is then informed of the patient to provide appropriate follow-up plans.

3. **Admittance to an open psychiatric ward.** This option is appropriate for the patient who no longer represents an acute suicidal risk and would tell staff if there is a recurrence of suicidal ideation. Such a decision can be a valuable therapeutic tool, emphasizing the individual responsibility of a patient in maintaining some independent control over his/her life.

4. **Admittance to a closed psychiatric ward.** Most often a patient who is judged acutely suicidal and impulsive is placed on a closed psychiatric unit. Admission is generally involuntary; even when the patient agrees to admission, the presence of impulsivity suggests the possibility of a change of mind and a subsequent decision to leave the ward. For the impulsive

suicidal patient, involuntary admission underlines the serious nature of a suicidal threat and need for careful surveillance on ward.

III. **Acute grief and bereavement.**

A. **Normal response to death.** Stages of the normal grief response.

1. Affective anesthesia (numbness).

a. Generally lasts minutes.

b. Occurs immediately on learning of death of significant other.

c. When told of death of loved one, person may appear to be unresponsive and/or detached. The therapist may need to repeat the information gently several times.

2. Protest.

a. Lasts minutes to hours.

b. Often a period of denial, with loud protestations. The therapist should maintain a calm, empathic manner.

3. Disorganization.

a. Lasts hours to days.

b. Survivor may be dysfunctional, i.e., unable to continue the usual pattern of daily living.

c. Often a preoccupation with the deceased. Survivor may "talk to" the deceased.

d. This state is important to incorporate the loss into reality.

B. **Pathologic grief.**

1. By definition, severe mourning and a lowered level of functioning that persist for over a year following the death of loved one.

2. May be prevented by therapeutic intervention in an emergency setting, followed by appropriate psychiatric care.

C. **Representative patients faced with an acute grief reaction who may present in emergency room setting.**

1. Family and friends of newly deceased patient in emergency room.

2. Family and friends of critically ill patients in emergency room.

3. Disaster victims.

4. Victims of rape.

D. **Care of family (or close friends) of dying or newly deceased patient.**

1. Contact the family.

a. If present in the emergency room, escort the family to a comfortable private room. In privacy, they can be apprised of situation.

b. If family is not present, contact by telephone. Inform the family member that a loved one is very ill and he/she should come to the hospital. Encourage the family member to come with a close friend who will drive the car. If the family member is so far away that he/she must be informed of the death or grave prognosis over the telephone, be sure that there is an adult nearby who can assist the relative should the news be severely compromising.

c. At all times, identify yourself, be calm, courteous, respectful, and gentle.

2. Telling the family.

a. Allow for an initial time, perhaps 5 minutes, to talk with the family about the issues.

b. Often, it is helpful to ask the family what they may know, or believe, about their loved one's condition. For example, "I wonder if you could tell me what you feel about your dad's condition over the past 4 days." This gives the physician a sense of the reality base of the family and their emotional condition.

c. The physician should explain the condition of the loved one. This may need to be done several times, always in a patient and an understanding manner. The family may become overtly distraught or may react with detachment and silence. The physician should remain with the family and be patiently supportive and ready to respond to further questions or discussion.

3. Seeing the dying or dead patient.

a. The family should not be denied an opportunity to see their loved one.

b. Allow the family to utilize its own cultural mechanisms for dealing with illness or death.

c. The body of the dead patient should be covered, with face and hands exposed, and where mutilation is evident, the family should be forewarned.

4. When a loved one is critically ill and dying:

a. Allow the family a private waiting area.

b. Staff needs to be available to answer questions and provide support.

c. Family should be permitted to see their loved one.

d. Should it be desired, clergy should be called.

5. The surviving family: disposition and follow-up.

a. Someone should remain with the survivor(s) for 24 to 48 hours. This person should be a friend or other family member who was less intimately involved with the deceased, if possible.

b. Consider admission of surviving family member(s) if it appears that acute grief reaction is so severe that suicide is a possibility. This is especially so if a survivor will be alone on leaving the hospital.

c. Follow-up calls should be made for severe cases. Optimally, these should be made 24 hours later, after 3 days, after 1 week, and after 1 month.

d. Use of continued long-term medications is discouraged. The process of mourning is normal and functions as a mechanism whereby the normal grief response can be resolved. Occasionally, if indicated, mild sedation may be prescribed, i.e., lorazepam (Ativan) 1 mg by mouth twice daily as needed for 1 week.

E. **Disaster victims.**

1. The victims themselves.

a. Answer questions about events of disaster; be calm, clear, and gentle.

b. Remain with victims as new, perhaps severely traumatized, victims of disaster are brought in. Psychiatrist in this setting should function as a calm, supportive member of the emergency room team.

2. Relatives of disabled or dead victims.

a. Relatives often rush to the hospital, searching for information about their loved ones.

b. Provide information in a gentle and supportive manner.

c. Relatives should be cared for as any loved one who suffers the impact of an acute grief reaction.

d. Where many relatives are involved, the psychiatrist may need to designate others to psychosocial work in the emergency room; call for backup help where necessary.

3. Disaster workers.

a. Often these people "postpone" the initial grief reaction during active time spent dealing with disaster.

b. These people may suffer a grief response complicated by feelings of guilt and helplessness.

4. Remember follow-up procedures may be necessary to deal with sequelae of disaster.

Acute Crisis and Intervention

F. **Victims of rape.**

1. Immediate interventions should necessarily involve the following:

a. Medical/surgical care where necessary.

b. Supportive "listening" on the part of the psychiatrist. Be aware that a woman who has been raped may suffer shame, humiliation, confusion, fear, and/or rage.

c. Be sensitive to fact that a woman who has been raped is often so physically and psychologically traumatized that the understandable needs of the police to review the details of the episode may exacerbate trauma for the victim.

d. Frequently, societal pressures result in a rape victim's being placed in the role of the guilty party who somehow "invited the attack."

e. The therapist may be called on to deal with significant others of the rape victim; in such cases, "identified patients" may include the woman and those close to her.

f. Not surprisingly, rape victims, both immediately and over the long term, have fears of repeated attacks. The therapist will need to reassure the patient, while, at the same time, ascertain that the patient will be returning to a safe and supportive environment.

2. Follow-up management should be discussed with the patient.

a. Arrange for accompaniment to court, if desired, with psychosocial assistance in taking needed steps with social agencies.

b. Provide follow-up counseling, including further supportive psychotherapy on an outpatient basis. The focus should include attempts to "work through" traumatic memories.

3. Psychodynamic psychotherapy is not the treatment of choice for rape victims acutely, although issues associated or triggered by rape may come up obliquely in therapy many years later.

REFERENCES

1. Albrizio M: The client who is bereaved, in Gorton JG, Partridge R (eds): *Practice and Management of Psychiatric Emergency Care*. St Louis, CV Mosby Co, 1982.
2. Greenblatt M: The grieving spouse. *Am J Psychiatry* 1978; 135:43–47.
3. Hanke N: The suicidal patient, in *Handbook of Emergency Psychiatry*. Lexington, Mass, DC Heath & Co, 1984, chap 7.
4. Hatton CL, Wustman E: The client with suicidal behavior, in Gorton JG, Partridge R (eds): *Practice and Management of Psychiatric Emergency Care*. St Louis, CV Mosby, 1982, chap 8.
5. Lindemann E: Symptomatology and management of acute grief, in Wilcox SG, Sutton M (eds): *Understanding Death and Dying: An Interdisciplinary Approach*. New York, Alfred Publishing Co, Inc, 1977.
6. Mayerson AT, Glick RA, Kiev A: Suicide, in Glick RA, Mayerson AT, Robbins E, et al (eds): *Psychiatric Emergencies*. New York, Grune & Stratton, Inc, 1976.
7. Motto JA: Identifying and treating suicidal patients in a general medicine setting. *Resident Staff Physician*, March, 1983, pp 79–87.
8. Robins E: Suicide, in Kaplan HI, Sadock BJ (eds): *Comprehensive Textbook of Psychiatry/IV*. Baltimore, Williams & Wilkins, 1985.
9. Rothschild AJ: Acute grief: Disaster victims, in Hyman SE (ed): *Manual of Psychiatric Emergencies*. Boston, Little Brown & Co, Inc, 1984.

10. Rose DS: Worse than death: Psychodynamics of rape victims and the need for psychotherapy. *Am J Psychiatry* 1986; 143:817–824.
11. Rund DA, Hutzler JC: Psychiatric emergencies associated with death, in Rund DA, Hutzler JC (eds): *Emergency Psychiatry*. St Louis, CV Mosby Co, 1983.
12. Vaillant GE: Attachment, loss and rediscovery. *The Psychiatric Times* 1986; 8:1, 10–16.

36 | Short-Term Individual Psychotherapies: An Overview

I. **Introduction.** Brief psychiatric interventions include emergency treatment, crisis intervention, and short-term or "brief" individual psychotherapy.

A. *Emergency care* is given to those individuals who have become acutely psychologically disturbed and require immediate attention. Examples include the acutely suicidal, homicidal, recently traumatized, or severely psychiatrically disabled individual. The goal is to protect the safety of the patient and others and attempt to stabilize the acuity of the situation.

B. *Crisis intervention* is a treatment model indicated for patients who are not in an emergency status but who may acutely decompensate if not treated promptly. The goal is to restore the patient's ability to function, often by bolstering his/her coping mechanisms and defenses or by helping him/her to reduce an external stressor. Crisis intervention generally occurs within six sessions, and its end point is determined by the therapeutic progress.

C. *Brief (short-term) individual psychotherapy* is a third category of short-term intervention that is designed with a specified length of treatment and is *not* intended for *acutely* unstable patients. The *time restriction* is usually between ten and 20 sessions. This time limitation creates a pressure on the patient's sense of motivation for change and can require the therapist to play a more active role in the therapeutic session. Please see Chapters 35 and 37 on crisis intervention and psychotherapy for the difficult patient, respectively, for a discussion of emergency and crisis therapy. This chapter will discuss brief treatment.

II. **Exploratory vs. directive therapy.**

A. **Major divisions.** The brief psychotherapies fall into the two general categories of *exploratory* or psychodynamically oriented brief psychotherapy and the *directive* group of interpersonal and cognitive therapy. In general, the experiential schools and the purely supportive therapy approaches are, by nature, open ended and not highly focused on a specific problem area.

B. **Goals and general approaches.** All of the brief individual psychotherapies overlap in their *goals and general approaches* as follows: time-limited nature of therapy, focused orientation of techniques, relatively active therapist, and specific selection criteria. There are considerable differences in the conceptualization of the patient's problem areas and, therefore, what technical interventions should be used to treat them.

C. **Exploratory therapy.** The *psychodynamic therapies* tend to utilize psychoanalytic techniques, especially the "therapeutic triad" of transference, past and present relationships, and the clarification of unconscious defense mechanisms in use to reduce anxiety from inner conflicts. These interventions are based on psychoanalytic concepts of developmental etiology and therapeutic efficacy.

D. **Directive therapy.** The *directive brief psychotherapies* described here both attempt to teach new behavioral skills actively. The *interpersonal* school emphasizes present social relatedness, present and past models, focusing on the patient's symptoms as related to issues of attachment and withdrawal. The parallel to the psychodynamic view of object relations theory is the evidence of one area of overlap in the two views.

Cognitive therapy examines faulty cognitions as etiologic in producing dysphoric symptoms. These negative cognitions may stem from hidden (unconscious) mind-sets or "schemata" that may originate from early experience. Thus, the conceptual and therapeutic process here also has a parallel to the psychodynamic approach of genetic reconstruction and the elucidation of unconscious patterns of behavior.

Despite these overlaps, the cognitive and interpersonal therapies differ in their use of more directive teaching and advising regarding the acquisition of new behaviors. The psychodynamic therapies utilize active interpretation and clarification but require that the patient rely on his/her own motivation in actualizing these insights into behavioral change.

All of the brief psychotherapies aim for *symptom reduction* and not for characterologic change. Patients in this form of therapy need to be able to tolerate a preset date of termination or specified number of sessions. Brief therapy aims for a modification of a person's behavioral responses but does not attempt to restructure his/her long-standing defense structure. A major issue is, thus, which kind of patient is appropriate for open-ended vs. brief therapy. Clinically, the brief therapies are used for the kind of patient who is thought to be suitable for this type of intervention. *Selection criteria* for each therapy are reviewed below.

III. Directive brief psychotherapies.

A. **Overview.** *Interpersonal therapy* and *cognitive therapy* have several characteristics in common: short-term duration, manual-based theory and clinical technique, and initial application to a specific disorder, e.g., depression. Both treatment approaches have been shown to be effective in depressed patients in several randomized clinical trials that have included pharmacotherapy and placebo. The use of treatment manuals that specify techniques has allowed for standardization of training procedures, has increased consistency among certified therapists, and has enhanced the ability to study the efficacy and reliability of the therapeutic intervention. The therapies differ in their conception of the patient's problem and in the techniques applied and will therefore be reviewed separately.

B. **Interpersonal therapy.** Klerman et al. (1984) have described the use of interpersonal therapy as an approach to the treatment of depressed patients, by focusing on current social and interpersonal problems: "IPT [interpersonal therapy] is based on the assumption that depression, regardless of symptom patterns, severity, biological vulnerability, or personality traits, occurs in an interpersonal context and that clarifying and renegotiating the context associated with the onset of symptoms is important to the person's recovery and possibly to the prevention of further episodes."

1. **Selection criteria.** Ambulatory, nonpsychotic, nonbipolar, depressed patients.

2. **Theory.** Interpersonal and social context of symptoms (Sullivan and Meyer were early proponents).

3. **Goals.** Reduction of symptoms and improving functioning during the acute phase of a depressive episode.

4. **Techniques.** Symptom review; teaching about natural course of depressive illness; reassurance; assessment of interpersonal problem areas, including grief reaction, interpersonal disputes, role transition, and interpersonal deficits; focus of attention is on the "here and now" problems and primarily on current interpersonal relations; resolving problem areas with clarification of feeling states and perceptions; and identification of past models for relationships and guidance and encouragement by the therapist to choose alternative interpersonal behaviors.

The therapist's focus on the patient's interpersonal

experiences, expectations, perceptions, and reactions may thus provide new social options for providing an exit from the cycle of depressive symptoms.

5. **Duration.** Twelve to 16 weeks.

C. **Cognitive therapy.** Cognitive therapy is a short-term psychotherapy that was developed primarily by Aaron Beck and A. John Rush. Its premise is that certain cognitions (thoughts, images, and/or assumptions) lead to the onset and persistence of symptoms, especially of anxiety and depression. Treatment is focused at revealing these overt and covert processes to patients, and then teaching patients to recognize them and to use alternative cognitions to alleviate symptoms.

1. **Selection criteria.** Patients with various diagnoses, including generalized anxiety disorders, phobic disorders, depression (mild to moderate, acute, and nonpsychotic), substance abuse disorders, and chronic pain syndromes. Patients must be suitable for active but time-limited therapy. Unlikely to respond are patients with marked cognitive or memory impairments, organic affective disorders, acute psychotic states, or severe personality disorders.

2. **Theory.** Specific situations produce certain cognitions; specific cognitions produce symptomatic affect or behaviors; "schemata" or silent assumptions effect the content of cognitions (i.e., distortion of perception, categorization, and generalization of experience); early experience shapes nature of "schemata"; and "negative" or symptom-producing cognitions lead to "logical errors" (i.e., incorrect inferences about experiences, including overgeneralization, personalization, and/or selective perception).

3. **Feedback loop.** Logical errors and an associated increase in symptoms may reinforce inaccurate perceptions and lead to a strengthening of negative cognitions produced by early schemata in specific symptom-connected situations.

4. **Goals.** Identify repeated "cognitive sets" that are brought to situations; develop ability to recognize and correct negative cognitions and logical errors; gain awareness of schemata underlying cognitive processes; develop and apply new cognitive approaches to situations; and develop new schemata and learn to apply them to situations.

5. **Techniques.** (Please see Chapter 31 on cognitive therapy for more detailed explanations.)

6. **Behavioral.** Activity scheduling, mastery and pleasure ratings, graded task assignment, cognitive rehearsal, assertive training/role-playing, and mood graph.

7. **Cognitive.** Recording automatic thoughts, attrition techniques, responding to negative cognitions, counting automatic thoughts, identifying assumptions, modifying "should's," pro/con refutation of assumptions, homework to test old assumptions, and homework to test new assumptions.

8. **Duration.** May vary depending on diagnosis and severity of illness; for mild to moderate depression: once to twice per week for up to 14 sessions in the short-term treatment phase and then once or twice monthly maintenance therapy for 6 to 12 months to decrease the probability of relapse.

IV. **Exploratory brief psychotherapies.** There are *four major schools* of brief dynamic psychotherapy: focal therapy (Malan), short-term anxiety-provoking therapy (Sifneos), broad-focus therapy (Davanloo), and time-limited psychotherapy (Mann). These therapies are all based on psychoanalytic principles in their theory, goals, and techniques. Their selection criteria overlap considerably as do their durations of treatment. All maintain a specific focus during therapy that tends to be established during an initial evaluation phase and discourages overinclusiveness in the goal setting by the therapist and patient.

Central to all psychodynamic therapies, and especially highlighted in the brief forms, is the concept of the therapeutic triad of transference and past and present relationships. In essence, what the patient provides are the data regarding present interpersonal relationships. In the course of therapy, reactions to the therapist (the transference) may parallel these relationships and help to shed light on the "genetic" (i.e., family of origin developmental history of the patient) origins of the patient's present difficulties. Using the time-honored techniques of interpretation of the transference and resistances, the psychodynamic therapist can aid in the gaining of insight that can thus be coupled with emotional growth and freeing the patient from developmentally anachronistic and presently maladaptive defensive styles. Thus, psychodynamic therapy can help patients develop more flexible coping mechanisms and not merely re-enact the survival options chosen in childhood.

1. **Selection criteria.** Patients generally must have good psychosocial functioning (the ability to assume responsibility, work history, and absence of a major psychopathology); the ability to establish good interpersonal relationships (good initial working relationship with the evaluator and a history of at least one "meaningful" relationship in the past); psychologic mindedness and motivation to understand themselves, good response to early interpretations, ability to mobilize, express, and experience emotions, and an interest in learning to tolerate them; ability for the evaluator to identify a specific "core" problem or "focal conflict" from the patient's initial interview; ability to tolerate quick engagement and disengagement from therapy and the limited nature of therapeutic goals; and motivation for change and desire to work toward goals.

2. **Theory.** Essentially all schools based on the analytic principles outlined above, with the difference primarily in their emphasis on the application of techniques. Thus, early conflicts are resolved by defenses to diminish anxiety in consciousness. Rigid defenses from

childhood lead to inflexibility in adulthood which then produce symptoms.

3. **Goals.** To identify the unconscious conflicts underlying the rigid maladaptive defensive structure; insight into defensive inflexibility leads to a freeing of the emotional restrictiveness and an increase in the possible internal and external responses and a diminution in the presenting symptoms.

4. **Techniques.** (Please see Chapter 30 on psychodynamic psychotherapies for more details.) The timing and emphasis of different techniques described above will be highlighted for each proponent:

a. **Malan.** Transference interpretations are given only when the transference becomes a resistance; the therapist's role is to maintain the focus throughout the therapy (identifying the precipitating factors, early traumatic experiences, and patterns of behavior); to contrast the current problem with the developmental conflict as it manifests itself in the transference; and to clarify defenses, anxiety, and impulses.

b. **Sifneos.** Major focus is on the oedipal conflict as the origin of current difficulties; use of anxiety-provoking confrontations to clarify connection between past and present issues; and use of early, aggressive transference interpretations.

c. **Mann.** Focuses are on "fears and pain" and issues of dependency, loss, and attachment; initial phrasing of central issue of crucial importance to specify goals; use of nonconfrontational psychoanalytic techniques with interpretations close to the literal statements of the patient; and a focus on the different phases of the treatment with and emphasis on separation and termination issues.

d. **Davanloo.** Psychoanalytic techniques focus on genetic reconstruction with early transference interpretations; confrontational style used especially with severe obsessional disorders to uncover aggressive impulses behind the obsessional isolation of affect.

5. **Duration.** There is a high degree of overlap in the general length of treatment. However, each school emphasizes a slightly different feature of the duration.

a. **Malan.** Definite date (with an average 20 sessions.).

b. **Sifneos.** No date or specified number given; patients told will last a "few months"; and average, 12 to 16 sessions with 20 maximum sessions at weekly frequency for 45 minutes per session.

c. **Mann.** Twelve treatment hours with two to four evaluation sessions.

d. **Davanloo.** Five to 40 sessions with 15 to 25 average lengths; no date given, and duration tends to be shorter for oedipal focus and longer for multiple foci.

REFERENCES AND SUGGESTED READING

1. Beck AT, Rush AJ, Shaw BF, et al: *Cognitive Therapy of Depression.* New York, Guilford Press, 1979.
2. Davanloo H (ed): *Short-term Dynamic Psychotherapy.* New York, Jason Aronson, Inc, 1980.
3. Horowitz MJ, Marmar C, Weiss DS, et al: Brief psychotherapy of bereavement reactions. *Arch Gen Psychiatry* 1984; 41:438–448.
4. Klerman GL, Weissman MM, Rounsaville BJ, et al: *Interpersonal Psychotherapy of Depression.* New York, Basic Books Inc Publishers, 1984.
5. Malan DH: *The Frontier of Brief Psychotherapy.* New York, Plenum Press, 1976.
6. Mann J: The core of time-limited psychotherapy: Time and the central issue, in Budman S (ed): *Forms of Brief Therapy.* New York, Guilford Press, 1981.
7. Rogawski AS: Current status of brief psychotherapy. *Bull Menninger Clin* 1982; 46:331–351.

8. Sifneos P: Short-term anxiety-provoking psychotherapy: Its history, techniques, outcome and instruction, in Budman S (ed): *Forms of Brief Therapy*. New York, Guilford Press, 1981.
9. Ursano RJ, Hales RE: A review of brief individual psychotherapies. *Am J Psychiatry* 1986; 143:1507–1517.

37 Psychotherapy With Difficult Patients

I. **Introduction.** Difficult patients arouse the psychiatrist's feelings of helplessness, guilt, anger, fear, and even boredom. They force us to examine our fantasies of healing all, knowing all, and loving all. With difficult patients, it is particularly important to address the patient's chief complaint and to reassess the diagnosis and goals continually.

II. **The somaticizers.** These are people who are alexithymic, i.e., without words for feelings, they express emotional pain through physical symptoms.

A. What to look for.

1. Underlying depression.

2. Fear of deprivation, of not being cared for.

3. Identification with significant family member or friend with similar symptoms.

4. Fear of abandonment.

5. Guilt over aggressive impulses.

B. What you can do.

1. Acknowledge the patient's distress.

2. Reassure the patient that he/she will receive care.

3. Avoid focusing on the cause of the patient's symptoms.

4. Set up a schedule for care, for inpatient daily 5-minute rounds with two to three 15-minute sessions a week and for outpatient two or three 30-minute sessions, during which the listing of symptoms is limited to 5 minutes. Note: As soon as patient is able to sustain a session without falling back on his/her symptoms, extend sessions gradually to the full length.

5. Work closely with the patient's internist and follow up his/her medical problem. If you suspect a medical illness, refer to an internist.

6. Protect against unnecessary medical intervention and/or hospitalization; whenever possible, arrange for outpatient care.

7. Hospitalize for suicidal plans, severe anxiety, and depressive and/or psychotic symptoms.

8. Encourage the family to direct all the patient's somatic complaints to the internist.

C. What to discuss.

1. Translate the patient's symptoms into feelings by teaching him/her to verbalize his/her own affect, first by validating it with labeling statements, e.g., "You seem…(sad, angry, etc.)."

2. Identify the patient's fears and help him/her to understand how his/her symptoms either confirm his/her fears and/or defend against his/her fears and offer alternatives to deal with those fears.

3. Teach relaxation techniques and alternate behaviors to avoid precipitants or aggravants.

III. **The organic patient.**

A. *What to Look for.* A person whose altered mental status is anatomic, physiologic, metabolic, or toxic in etiology, e.g., the delirious, the demented, the substance-abusing, or the postconcussive patient.

1. Medical causes.

2. Degree of impairment: perform the Folstein Mini-Mental State Examination.

3. Underlying depression or psychosis.

4. Feelings of loss, e.g., of self, autonomy, friends, family, hobbies, and skills.

5. Awareness without acceptance of the disease, leading to denial, anger, paranoia, and anxiety.

6. Disruption of the family.

7. Suicidality.

B. What you can do.

1. Treat medical causes.

2. Arrange for neuropsychologic and occupational testing, if needed.

3. Treat any underlying psychosis or depression with psychotropic drugs.

4. Hospitalize or commit, if the patient is severely impaired or suicidal or if the family's emotional and/or physical resources are depleted.

5. Work with the hospital staff to have the same personnel caring for the patient whenever possible, and set up schedules for meals and/or medications; allow the patient and his/her family to participate in his/her care as much as possible.

6. Initially, meet with the patient and his/her family separately, to identify their concerns. Family meetings with or without the patient may be needed to supplement individual sessions with the patient.

7. Support and educate the patient and his/her family; help identify his/her deficits and teach them to compensate with memory aids, such as list making, item labeling, and established daily routines.

8. Show them how to reorient the patient repeatedly, e.g., today is Monday and you wanted to do—."

9. Help the family, and when indicated, arrange for a home-health aid, visiting nursing care, meals-on-wheels, etc.

10. When indicated, provide recreational and occupational therapy to develop independent living skills.

11. Help the patient and his/her family to understand the prognosis and what can be done.

C. What to discuss.

1. Encourage the patient to mourn over such losses as self-esteem and physical and intellectual skills.

2. Let the patient tell you his/her life story; in reliving his/her life with you, he/she can rebuild his/her sense of self.

3. Help the patient identify his/her conflicts and guide him/her to find some meaning to his/her life by reinforcing his/her sense of self, or his/her likes and dislikes.

4. Explain to both the patient and his/her family how hard it is to determine the degree to which emotions are a consequence of the organic process. The family needs to understand that apparent selfishness may be an inability to recognize social amenities and impulsivity, i.e., a loss of self-regulation.

5. Encourage the family to accept their own limitations and to nurture themselves by maintaining social contacts and pleasurable pastimes.

6. Explore the meaning of death for both the patient and his/her family. Once understood, help them to confront the issues of how and where the patient wants to die.

IV. **The dying patient.** This is the person who is terminally ill in the end stages.

A. What to look for.

1. Dementia/delirium secondary to an organic process.

2. Underlying depression or psychosis.

3. Fears of dying.

4. Fears of abandonment, particularly in patients with acquired immunodeficiency syndrome.

5. Suicidality.

6. Guilt over past and present feelings, behaviors or impulses.

7. Anger at fate and loss of control.

8. Fears of helplessness.

9. Support system: Does one exist?

B. **What to do.** Refer to Section III./B.: What to do for the organic patient.

1. Perform serial mental status examinations to evaluate the degree of impairment.

2. Identify any support system (e.g., friends, family, and/or significant others) and arrange meetings with or without the patient, if indicated.

3. Encourage the patient to participate in group therapy to provide support and a sense of belonging if the advancing disease is producing isolation.

4. Encourage the family and staff to support the patient's defense mechanisms if they sustain his/her hope and sense of autonomy and are not interfering with his/her medical care.

C. **What to discuss.** Review Section III./C.: What to discuss with the organic patient.

1. Acknowledge fears of abandonment and of dying alone.

2. Allow him/her to ventilate his/her disappointments and his/her anger at being cheated of enjoying the harvest of his/her family or his/her work.

3. Identify and validate paradoxical feelings; with family and friends, the patient may be feeling just as

guilty and worthless because he/she is unable to help them as he/she does because they can cope without him/her, appearing not to need him/her.

4. Help him/her through his/her own process of dying; find out if he/she has seen friends or family die from his/her own illness.

V. **The noncompliant patient.** These externalizing patients have difficulty taking responsibility. They refuse to take medications as prescribed. As outpatients, they consistently miss or come late for appointments and, as inpatients, do not abide by hospital rules. Key concepts relevant to these people include alexithymia and projective identification.

A. **The entitled demanders.** These patients, whether they are initially charming or abusive, are the exploiters.

1. What to look for.

a. Attempts to intimidate, devalue, and make you feel guilty for not taking care of them.

b. Self-destructive behaviors, such as substance abuse, suicide attempts, chaotic relationships, job difficulties, and legal problems, including a history of assaults.

c. Fear of being neglected, helpless, abused, or humiliated.

d. Lability: These patients may be alternately charming and threatening.

2. What to do.

a. Acknowledge with the involved staff how infuriating this patient is to diminish resentment which may lead to acting out, e.g., ignoring the patient and reinforcing his/her fears of deprivation.

b. When seeing a patient for the first time, look for a secondary gain, i.e., legal problems, family conflicts, a lost job, a broken relationship, or a lack of funds and friends to provide shelter for the night.

c. Whenever possible, emphasize the need for a long-term solution to the patient's problems.

d. If the patient is genuinely suicidal or homicidal, admit the patient briefly.

e. When interviewing a potentially violent patient, have other staff or a security officer present with you.

f. These patients need a structure of regular appointment times that begin and end punctually. For an outpatient, define fee schedules and a procedure for canceling appointments. For an inpatient, establish a treatment plan that includes a set discharge date.

g. Limit and confront the patient's acting out. If the patient is repetitively unable to comply, consider a transfer from the ward or your practice with referrals.

h. Avoid ambiguity: Communicate clearly and regularly to avoid distortions.

i. On an inpatient ward, work closely with the staff to prevent the patient from pitting one staff member against another, by either labeling one as good or bad and recreating his/her own internal fragmentation or by manipulating one against the other to get his/her way.

j. Provide the patient with referrals for community resources.

k. Consider group therapy for these individuals who may assimilate new copying styles from those with similar problems and backgrounds.

3. What to discuss.

a. Help the patient to label his/her feelings or "reactions" in problem situations with other people.

b. Once having identified those feelings, help the patient to understand how he/she acts out or externalizes his/her feelings to avoid having to experience them.

c. Emphasize the detrimental consequences of such acting-out behaviors and their failure to resolve his/her conflicts.

d. Provide a vocabulary for ventilation of affect, assertion training, problem-solving skills, or even relaxation techniques.

e. Try to restore a sense of self-determination via participation in the treatment plan.

B. **Self-destructive deniers.** These are the obsessive-compulsive, paranoid, and avoidant patients.

1. What to look for.

a. Difficulty with dependency.

b. Isolation of affect: The patient's emotional experience is out of his/her awareness.

c. A fear of losing control if compliant with treatment.

d. A need to defend against being labeled as a psychiatric patient, or of being defective.

e. An inability to trust others, fearing that treatment may do more harm than good.

2. What to do.

a. Give the patient as much control as possible over own treatment.

b. Group therapy may make it difficult to deny or disavow illness in the face of peer pressure.

c. When appointments are consistently missed, gently confront the patient by saying you would like to help him/her, but you need him/her to tell you how to make it easier for him/her to come in for therapy and/or medications.

d. Allow the patient to determine his/her goals and criteria for improvement.

3. What to discuss.

a. Help to explore the patient's feelings.

b. Allow the patient to express both his/her need to fend off dependency and his/her need to be dependent.

c. Identify what makes the accepting of care so difficult for this patient, e.g., is it because a "good person" should be able to care for himself/herself, or an abhorrence of helplessness?

d. Support the patient's strengths while exploring his/her vulnerabilities.

VI. Violent and suicidal patients.

A. **The violent patient.** These patients act out aggressively often out of fear, shame, or confusion.

1. What to look for.

a. Possible organic causes.

b. Psychosis.

c. Threatening behavior, e.g., pacing, baring teeth, fist clenching, and/or posturing.

d. History of assaults.

e. History of having been abused.

f. Suicidality or homicidality.

2. What to do.

a. Act and speak in a manner that allows the patient to save face and maintain as much self-dignity as possible.

b. Always deal with an acutely violent patient as a team, including other staff and/or security. Avoid antagonistic confrontation; usually, a show of force is effective.

c. As a team, assess the patient and plan how to handle potential outbursts.

d. Have physical and chemical restraints available, along with a designated leader to coordinate.

e. Ideally, have the patient placed in a room as bare and open as possible.

f. If you choose to stand near such a patient, stand by him/her as an ally, not across from him/her as a possible assailant.

g. You may talk a patient down by addressing his/her basic needs.

h. Warn him/her of potentially upsetting questions that you must ask him/her.

i. Explain your actions repeatedly to avoid startling the patient.

j. Treat drug withdrawal or psychoses whether or not the patient requires restraints.

k. When no longer agitated, encourage group therapy for these individuals who often assimilate new copying styles best from those with similar problems and backgrounds.

3. What to discuss.

a. When a patient is acutely agitated, focus on containing his/her distress to the point that he/she can verbalize his/her feelings and describe the provoking precipitant.

b. Once the acute episode has resolved, address his/her tendency to act on feelings instead of verbalizing them.

c. Emphasize the detrimental consequences of such acting-out behavior and their failure to resolve conflicts.

d. Teach him/her to recognize aggravants and to respond with alternative behaviors.

B. **The chronically suicidal patient.** These patients act out their distress by suicide gestures or attempts, e.g., overdoses and self-mutilating acts, such as wrist slashing.

1. What to look for.

a. Intolerance for being either intimate or alone.

b. Emotional lability.

c. History of suicide attempts.

d. Lack of identity and a feeling of being "empty"

that is often relieved by self-inflicted pain or the sight of blood.

e. History of having been abused.

f. A belief that others hate them that leads to their being provoking and inciting anger and/or rejection, reinforcing that belief.

g. Substance abuse or affective disorder.

2. What to do. (Refer to Section V./A.: What to do for entitled demanders.)

a. Evaluate for acute suicidality.

b. Identify the precipitating event.

c. In some cases, hospitalization may be avoided by mobilizing support systems to maintain the patient as an outpatient, i.e., have the patient stay with a supportive family member or friend.

d. Carefully monitor your own defenses to avoid acting on them; avoid being either overly helpful by intervening in personal relationships on the patient's behalf (reaction formation) or indifferent and resigned to believing that this patient is beyond help (denial).

e. If you do hospitalize a patient, make it a brief crisis admission, if possible.

f. Provide a structure by setting up regular appointments and rules for cancellations and paying fees.

g. Notify this patient of any vacations that you plan to take well ahead of time and who the covering physician will be.

h. Teach the patient alternate responses to his/her feelings.

i. Arrange for sessions with the family or significant others, if indicated.

j. Consider psychotropic drugs; if you do decide to prescribe medications, provide less than lethal amounts.

3. What to discuss.

a. Identify the feelings that drive the patient to feeling suicidal.

b. Validate patient's "bad" feelings (e.g., anger, helplessness, and envy) by letting the patient know that what must be changed is how the feelings are acted on rather than the feelings themselves.

c. Explore the patient's reactions to you (transference) and clarify misconceptions, pointing out the similarity in his/her responses to others and to you.

d. Clarify how suicidal behavior is alienating to others, leaving the patient feeling only more isolated, empty, and misunderstood.

VII. **Conclusion.** The most powerful therapeutic tool is the relationship unique to each patient and therapist. This relationship is the source of hope that many difficult patients have lost. Within this relationship, the therapist provides the structure that enables the patient to reach his/her goals. The therapist provides the means for a patient to change by balancing discipline and confrontation with tolerance and acceptance.

REFERENCES

1. Groves JE. Taking care of the hateful patient. *N Engl J Med* 1978; 298:883–887.
2. Lezak M: Living with the characterologically altered brain injured patient. *J Clin Psychiatry* 1978; 30:592–598.
3. Maltsberger J, Buie D: Countertransference hate in the treatment of suicidal patients. *Arch Gen Psychiatry* 1978; 30:592–598.
4. Nichols SE: Psychosocial reactions of persons with acquired immunodeficiency syndrome. *Ann Intern Med* 1985; 103:765–767.
5. Nichols SE: Emotional aspects of AIDS—impli-

cations for care providers. *J Substance Abuse Treat* 1987; 4:137–140.
6. Perry S, Viederman M: Management of emotional reactions to acute medical illness. *Med Clin North Am* 1981; 65:3–14.
7. Rada R: The violent patient: Rapid assessment and management. *Psychosomatics* 1981; 2:101–105.
8. Reiser DE, Levenson H: Abuses of the borderline diagnosis: A clinical problem with teaching opportunities. *Am J Psychiatry* 1984; 141:1528–1532.
9. Rittelmeyer LF: Coping with the chronic complainer. *AFP* 1985; 211–215.
10. Schwartz DA: The suicidal character. *Psychiatr Q* 1979; 51:64–70.
11. Tupin J: The violent patient: A strategy for management and diagnosis. *Hosp Community Psychiatry* 1983; 34:37–40.
12. Vaillant GE: Sociopathy as a human process. *Arch Gen Psychiatry* 1975; 32:178–183.
13. Waldinger RJ: Intensive psychodynamic therapy with borderline patients: An overview. *Am J Psychiatry* 1987; 144:267–274.

38 | Psychotherapy With Children and Adolescents

I. Background.

A. The contrasts to psychotherapy with adults.

Children and adolescents are in the midst of *major developmental changes* in the realm of cognitive, emotional, and psychosocial functioning. Psychotherapy must take into account the developmental stage of the individual to provide the appropriate forms of communication and modes for therapeutic change. Psychotherapy is often aimed at allowing the normal forces of child and adolescent development to proceed beyond obstacles and pressures that inhibit this process. Adults also go through developmental stages, at times, that require therapeutic intervention, but these changes are primarily psychosocial and do not require different basic levels of communication on the part of the therapist.

By virtue of their stage in life, adolescents and children are *dependent on adults:* in the family and in school, they rely on others for much of what shapes their world. This reliance necessitates the therapist's involvement to various degrees with the family, parents, and school staff in both evaluation and treatment.

Children or adolescents *rarely seek psychotherapeutic intervention on their own* but are usually referred by parents or school officials. Thus, these individuals may be unaware of the specific reasons for psychotherapy, and their motivation to engage in therapy needs to be nurtured, especially if external behaviors, rather than internal distress, have brought them to professional attention.

Working with children or adolescents often requires the therapist to use "preadult," *alternative forms of communication* to relate on the specific developmental level of the patient. This can be especially demanding on the therapist in that it requires a simultaneous "professional regression" to recall earlier stages of thinking, feeling, and behaving (e.g., play therapy) while, at the same time, maintaining a sophisticated perspective on the therapeutic process.

The therapist is the child or adolescent's advocate. In cases of serious neglect or physical, sexual, or emotional abuse, the therapist may be morally and legally obligated to intervene between patient and family. Thus, the therapist may, at times, need to take an active role in protecting the child from external traumas that may have occurred or be presently occurring in the child or adolescent's home.

B. **General goals and characteristics of psychotherapy with children and adolescents.** To allow the normal, healthy forces in the child's development to prevail in the face of internal or external factors that inhibit them is the overall goal of therapy with individuals of this age. Internal factors include the focus on symptoms (depression and anxiety) or symptomatic behaviors (hyperactivity, impulsivity, and social avoidance). External factors include overstimulation (inappropriate parental overinvolvement or withdrawal in anger, sexual or physical abuse, and witnessing traumatic events) or empathic failures ("poor" parent-child bonding, misunderstanding of developmental needs, and lack of parents to see child as a separate but dependent person). Growth may also be impaired by major life stressors (divorce and death of a parent or sibling) and biologic deviance (birth defects, medical illness, and mental retardation) that may require psychotherapeutic intervention for healthy adjustment.

Each of these impairments to normal growth and development should be understood in the context of the various "lines" of active development that the child or adolescent is undergoing. The therapist for these patients needs to be cognizant of these stages to both facilitate the therapeutic process (i.e., age-appropriate communication and techniques) and to establish meaningful therapeutic goals. These efforts also need to encompass the patient's social world, i.e., the family and school; thus, family therapy, parental guidance, and, at times, school intervention are routine aspects of therapy with children and adolescents.

Therapy may occur in the setting of in-hospital, day treatment, or outpatient sessions, depending on the severity of the disorder. Formats include family, individual, group, and parental therapy. The combination of these modalities will be dependent on the nature of each case and the willingness and financial ability of the family to participate. Therapy may be short term or long term and often involves the family to varying degrees. Some therapists, in certain cases, support "family therapy only" as a mode of treatment, especially when the child or adolescent's "illness" is viewed as a symptom of a dysfunctional family.

Theoretical and technical approaches include psychoanalytic (including play therapy), behavioral, experiential, and supportive therapies. The application of these approaches to children and adolescents takes into account the developmental stage and parent-child relationship. The developmental level will determine the nature of the communication and therapeutic agent of change. Thus, for children under 9 or 10 years of age, play therapy is an important means of expression and working through of internal conflicts and past traumatic experiences. Young adolescents may be more likely to be influenced by their peers; thus, group therapy might be more effective for this age range.

Constitutional issues are also an important consideration in understanding potential "mismatches" between parent and child that may lead to low self-esteem and difficult early social relationships. Thus, the focus of therapy needs to consider the living, evolving relationship of the "patient" to his/her parent that may require intervention in parental counseling and family sessions.

C. **Three aspects of development.** Three views of development will be briefly outlined here as a reference point to help the reader conceptualize the various development tasks that children at various stages are mastering. A failure to progress may result in age-inappropriate abilities and behavior that, in turn, may present as "disorders." Reasons for the inability to master these stages, in general, span the range from the biologic (e.g., the psychotic disorders, severe mental retardation, and autism) to failures and overstimulation (including severe traumas and their psychologic sequalae and intrapsychic, internal conflicts leading to the inability to progress to more mature stages of development).

1. **Anna Freud's diagnostic profile and the concept of developmental lines.** Anna Freud (1965) has described a developmental profile of the child that focuses on the intrapsychic (psychoanalytically based) structures and dynamics as they evolve during the child's maturation. Clinically, this profile requires a good deal of familiarity with the basic psychoanalytic concepts. The reader is referred to Chapter 30 on psychoanalytic therapies and to the suggested readings. The portion of the profile supplied here as a reference is intended to give a sense of the depth with which the child's development can be understood. Many clinicians refer primarily to the "developmental lines" in this section of the outline as one of the most useful constructs of

the profile; therefore, the reader may find it helpful to focus on this portion of the following outline.

a. Diagnostic profile adapted from Anna Freud.

(i) Reason for referral.

(ii) Description of child (personal appearance, moods, manner, etc.)

(iii) Pediatric history and family background.

(iv) Significant environmental influences.

(v) Assessments of development.

(a) Assessment of drives, i.e., libido and aggression libido: level and dominance of phase of development (oral, anal, etc.); age-appropriate?; object investment (distribution); and level, quality, and dominance of object relatedness; and aggression: quantity, quality, and direction (self or outside world).

(b) Superego and ego development.

(1) Autonomous functions: perception, memory, speech, secondary process thinking, reality testing, and intelligence.

(2) Defense organization: adequate for age, effectiveness, and direction (toward which specific drives).

(3) Secondary interference of defense with ego function (e.g., depression-inhibiting ability to learn).

(c) Developmental lines: lines from dependency to emotional self-reliance and adult object relatedness; lines toward body independence (from suckling to rational eating, from wetting and soiling to bladder and bowel control, and from irresponsibility to responsibility in body management); lines from egocentricity to companionship; and lines from body to the toy and from play to work.

(d) Elaboration of one line of development: The most fully elucidated line is from dependency to emotional self-reliance and adult object relatedness; therefore, the details of this aspect of development will be outlined here:

Biologic unity with mother

Need-gratification as basis of dependency

Object constancy (positive inner image of object maintained)

Ambivalent relationship with parent ("preoedipal anal-sadistic stage)

Object-centered phallic-oedipal phase (possessiveness of parent of opposite sex)

Latency period (transfer of libido from parental figure to contemporaries and adults outside of the family and postoedipal lessening of drives)

Preadolescent period with return to "part-object, need-fulfilling ambivalent-type relations" of the preoedipal stage

Adolescence: large shift in ties to infantile objects and toward objects of the opposite sex outside of the family

(vi) Genetic assessment. (Refers to "genesis" of problems, not chromosomal inheritance.) Analysis of fixation points and regression through viewing of behavior, fantasy life, and symptoms.

(vii) Dynamic and structural assessment.

External conflicts ("ego vs. the outer world")

Internalized conflicts ("ego vs. the superego" as in guilt)

Internal conflicts (centered within the ego itself as in unresolved ambivalence or conflicts)

Assessment of severity of disturbance in the context of the level of independence and maturity

(viii) General assessment.

Frustration tolerance

Sublimation potential

Overall attitudes to anxiety (withdrawal vs. mastery)

Assessment of balance between the progressive and regressive developmental forces

(ix) Diagnosis. (not *DSM III-R!*).

Variations of normal

Transitory symptoms leading to developmental strain

Permanent developmental regression and fixation (neurotic conflicts, infantile neurosis, and character disorders)

Developmental ego/superego regression (borderline children and psychotic children)

Primary deficiency of organic nature or early deprivation, distorting development and structuralization (of the psyche)

Onoing destructive processes (progressive deterioration due to organic, toxic, or psychic factors)

2. Erik Erikson's Eight Ages of Man. In Erikson's classic work, *Childhood and Society*, he eloquently elaborated his conceptualization of the psychosocial development of the individual from infancy through maturity. This perspective has been found to be helpful in understanding the underlying developmental themes at various ages. Erikson emphasized that while each of these stages is "mastered" before the subsequent stage is realized, elements of the preceding themes persist in various forms throughout the life cycle. Thus, the stages are integrated and characterized by encounter and crisis, with a sense of progression and building on one another. Furthermore, he described the "stages" as broadly defined periods and not as sharply demarcated chronologies. In his revised edition, he has added the "essential strengths and basic values" that correlate with the struggle described by the name of each stage. For the readers' benefit, the following outline (Table 38–1) will condense the developmental stages with their approximate chronologic age range, essential strengths and basic values (respectively, in parentheses), and essential developmental struggle.

3. **Piaget's Concept of Intellectual (Cognitive) Development.** Jean Piaget devoted his scientific life to the elaboration of the evolution of intellectual ability in the individual. He described a series of periods, stages, and substages that are characterized by the qualities of succession and integration with the need for preparation and completion of previous stages. He distinguished the process of formation of certain cognitive abilities from the final forms of equilibrium between these functions. Lags in development were seen as the obstacles to achieving further developmental stages. Piaget divided intellectual development into three important "periods" that were then characterized by stages and substages outlined below. The clinical utility of this reference outline is in the view that it provides of how children at different ages are able to conceptualize the world around them. This can then serve as a general guide to the nature of the therapist's level of communication and expectation for how the child may integrate the therapeutic interventions. The following outline of Piaget's conceptualization of cognitive development is adapted from Piaget (1976) and Ginsburg (1985).

(i) *Sensorimotor Period: (Birth to 2 Years).* Reflexes (0 to 1 month); first habits (1 to 4.5 months); coordination of vision and prehension (4.5 to 9 months); coordination of secondary schemes (8 or 9 to 11 or 12 months); differentiation of schemes of action by tertiary circular reaction and discovery of new means (11 or 12 to 18 months); and beginning of interiorization of schemes and solution of a few problems with action stopping and sudden understanding (18 to 24 months).

Summary: Infant progresses through these stages from reflexes to learning from basic experience and im-

TABLE 38–1.

Erickson's Psychosocial Stages of Development*

Eight Ages of Man

Basic trust vs. basic mistrust
  (Drive and hope)
  0–18 mo; oral-sensory
Autonomy vs. shame and doubt
  (Self-control and willpower)
  18–36 mo; muscular-anal
Initiative vs. guilt
  (Direction and purpose)
  4–6 yr; locomotor-genital
Industry vs. inferiority
  (Method and competence)
  7–11 yr; latency
Identity vs. role confusion
  (Deviation and fidelity)
  12–18 yr; puberty-adolescence
Intimacy vs. isolation
  (Affiliation and love)
  young adulthood
Generativity vs. stagnation
  (Production and care)
  middle age
Ego integrity vs. despair
  (Renunciation and wisdom)
  maturity

*Adapted from Erickson E: *Childhood and Society, ed 2.* New York, WW Norton & Co, Inc, 1963.

itation toward the development of mental representations (symbols that signify abstract items).

(ii) *"Preparatory" Period: (2 to 11 Years).* This large period is of preparation and of organization of concrete operations of categories, relations, and numbers. It can be divided into three subperiods (although Piaget combined the first two) as follows.

(a) *Preconceptual Stage (2 to 4 Years).* Appearance of the symbolic function and beginning of the interiorization of the schemes of action in representations (as seen in symbolic play and the development of language). This period involves the development of basic mental representations through imitation, formation of mental symbols, preliminary stages of reasoning, and "egocentric" forms of speech (this "egocentrism" overlaps into the ages of 6 or 7 years and involves a limited viewpoint, realism, and lack of introspection).

(b) *Preoperational Stage (4 to 7 Years).* Representative organizations, founded either on static configurations or on an assimilation to the action itself; articulated representative regulations (examples include the use of classifications, order relations, and the beginning of the ability to recognize conservation principles); and the pattern of thought is distinguished by "centration," i.e., the focusing on only one aspect of a real problem.

(c) *Concrete Operations Subperiod: (7 to 11 Years).* "Concrete operations" are characterized by reversibility and flexibility, recognition of space and time relationships, and the understanding of simultaneous events (temporally and dynamically); this opening of a viewpoint can be thought of as a "decentration" process.

(iii) *Formal Operational Period: (11 Years to Adulthood).* This period has been described as beginning abruptly with a first stage and reaching an equilibrium by 13 or 14 years ("second stage"). This period is characterized by thinking that is flexible and effective, able to focus on complex problems of reason in a comprehensive manner, sees reality as secondary to possibility (i.e., considers the possible first before the concrete), and can reason about hypothetical ideas.

This cognitive ability to distance oneself from the concrete reality and consider alternate possibilities has clear implications for therapeutic work that involves introspection and the use of complex psychologic constructs in communicating to children who have not yet reached this period in their development.

II. Assessment.

A. **Gathering information.** Before deciding to initiate psychotherapy, a thorough assessment should be performed. This evaluation should include a clinical history, examination of the child and family, and a history from the school. Rating scales (e.g., Connors' Scale for hyperactivity) are helpful, along with parent questionnaires filled out by both child and parent. Educational testing is often important to rule out learning dysfunction and assess the level of intelligence. Psychologic testing may be helpful to support clinical impressions of mood or thought disorders and underlying themes in the patient's subjective world. Formal diagnostic interviews are available for children as with adults.

Initiating the assessment is approached in different ways by different clinicians, depending on the case or their theoretical orientation. Thus, some therapists will start by seeing the entire family; others will begin by interviewing the parents alone and then the child individually or with the parent. Trainees might try different approaches and decide for themselves how best to approach the assessment initiation.

The assessment period should address parental concerns about their child's dysfunction and should approach parents as helpful informants and colleagues rather than as patients. It is crucial to elicit the support of important care givers and family members to engage the child in the evaluation and possible therapeutic interventions.

Information from the direct interview of the child is important, but the clinician should remember that the patient may behave dramatically different at home or in school; therefore, multiple "informants" from these settings are crucial for a thorough evaluation.

B. **Summarizing the data.** The result of the assessment should summarize the following.

1. Presenting problem and history of the present illness (degree of functional impairment in the realms of family relations, school behavior and performance, peer relations and leisure time activities, and personal distress).

2. Past psychiatric illness and treatment.

3. Medical history, including immunizations, neurologic or communicative deficits, and congenital defects.

4. Family genetic history.

5. Developmental history, including pregnancy, delivery, infancy, early temperament, developmental milestones (fine and gross motor, speech, social, and bladder/bowel control); developmental lags include delays in achieving age-appropriate abilities and the persistence of more immature behavior as other stages evolve.

6. Educational history (grades, favorite and disliked subjects, special classes, and tutoring).

7. Social functioning (close friends, ability to play with other children, and nature and quality of peer relations).

8. Family description (members and relationship of patient to others: see details in Chapter 32 on family therapy).

9. Review of psychiatric symptoms.

10. Mental Status Examination.

11. Rating scales and formal testing results.

12. Laboratory test and physical examination results.

13. Case summary (discussing the pertinent positives, the psychodynamic formulation and developmental profile, and their relationship to family functioning and the presenting "illness").

14. Diagnostic axes.

15. Treatment recommendations.

C. **Diagnosis.** The diagnostic process in evaluating children and adolescents is more than finding the essential number of criteria that are met for a *DSM III-R* category's requirement. A developmental approach is essential and requires the ability to distinguish normal vs. abnormal development, to assess the severity of a disorder as viewed by its interference with development, and to recognize the different vulnerabilities of individuals at different ages.

Dr. Dennis Cantwell (verbal communication, 1987) has outlined a helpful view of the steps of the diagnostic process as follows:

1. Is there a psychiatric disorder? (Is there *functional* impairment in behavior, cognition, interpersonal relations, or subjective distress?

2. Is there a known, recognized clinical syndrome?

3. What are the roots of the disorder in *this* child?

4. What are the forces (internal or external) maintaining the problem?

5. What are the forces facilitating normal development?

6. What are the child's strengths and competencies?

7. What is the natural history of the untreated syndrome?

8. Is intervention necessary? (How urgent or significant does intervention need to be? What will the goals and measures of effectiveness of the intervention be?)

9. What types of intervention are needed?

D. **Treatment recommendations.** Treatment recommendations should include suggestions in the following general categories.

1. Medical (i.e., the need for further evaluation or treatment).

2. Psychiatric: (1) Is there a disorder in which psychopharmacologic intervention is indicated? (2) How does the case summary suggest which types of psychotherapeutic interventions, if any, are indicated? (3) If no clear disorder is present, is there evidence for a prodromal presentation that requires close follow-up but not intervention presently?

3. Family: Is further family assessment or intervention indicated? How has this "illness" affected the family, and what family supports or interventions are needed?

4. School: Is there a learning disorder present? Is there a need for special classes or a tutor?

5. Legal: Is there a history of abuse (requiring reporting)? Is this a high-risk situation (requiring further on-site evaluation)?

III. **Indications for psychotherapy with children and adolescents.** Patients of this age range may benefit from a relationship with a caring, respectful person who is able to acknowledge their individuality and support their development. Given the expense in time and money and the potential identification as an "ill" person, psychotherapy needs to be prescribed only as needed. The nature of the core "problems" of the child/adolescent need to be understood in relation to their developmental stage (as described above) and to their family system (see Goldner, 1985; and also Chapter 32 on family therapy for discussions of assessment and intervention).

Psychotherapy may be indicated, regardless of the

specific *DSM III-R* diagnosis. Therapy may include various combinations of individual, family, parent, and group therapy. Some general indications for therapeutic intervention include the following categories of presenting difficulties.

A. Internally distressful symptoms (anxiety and depression).

B. Externally dysfunctional behavior (poor impulse control, lack of interpersonal skills, and impaired reality testing).

C. Adjustment difficulties (after divorce and death of a relative).

D. Post-traumatic sequalae (witnessing severely violent acts, direct physical or sexual abuse, and chronic parental mental illness).

E. Developmental crises (separation anxiety and school phobia).

F. Specific diagnoses (eating disorders, chronic medical illness and its psychosocial sequalae, and some cases of attention deficit disorder and autism).

Contraindications or limitations to psychotherapy in treating children or adolescents focus primarily on the need to avoid the potentially "pathologizing" effect of individual therapy on the patient that may isolate him/her from the family and, in cases of severe family psychopathology, may serve to solidify the negative identity as the "ill member." In other cases, the individual strengthening of the patient without intervention in the family system might produce negative consequences on a precarious dysfunctional family balance.

Certain individuals, especially during adolescence, may be filled with distrust of adults and might better be served by group therapy rather than a dyadic individual therapy setting.

IV. Special considerations.

A. Initiating therapy.
Whatever form of psychotherapy is to be started, it is helpful to clarify the reasons for and the nature of the therapy. For example, the therapist might state to a depressed 7-year-old child whose mother died several months earlier: "I'm the kind of doctor who talks and plays with kids so that whatever they are feeling or thinking is something that is OK to bring up in therapy." Issues around the child's conception of why therapy is being prescribed ("I was bad") should be explored in therapy. Both the child and family members may be feeling guilt and worry about the need for therapy; these concerns should be explored with all participants early on in therapy. In adolescents, the issue of "who" initiated therapy may be an important area to explore.

B. Play therapy with children.
Children below the age of 10 years may have difficulty with a purely verbal form of communication. Their subjective world may be better expressed through their own media of drawing, playing games, or storytelling. These modes of communication are integral to "play therapy." They should be seen as direct forms of expression and not as inadequate substitutes for talking. Thus, children can express their feelings or tell the details of their experience through these forms of play.

Therapy relies on a supportive, respectful therapeutic relationship with a caring adult who shows respect for the child as an individual. Children have a natural tendency to enact their internal experience through play. Children with past traumatic experience (direct abuse or witnessing violent events) may be able to "work through" their traumatic experience by play therapy directly, even though they may never put their feelings or experiences into "actual words."

Most children have a progressive force toward healthy development. The therapeutic setting of support basically puts communication at their level and allows them to deal with their difficulties. Understanding, empathic statements, or clarification and interpretation can facilitate this process. For children, these interventions may be more concrete and educational and, at times, enacted in play itself. The child's limited cognitive/conceptual capabilities need to be accepted and understood, but some degree of self-observation may be achieved and useful with some children.

Play therapy can be physically and emotionally demanding on the therapist. Children are highly physically active. They also utilize emotionally age-appropriate defenses of denial, projection, and isolation that tend to work against an integrative functioning. The therapist has the task of recognizing these developmental factors, conceptualizing the psychologic issues, and "professionally regressing" to "be with" the child at their level. All of this can be very draining, as well as deeply rewarding for the therapist.

C. **Psychotherapy with adolescents.** Developmental issues specific to adolescence play a major role in the nature of psychotherapy with individuals of this age range. The adolescent is in the midst of major changes in the areas of their social worlds (with family and peers), cognitive abilities, emotional, physical and sexual experiences. The outline below will highlight the changes for the different phases of adolescence and their therapeutic implications. The key clinical points focus on engaging the adolescent in the therapeutic process and which forms of intervention are likely to be effective.

1. **Early adolescence (11 to 14 years).**

a. **Characteristic changes.** These include the initiation of puberty and powerful bodily changes with subsequent changes in self-image, sexual feelings, and interpersonal relations. As described in Anna Freud's profile, maintenance of this shaky sense of identity is achieved through the defenses of projection, rationalization, and ambivalent relationships to adults. There is thus a reliance on peers for support. Cognitively, they may be just emerging into the first stage of the formal operational period; thus, their thinking may still be primarily "egocentric." Self-involvement and a focus on the here and now as opposed to a future orientation are frequent.

b. **Therapeutic implications.** Early adolescents are difficult to engage in therapy of any nature. The therapist may need to be less intense and more informal and active; at times, the therapist may have to play age-appropriate games or the patient's favorite activity (e.g., basketball, chess, etc.), especially when verbal communication has come to a stalemate. Groups may be effective settings to utilize peer support and pressure for therapeutic change.

2. **Midadolescence (14 or 15 to 17 or 18 years).**

a. **Characteristic changes.** Physically, the adolescent is reaching equilibrium with pubertal changes and sexually may be furthering or initiating experimentation. Socially, there may be increased interaction and dependence on peers while a stabilization is also achieved in their relations to adult figures. Cognitively, most adolescents at this age have reached the stable phase of the formal operational period and thus may have less egocentric, more global time-oriented perspectives. They are able to think about others, the past, and the future more readily.

Emotionally, there may be less intense sudden changes in their mood and affect and a lessening in the rigidity of their defenses.

b. **Therapeutic implications.** Patients at this phase may be more accessible to therapy and more readily able to accept the roles of "patient" and adult therapist. There is an increased ability to reflect on their internal experience, as well as on their external behavior. Individual and group therapy may thus rely more on insight-oriented modes of change as needed.

3. **Late adolescence (17 or 18 years to early 20s)**

a. **Characteristic changes.** Physical stability is reached; sexually, there is continued exploration but in the setting of more dyadic social relationships. Relationships with parents may continue with a delayed dependency mode secondary to formal educational/financial responsibilities. Emotionally, there may be a focusing of energy toward sexual-romance partners. Identity issues reach toward equilibrium but may be an important area of stress in social, financial, and family arenas.

b. **Therapeutic implications.** At this phase, there may be developmental issues of identity and family relations that require intervention. Modes of therapy can often be those used with adults, with a special focus on these important developmental tasks. Financial ties to the family may remain and become significant therapeutic issues conflicting with the emotional desire for independence.

REFERENCES AND SUGGESTED READING

1. Bird HR: Individual psychotherapy with young children, in Shaffer D, Ehrardt A, Greenhill LL (eds): *The Clinical Guide to Child Psychiatry.* New York, The Free Press, 1985, pp 554–565.
2. Cantwell DP: The diagnostic process and diagnostic classification in child psychiatry—*DSM III. J Am Acad Child Psychiatry* 1980; 19:345–355.
3. Erikson EH: *Childhood and Society,* ed 2. New York, WW Norton & Co, Inc, 1963.
4. Freud A: *Normality and Pathology in Childhood.* New York, International Universities Press, Inc, 1965.
5. Ginsberg GP: Jean Piaget, in Kaplan HI, Sadock BJ (eds): *The Comprehensive Textbook of Psychiatry,* ed. 4. Baltimore, Williams & Wilkins, 1985.

6. Goldner V: Family therapy, in Shaffer D, Ehrardt A, Greenhill LL (eds): *The Clinical Guide to Child Psychiatry*. New York, The Free Press, 1985, pp 539–553.
7. Harrison SI, Robbins D, Esman AH: Children and adolescents, in Karasu TB (ed): *The Psychiatric Therapies: II. The Psychosocial Therapies*. Washington, DC, American Psychiatric Association, 1984, pp 347–381.
8. Lidz T: *The Person*, revised ed. New York, Basic Books Inc Publishers, 1976.
9. Piaget J: *The Child and Reality*. New York, Penguin Books, 1976.
10. Robson KS: *Manual of Clinical Child Psychiatry*. Washington, DC, American Psychiatric Press, Inc, 1986.
11. Rutter M: Resilience in the face of adversity: Protective factors and resistance to psychiatric disorder. *Br J Psychiatry* 1985; 147:598–611.
12. Slavson SR, Schiffer M: *Group Psychotherapies for Children*. New York, International Universities Press, Inc, 1975.

39

Psychotherapy With the Elderly

I. Introduction.

> "...near or above the fifties the elasticity of the mental processes, on which treatment depends, is as a rule lacking—old people are no longer educable..."
>
> Sigmund Freud, *Collected Papers* (vol 1, p 258)

This seems a curious thing for a man of 68 years to say, as this was a man who would continue to make important contributions to his field into his early 80s. While he was, by no means, the first to take an "ageist" stance toward psychotherapy with the elderly patient, he did play a major role in entrenching the attitudinal bias of the mental health profession. That legacy has been faithfully passed from generation to generation, and its all-too-clear remnants persist even to the present day. It is lamentable that such statements as, "They are incapable of changing," and "They are not interested in understanding their inner worlds," are commonly heard in reference to the elderly patient.

The record of our profession in this arena throughout the 65 years since Freud wrote those words has not been uniformly bad. It is probably fairest to say that we have just been inexcusably slow. This last decade, though, has seen a satisfying proliferation of interest in research, theory, and practice. Articles on the needs and problems of the elderly have appeared in major psychiatric journals and curricula, including specialized postresidency fellowships, which have been established to increase the geriatric expertise of future psychiatrists. This recent upsurge in interest can, in part, be explained by the progressive aging of our population (i.e., the elderly cohort is increasing out of proportion to the overall population rise), but it can also be seen as a compensatory reaction to historical sluggishness.

The purpose of this chapter will be twofold: (1) to delineate and categorize the more common resistances of psychotherapists to working with the elderly and (2) to make some general suggestions on modifying the psychotherapeutic approach to these patients.

II. **The therapeutic relationship.** The process of psychotherapy can be parsed, from the therapist's perspective, into two very different postures or ego states. The first ego state, the cognitive position, characterizes those times when the therapist is doing the cognitive work of psychotherapy (observation, hypotheses building, synthesis, etc.) and is the cool, detached clinician. The second ego state, the empathic position, is evidenced when the therapist is aroused affectively and is sharing something of the patient's feelings. During these times, there is a diminution of the interpersonal distance between the therapist and the patient, i.e., a process that has been termed "a temporary regression in the service of the therapy." Generally speaking, the therapist moves back and forth between these two states. Therapist resistance to psychotherapy with the elderly then develops whenever there is a deficit in either of these two states.

A. **Resistance to cognitive work.** When working with the elderly, deficits in the cognitive position can occur whenever there is an inadequate understanding of the processes of normal aging. Familiarity with the phenomenology of normal aging greatly helps to minimize the tendency toward cognitive resistances. Among these general processes of normal aging are the following types.

1. The tendency of older individuals to become focused on inner life with diminished cathexes to persons and objects in the outer world. This process that has been termed "interiority" can be misinterpreted by the therapist as a lack of motivation for change through therapy.

2. The tendency to think in terms of time left to live rather than time since birth. This is contrary to the anamnestic orientation by which the therapist usually works with younger patients. Associated with this altered perception of time is the increased need to come to terms with his/her own past, present, and future life and death without despair.

3. The inclination toward a diminished capacity for the spontaneous expression of emotional warmth. This move toward "affective stinginess" has been seen to involve the fear of the lack of reciprocation by a younger unempathic world.

4. The reversal of culturally determined sex role patterns, as men become less aggressive and more tolerant of their nurturing, affectionate, and dependent impulses and women become less dependent and more tolerant of their aggressive and competitive impulses.

5. The experience of grief as the older person comes to grips with the, at least, partial nonrealization of their earlier, normal, heroic aspirations.

B. **Resistance to empathic work.** Because the resistances associated with the empathic position of the therapist are, by definition, localized to the affective realm, they can be less amenable to scrutiny, more pervasive, and potentially more disruptive to the psychotherapeutic process than those associated with the cognitive position. A complete delineation of the possible sources of resistances to empathic work with the elderly is impossible, but the following list includes some of the more commonly experienced sources.

1. The physical signs of aging and the obviously limited life span of the patient can stimulate interpersonal distancing because they foreshadow the therapist's own future physical decline and death. Said another way, the weakening of the therapist's own denial of his/her death by the intimate proximity of the aging patient may provoke avoidance of empathic work.

2. Helping the older person work through the grief of partially or completely failed heroic aspirations may provoke anxiety in the therapist if the therapist senses that his/her own heroic aspirations are also destined to failure.

3. Working with the elderly patient may kindle feelings in regard to the relationship to aging and death of the therapist's parents. These feelings can be painful, especially when associated with unresolved conflicts that the therapist has with his/her parents and can undermine a good portion of the empathic work.

4. The older patient's age may provoke dependent feelings in the therapist. These dependent feelings, present to some degree in even the most mature of therapists, may be so conflicted that the intimacy associated with empathic work is avoided.

5. The older patient's known limited life span may emotionally distance the therapist who fears the pain of a "heavily invested" patient.

Each of these areas has the potential of emotionally distancing the therapist and effectively precluding the progression of the empathic work. Some of the more common manifestations of this distancing are feelings within the therapist of anger, hopelessness, depletion, and futility. These feelings, when recognized, should lead to a search for their "countertransferential" roots within the therapist's own personality and experiences.

C. **Modifications for the elderly.** Once a therapist recognizes the pitfalls of resistances to cognitive and empathic work with the elderly patient there are still some general modifications to the usual psychotherapeutic technique which should be made. Like so many areas of psychotherapy a consensus of opinion is impossible to obtain. Impression and opinion make up the bulk of our knowledge in the area of psychotherapy with the elderly. Nonetheless, current clinical impression favors the following modifications.

1. Set specific, time-limited goals. The elderly patient can tolerate briefer therapy because, as has been said, "The prospect of execution concentrates a man's mind wonderfully." The older patient does not have time to sit about contemplating the minutiae of life's mysteries; he/she wants to get on to other things. Goals should be established at the outset of the therapy, and plans should be laid out for their expeditious attainment.

2. Assume greater initiative in probing and identifying areas of conflict and emotional disturbance to facilitate the establishment of immediate specific therapeutic goals. Direct intervention into a patient's life may also be attempted.

III. **Conclusion.** In conclusion, in doing psychotherapy with the elderly, one has to be aware of one's own issues regarding health, death, parents, and aspirations, as well as the phenomenology of normal aging. In addition, one has to be tolerant of a more active and personally intrusive style of therapy. With these tenets in mind though, many therapists find treating the elderly patient to be clinically rewarding and fascinating.

SUGGESTED READING

1. Pfeiffer E: Psychotherapy with the elderly patient, in Bellak L, Karasu TE (eds): *Geriatric Psy-*

chiatry. New York, Grune & Stratton, 1976, pp 191–204.
2. Rechtschaffen A: Psychotherapy with geriatric patients: A review of the literature. *J Gerontol* 1959; 14:73–84.
3. Butler RM, Lewis ML: *Sex After Sixty*. New York, Harper & Row Publishers, Inc, 1978.
4. Lewis JM, Johansen KH: Resistances to psychotherapy with the elderly. *Am J Psychother* 1982; 36:497–504.
5. Bussee EW, Barnes RH, Silvermann AJ, et al: Studies of the process of aging: X. The strengths and weaknesses of psychic functioning in the aged. *Am J Psychiatry* 1955; 11:896.
6. Berezin MA: Psychodynamic considerations of aging and the aged: An overview. *Am J Psychiatry* 1972; 128:12.
7. Meerloo JAM: Psychotherapy with elderly people. *Geriatrics* 1955; 10:583.

V
Special Topics

40

Forensic Psychiatry

I. **Introduction.**

A. Forensic psychiatry is constantly changing in response to patient's rights issues and "due process."

B. The psychiatrist's dealings with patients are markedly constrained by case law and statutes.

C. Laws differ markedly from state to state.

D. Forensic psychiatry now includes child custody and visitation, child abuse, juvenile crime, involuntary commitment of patients to mental hospitals, patient's rights, competency procedures, workman's compensation, traumatic experiences, general disasters, and malpractice.

II. **Involuntary treatment and commitment.** Treatment is the sole asserted ground of depriving personal liberty. This is so because civil commitment for any purpose constitutes a significant deprivation of liberty that requires due process protection.

A. **Involuntary civil commitment/dangerousness standards.**

   1. *O'Connor vs. Donaldson* (1974) states "a State cannot constitutionally confine a nondangerous individual who is capable of surviving safely in freedom by him-

self/herself or with the help of willing and responsible family members or friends," declaring the existence of a "constitutional right to freedom."

2. Dangerous conduct (vs. criminal conduct) "involves not merely violation of social norms enforced by criminal sanctions, but significant physical or psychological injury to persons or substantial destruction of property."

B. **Criteria for involuntary commitment or probable cause for hold.**

1. **Mental illness (presence thereof).** Psychosis is included, but a personality disorder is not. Drug and/or alcohol abuse may be accepted. Probable cause is acceptable. In addition, one of the following two is required.

a. Dangerousness to self or others; imminent (24 hours) vs. relative problems.

(i) Psychiatrists cannot predict the future, except in the most obvious case.

(ii) The law requires a level of certainty that there is clear and convincing proof or evidence (civil) that the person is dangerous vs. beyond a reasonable doubt (criminal).

b. **Gravely disabled.** The patient is unable to provide food, shelter, or clothing and is in need of treatment, although some states allow commitment solely on the grounds that a person is significantly handicapped and in need of treatment.

Most states allow a brief involuntary hold of 3 to 14 days, with the patient having the right of a hearing by a writ of habeas corpus to reverse the hold.

As fewer patients are treated involuntarily, there is a trend where mental patients are shifting from the civil to criminal system, i.e., mental illness causes them to break a law that they ordinarily would not have broken. In addition, patients are released from both the mental health system, as well as the penal system, much earlier than they would have in the past. This places many marginally functioning persons into the community that is ill equipped to deal with their problems.

c. **Regarding institutionalization.**

(i) Errors in parental decision making concerning institutionalization of their children was significant enough to mandate an independent inquiry by a neutral fact finder.

(ii) The inquiry must "carefully probe the child's background using all available services."

(iii) The decision maker has the authority to refuse to admit a child who does not meet ethical standards of treatment.

(iv) The need for continued commitment must be periodically reviewed by an independent procedure.

d. Prisoners are entitled to a notice, a hearing, and an opportunity to present evidence and cross-examine witnesses, and to a written statement by an independent decision maker concerning whether a prisoner may be transferred from a jail to a psychiatric hospital.

e. **Right to treatment.**

(i) A person who is committed involuntarily must receive a level of effective treatment adequate to encourage improvement (*Wyatt vs. Stickney*, 1912; *Donaldson vs. O'Connor*, 1974). With a patient who is unlikely to improve, the patient is admitted and given a trial of treatment of choice.

(ii) Minimal requirements in treatment milieu requires the following.

(a) Humane physical and psychologic environment.

(b) Qualified staff personnel in sufficient numbers.

(c) Individualized treatment plans for each patient.

(iii) Persons have substantive constitutional rights

to "adequate food, shelter, clothing and medical care, personal security, freedom from bodily restraint and to minimally adequate or reasonable training to ensure safety and freedom from undue restraint" (*Youngberg vs. Romeo*, 1982).

f. **The right to refuse treatment.** This is the most controversial area of forensic psychiatry.

(i) Involuntary commitment is NOT prima facie evidence that the patient is incompetent to decide what treatment he/she is to receive.

(ii) A patient has a qualified right to refuse treatment and have an appeal process (*Rennie vs. Klein*, 1979).

(iii) A patient has a right of absolute refusal but provides for treatment by an authorized guardian if the patient is incapable of deciding for himself/herself. Local laws control the remainder of specific treatment protocols. These are clarified by the Supreme Court unless "a state is free, under its own constitution or common law, to create liberty or due process interest broader than those mandated under the Federated Constitution" (*Rogers vs. Okin*, 1981).

(iv) Very cautious and legal precautions must be taken when a patient is to receive electroconvulsive therapy or medication against his/her will, even when indicated. It must be emergent, or the patient must be involuntarily committed. Presently, there is a movement under way that, even when a patient is involuntarily committed, he/she may not be able to receive psychoactive medicine, except when it is emergent.

III. Informed consent.

A. Informed consent is needed from all patients.

B. Written consent must be obtained for physician procedures (i.e., electroconvulsive therapy and psychoactive medication).

1. It must include reasons for the treatment, nature, likelihood of success and danger, and likelihood and nature of side effects and alternative treatments.

2. Problem: Patients who are "incapable of understanding informed consent."

a. Emergent decisions may be made while a person is on hold.

b. A guardian is appointed to make decisions for the patient.

IV. **Confidentiality.**

A. This is maintained, except when waived by a competent patient.

B. *Tarasoff vs. UC Regents* (1975) obligates a therapist to protect and warn a third party who is threatened harm by a patient even if the therapist or health care worker violates confidentiality. The therapist must do what is necessary to prevent harm.

C. Utilization review and third party payers have the right to privileged information.

V. **Competence.** This legal concept is defined as the mental capacity or ability of a person to perform an act (Table 40–1). The medical concept of competence is described as the level of judgment sufficient to make decisions that may deprive a person unnecessarily of his/her authority to exercise his/her choice legally and practically. Most importantly, only a judge can decide competence.

A. **Legal principles.**

1. Evaluation of competence safeguards the accuracy of any criminal judication.

2. An evaluation of competencies is important, to guarantee a fair trial.

3. A patient must be competent to preserve the integrity and dignity of the legal process; the defendant must be a conscious and intelligent participant.

4. A person must be competent to be certain that the defendant, if found guilty, knows why he/she is being punished.

b. *Dusky vs. US* describes the need to define better the mental competence required to withstand trial. The America Law Institute (ALI) interpreted this as follows: "No person as a result of mental disease or defect who lacks capacity to understand the proceedings against him or to assist in his own defense shall be tried."

C. **Two questions to assess competence.**

1. Is there a mental disease or deficit that affects judgment, decision making, or behavior?

2. If there is, is it such that it meets the criteria of the law regarding these specifications?

D. **McGarry scale to operationalize the competence assessment.**

1. Ability to appraise available legal defenses.

2. Level of unmanageable behavior.

3. Quality of relating to an attorney.

4. Ability to plan legal strategy.

5. Ability to appraise the various roles of participants in the courtroom.

6. Understanding of court procedures.

7. Appreciation of the changes.

8. Appreciation of the range and nature of possible penalties.

9. Ability to appraise the likely outcome.

10. Capacity to disclose to an attorney available pertinent facts that surround the offense accused of.

11. Capacity to challenge the prosecution of a witness realistically.

12. Capacity to testify.

13. Ability to manifest a self-serving vs. self-defeating motivation i.e., the capacity to protect oneself through legal safeguards.

TABLE 40–1.
Representative Tests of Some Common Capacities

Capacity	Definition of Tests
Making a will	Knows what property he/she has and those relatives who would be his/her natural objects of bounty and understands the nature of the disposition of the property that he/she has made and does not suffer from a delusion that influenced the disposition of the property
Making a contract	Possesses sufficient mind or reason to enable him/her to comprehend the nature, terms, and effect of the particular transaction in which he/she is engaged
Being not responsible for a criminal act (to be excused)	Unable to distinguish between right and wrong and incapable of resisting an impulse that led to the commission of a crime
Standing trial	Possesses sufficient present ability to consult with his/her attorney with a reasonable degree of rational understanding and has a rational understanding of the nature of the proceedings against him/her
Being married	Able to understand the nature of the marriage relation and the duties and obligations involved

Being divorced	Suffering from incurable insanity as evidenced by medical testimony and 3 years of continuous institutionalization
Having a guardian or committee appointed	Not necessarily insane but by reason of old age, disease, or weakness of mind, unable to manage property and affairs unassisted or likely to be deceived by some artful person
Being committed to an institution	Rendered by mental illness so deficient in judgment or emotional control that he/she is in danger of causing physical harm to himself/herself or others or may cause the destruction of valuable property
Being discharged from an institution	Recovered his/her sanity and will not in the reasonable future be dangerous to himself/herself or others
Being a witness	Able to understand the moral obligation to speak the truth and the nature of the question asked and be able to form and communicate an intelligent answer

642 Special Topics

E. **Special issues in competence evaluation.**

1. Amnesia in competence hearings is only relevant if the person is amnestic at the time of the act and does not understand the nature of the act or that it was wrong.

2. Synthetic sanity refers to the use of drugs in preparing a defendant for a sanity trial. If a person is only competent with medication, the implication is that having a defendant medicated is the only way that the defendant can calmly go through a trial for a crime committed; therefore, is the defendant responsible for his/her acts while noncompliant off medicine?

3. Courtroom decorum must be maintained, even if it includes barring the defendant.

4. Whether a person is competent enough to be executed is usually determined by a warden in conjunction with a psychiatrist. If a person is temporarily or permanently insane, he/she may not be executed.

VI. **Patient's rights.**

A. Visitation.

B. Mail.

C. Vote.

D. Control assets.

E. Distribute a newsletter.

F. Telephone use.

G. Wear own clothing.

H. Exercise regularly.

I. Participation in voluntary therapeutic vocational rehabilitation.

J. Due process and disciplinary hearings.

K. Religious services.

L. Individualized community living arrangements or less

restrictive environments for aftercare unless these are clearly unsuitable.

M. Obtaining informed consent for research with psychiatric patients.

VII. **The insanity defense.**

A. In 1843, the *McNaghten* case established "rules" for what establishes insanity as follows.

1. "At the time of committing the act, the party accused was labouring under such a defect of reason, from disease of the mind, as not to know the nature and quality of the act he was doing."

2. "If he did know it, he did not know what he was doing was wrong."

B. *The ALI Test.* During the last 150 years, the *McNaghten* rules have been the predominant test, although alternatives have been proposed most notably, by the ALI test as follows: "A person is not responsible for criminal conduct if at the time of such conduct as a result of mental disease or defect, he lacks substantial capacity to appreciate the criminality (wrongfulness) of his conduct or to conform his conduct to the requirements of law."

1. "Appreciation" substitutes for cognitive understanding.

2. Requires only "substantial capacity" to be lacking.

3. Inability to control one's actions is added.

The ALI approach has been adopted in all federal jurisdictions and in approximately half of the states. The *McNaghten* rules are used in approximately one third of the states.

The Supreme Court has not addressed whether the Constitution requires the availability of any sort of insanity defense option.

The insanity defense has only been successful in

less than 1% of all felony cases. When successful, the defendant has traditionally been locked up for long durations in institutions for the criminally insane; usually, this has resulted from an agreement between the prosecution and defense.

During the last dozen years, however: (1) There have been several rulings that limit the confinement of defendants with successful insanity defenses to rules used for civil patients who have not committed a crime. (2) Psychopharmacologic agents have been increasingly effective in "restoring" sanity during very brief periods of time.

As a result, the average length of hospitalization of insanity acquittees has dramatically decreased, and the attractiveness of the insanity plea has increased. Along with public concern over increases in crime, this has led to increased public concern that the insanity defense is unfair and dangerous.

Many proposals have been made regarding the rewording of the definition of insanity, trial procedures, rules for continued hospitalization of the criminally insane, or even outright abolition of the insanity defense; however, no uniform system has been agreed to by the various states, federal courts, and Congress.

VIII. Family law/child custody.

A. Divorce and custody.

1. One of every five children live with a single parent.

2. Child psychiatry is therefore engaging in custody evaluations, primarily regarding which rational parent the child would do best with.

If the parents are both significantly disabled, so that it is detrimental to the child, by clear and convincing evidence, and this situation seems likely to continue indefinitely, the appropriate agencies have to be contacted to make efforts to help the parents remediate their problems, and the children are then placed with other more suitable arrangements.

B. Juvenile law.

1. Parents and guardians voluntarily admit their children for psychiatric inpatient treatment, but an "independent examination of the child's need for institutionalization must be provided." California, for example, requires precommitment and postcommitment hearings.

2. **Joint custody of children in divorce.**

a. Each parent assumes equal responsibility for the child's physical and emotional development.

b. Rights and responsibilities for making decisions are shared.

c. The child must live with each parent for a substantial amount of time.

3. **Juvenile delinquency.** A mental status evaluation helps to rule out a psychopathologic condition as a reason for delinquency.

4. Competency/malpractice rulings for children are similar to adults.

IX. Malpractice in psychiatry.

A. The risk is low.

B. Most suits involve complaints of ineffective or inappropriate treatment, wrong diagnosis, or failure to restrain a suicidal patient properly. Informed consent, abandonment, and faulty commitment are less common.

C. Negligence.

1. The plaintiff must show the following to recover damages.

a. Proof that the physician-patient relationship existed which created a duty on the part of the physician to the patient.

b. Show harm.

c. Show a causal connection between the breach of standards of care and the harm.

D. Primary causes of malpractice.

   1. Inadequate use of consultation.

   2. Failure to inquire into previous treatment.

   3. Failure to follow up on patient's progress.

   4. Failure to advise concerning medication use, including side effects.

   5. Failure to diagnose treatable medication side effects or complications of treatment.

   6. Failure to assess potential dangerousness of patients to themselves or others.

   7. Failure to provide sufficient information to the risks of procedures or treatment.

   8. Having sexual relations with a patient or former patient.

X. **Psychiatrist as an expert witness.**

A. Clinical testimony participation requires the following.

   1. Willingness.

   2. Proper preparation for court appearance.

   3. Adequate records.

   4. Reasonable objectivity.

   5. Honesty.

B. Forensic expert testimony is used to ascertain whether a person is stable enough to stand trial.

41

Seclusion and Restraint

I. **History.** The history of seclusion and restraint in some ways parallels that of psychiatry. Not surprisingly, as our understanding of psychopathology has grown, more specific or more effective means of treatment have supplanted the use of seclusion and restraint. In the Age of Enlightenment, Pinel is credited with striking the chains from patients at the hospital Bicetre in 1794. Pinel reserved the use of punitive imprisonment, however, for patients who disobeyed orders, who incited disobedience in others, and who would not work and women who would steal. Parallel reformation was conducted by Chiarugi of Italy and the Tukes of England, who advocated the moral treatment of mentally ill patients based on principles of humanity and education and their belief in nonrestraint. The nonrestraint movement perhaps culminated in 1856 with the publication of Robert Gardiner Hill's paper that advocated the total abolition of seclusion and restraint in the treatment of the insane. Hill's proposal was experience based at England's public asylum of Lincoln, where the effectiveness of nonrestraint was demonstrated by a reduction in the incidence of restraint from 2,364 per annum to zero in 2 years. Nonetheless, at the initial meeting (in Philadelphia in 1844) of the Association of Medical Superintendents of Asylums for the

Insane, later to become the American Psychiatric Association (APA), Isaac Ray articulated the resolution that "it is the unanimous sense of this convention that the attempt to abandon entirely the use of all means of personal restraint is not sanctioned by the true interests of the insane." It is perhaps a testament to the ongoing utility of seclusion and restraint as treatment modalities that the Massachusetts Psychiatric Society 132 years later addressed the federal court with the following endorsement: "Seclusion is a highly respected form of treatment of great value to many severely disturbed patients and essential to the preservation of order and safety during psychiatric emergencies."

II. **Definitions.** A survey of state mental health directors regarding the current practice of this treatment modality revealed considerable variation with respect to the length and specificity of regulation. In fact, of the 36 responses from state directors reviewed, 19 had no definition for seclusion, and 23 had no definition for restraint in their regulations. The *Adult Services Manual of the UCLA Neuropsychiatric Hospital* defines seclusion as the involuntary isolation of a patient in a locked room and restraint as any tying of hands or feet. A distinction is made between behavioral restraint, that described above, and medical restraint that consists of the temporary application of restraints to assist with a treatment procedure, such as arm immobilization for intravenous access. "Supportive" restraint is also distinguished as intervention when necessary for otherwise helpless patients to ensure their safety or to attend to hygienic needs. Examples would be the application of a posey jacket to prevent likely harm from falling out of bed or out of a chair or to allow feeding. Although a distinction is not formally made at UCLA, and in fact, medications are often given in conjunction with restraint, some locations further distinguish "chemical restraint," as being the use of medication for the purpose of controlling dangerous behavior.

TABLE 41–1.

Indications for Seclusion and Restraint

1. Prevention of imminent harm to patient or others if it is the most effective or appropriate means of control
2. Prevention of serious disruption of treatment programs or damage to the physical environment
3. As part of an ongoing plan of behavior therapy
4. To decrease patient stimulation
5. At the patient's request, barring contraindication.

III. **Incidence and prevalence.** Approaches to the estimation of the prevalence of modern-day use of seclusion and restraint have been difficult because of the variance in methodology, treatment setting, and patients. In only a very few studies, for example, are days at risk incorporated into data analyses in attempts to control for the likelihood that a longer hospital stay increases the time available during which seclusion may occur. Additionally, the use and effect of medication, either on the need for seclusion or the duration of the episode, are not always described. Consequently, the incidence reported varies from 1.9% among patients hospitalized on a long-time basis in a public state hospital setting to 66% among patients on a National Institute of Mental Health research unit where a treatment philosophy of medication-free maintenance is part of a research strategy.

IV. **Indications and contraindications.** The APA task force delineated five indications for the use of seclusion and restraint that were offered in deference to clinical judgment. These indications are listed in Table 41–1. As part of the decision to seclude or restrain a patient, clinical contraindications must be considered. The APA task force recognizes some neurologic conditions, including encephalitis, delirium, and dementia, wherein patients are vulnerable to sensory deprivation as a pathogenic force, as situations in which seclusion may lead to a worsening of the total clinical state and thus be contraindicated. Other situations denoted as relative contraindications to seclusion include paradoxical excitement reactions to phenothiazine medications, patients who (because of overdose attempts) require close monitoring, and patients with histories of serious and uncontrolled self-abuse and mutilation, or patients with impaired thermoregulation in cases where seclusion rooms cannot be sufficiently cooled on hot days. Seclusion is specifically proscribed as a purely punitive response or for the pure comfort or convenience of staff, or for mild obnoxiousness or rudeness on the part of the patient toward others, or staff anxiety or solely because of factors of ward dynamics. Additionally, seclusion or restraint should not be employed when inadequate resources or staffing preclude its efficient and safe implementation. Hospital policy should dictate not only the time interval between when a patient is secluded or restrained and when the treating physician should be notified to assess the patient, but also the frequency with which the patient should subsequently be reassessed, and the maximum duration of continuous seclusion.

V. **Technique.** A model technique for the implementation of seclusion and restraint is summarized in Table 41–2. While the staff should not approach the patient like a SWAT team, they should exhibit assurance in their ability to carry out the planned seclusion and/or restraint. The leader, who may be the treating resident physician, should articulate clearly the reasons seclusion is necessary and the patient's options, for example, "you need to walk to the seclusion/quiet room; if you are uanble to do so, we will have to assist you." There should be neither bargaining nor psychodynamic interpretation as these tend only to increase patient agitation and the likelihood of violence.

TABLE 41–2.

Specific Techniques of Seclusion and Restraint

1. The decision to implement seclusion or restraint is made on clinical grounds
2. Seclusion leader and monitor are designated
3. Monitor clears the path to seclusion room of patients/obstructions
4. Sufficient personnel are mobilized for a show of force (one staff for each extremity and head, excepting leader and monitor)
5. Leader, with team at hand, confronts patient with a clear statement of the purpose and rationale for seclusion
6. At leader's designation, staff seize predetermined extremities and secure their movement in a noninjurious manner
7. Patient is either escorted to a seclusion room or taken down to the floor for immediate control before being carried to the seclusion room
8. Patient is rid of potentially dangerous personal effects and items of clothing and placed in restraints if necessary
9. Medication may be administered if indicated
10. Seclusion monitor reviews overall technique with team in a debriefing session that follows event

VI. **Summary.** Seclusion and restraint are important means of providing for the safety of patients and staff and should be employed when clinically indicated. Special guidelines exist for the application of this procedure to children, the developmentally disabled, and the elderly, for which the reader is referred to the sources listed below.

REFERENCES

1. Tardiff K (ed): *The Psychiatric Uses of Seclusion and Restraint*. Washington, DC, American Psychiatric Press, Inc, 1984.
2. American Psychiatric Association: *Seclusion and Restraint*, task force report 22. Washington, DC, American Psychiatric Association, 1984.

42
Abuse

I. **Overview.** In general, abuse may be of a child, a spouse, a parent, an acquaintance, or a stranger. Dynamic factors, such as identification with the aggressor, cultural factors, such as victim blaming, and the necessity of providing victims with diverse forms of assistance (beyond simple medical/psychiatric treatment), are a few of the factors that make treatment of these victims difficult. Fetal abuse, child abuse, spouse abuse, elder abuse, and rape are discussed in the following sections.

II. **Fetal abuse.**

A. **Introduction.** Advances in prenatal care and monitoring demonstrate specifically that maternal health behaviors can adversely affect the fetus. If a pregnant woman behaves in such a way as to jeopardize fetal development despite being educated about the consequences, then the question of fetal abuse must be raised. Because fetal abuse has only recently been recognized, there are no legal definitions, no guidelines, nor any epidemiologic data. Intervention has been on a case-by-case basis.

1. **Syndromes.**

a. **Psychosis.** A psychotic woman may be unpredictable or irresponsible in her behavior toward the pregnancy or the fetus, e.g., she may deny that she is pregnant or have delusional thoughts about her growing belly and may not seek prenatal care.

b. **Medical noncompliance.** Certain maternal illnesses can negatively affect the fetus, especially if untreated. If such an illness is recognized in a pregnant mother, she must be informed about treatment and of the possible consequences if she neglects both her own health and the fetus.

c. **Drug abuse.** Many chemicals, including alcohol, cocaine, and opiates, have been implicated in causing prenatal and postnatal difficulties.

d. **Refusal of treatment for religious reasons.** The courts have not upheld the religious convictions of parents over the fetus' right to health under the doctrine of *parens patria*.

e. **Repeated exposure to physical assaults.** Pregnant mothers who show evidence of physical trauma, such as broken bones and bruises, may also be exposing the fetus to trauma. Maternal behaviors that might contribute to trauma, as well as other persons who might be inflicting injury, need to be assessed. For example, a mother may need to be isolated from an abusive spouse.

2. **Treatment.**

a. The physician must consider the right of the unborn fetus to be well born, while also considering the rights of the woman. If the fetus is seriously threatened, consider intervention.

b. A civil commitment can be pursued to restrain and treat the mother.

c. Under the child protection statutes, custody of the fetus can also be sought by the child protection services as neglect or abuse of children. This may be feasible and give better longitudinal care, although the service must be willing to take on the case.

III. Child abuse.

A. Epidemiology.

1. Violence against children has occurred throughout history; although societies against child abuse and neglect were formed in the 19th century, the syndrome of child maltreatment, i.e., "the battered-child syndrome," was only described in 1962 by Kempe in reference 3. Studies of the causes, prognosis, treatment, and prevention are still in the nascent stage, despite growing public awareness. Child abuse is still grossly under-reported; as such, about 1 million children are maltreated yearly, including 200,000 cases of sexual abuse and 200,000 to 300,000 cases of psychologic abuse, resulting in 2,000 to 5,000 deaths a year and permanent physical or psychologic sequelae.

2. Child abuse has no predictability; it knows no socioeconomic, intellectual, religious, or ethnic boundaries, but usually occurs in a triad of vulnerable families, vulnerable children, and a crisis—three factors that should raise a red flag.

3. Vulnerable families include the following types.

a. Socially isolated families.

b. Families with a history of violence, e.g., the parents themselves were battered when they were young, or parents who resort to violence on one another.

c. Families with stressors, such as alcohol or drug abuse, mental illness, low income, and poor living conditions. (Abuse is reported more frequently in low-income families, although under-reporting in middle- and high-income families may occur.)

4. Vulnerable children include the following types.

a. Premature or ill babies who require extra efforts at care and soothing.

b. Children with congenital abnormalities.

c. Children who have been hospitalized, which prevents early parent-child bonding.

d. Children with psychiatric illness, such as autism, developmental delay, and attention deficit disorder with or without hyperactivity.

5. The profile of the child abuser tends to be that of a low-income young woman with low-average intelligence, although the partner may be passively condoning maltreatment. The abuser often has difficulty with issues of self-esteem, independence, and maturity and was likely abused as a child. The abusing parent may have unusually high expectations from the child and may turn to the child for comfort and reassurance (role reversal) to meet dependency needs, only to be frustrated by the child's dependence on her. The abuser may interpret the child's crying as a lack of love and react aggressively, only to repeat the pattern of violence from generation to generation.

B. **Syndromes.** Child abuse constitutes a range of maltreatment from active abuse to neglect. The following are general categories that should alert the health team to the suspicion of abuse.

1. Physical abuse is a nonaccidental injury of a child. It is most easily recognized from bruises, welts, and burns, especially those forming a pattern, such as belt buckles, irons, and grills, or from fractures, lacerations, and abrasions. Other common injuries are abdominal trauma or head injuries with unlikely explanations.

2. Sexual abuse of children can range from fondling to intercourse to the use of children in pornography, with the common factor of exploitation for the gratification of adults. The perpetrator is usually known to the child. Though more difficult to detect than physical abuse, signs of sexual abuse are any venereal disease in a child, such as gonorrhea, syphilis, genital warts, recurrent UTIs, bruising or bleeding in the genital, perineal, or perianal areas, pain on walking or sitting, and/or torn, stained, or bloody undergarments.

3. Physical neglect occurs when a parent or guardian fails to provide for basic physical needs and care, such as nutrition, clothing, shelter, medical care, safety, and education. Signs of neglect are malnutrition, failure to thrive, poor hygiene and clothing, poor school attendance, repeated pica, or repeated stealing of food or clothing.

4. Psychologic abuse is the most subtle type of abuse and includes excessive verbal belittling and teasing, unreasonable demands or responsibilities for the child's age, exclusion of a child in family activities, and being locked in seclusion for prolonged periods of time.

C. **Diagnosis.**

1. Behavioral abnormalities that result from abuse or neglect may be the first clue. Many children display conduct disorders: they can be angry, defiant, and destructive and try to run away or be truant from school. Or, they might become isolated, withdrawn, anxious, and depressed with suicidal ideation. Younger children can have developmental delays.

2. Sexually abused children may be sexually aggressive at play, engage in excessive or exhibitionistic behavior, have feelings of guilt and shame, or have an overly attached relationship with the abuser. Many children will be afraid of adults or have a sudden deterioration in schoolwork.

3. Once an injury has occurred, the first objective is to assure the health and safety of the child. When medical care is completed, an investigative interview should take place. The aim is to understand and alleviate a stressful situation and not to blame or antagonize the family or even to prove neglect or abuse.

4. The child may be interviewed separately from the parents, depending on the circumstances. If possible, the local child protection worker might attend to avoid repeating the interview process. In interviewing children, after rapport is established, the following techniques should be used.

a. Use age-appropriate words.

b. Sit at eye level near the child rather than across the room.

c. Ask "how come?" rather than "why?"

d. Explain to the child if and why hospitalization or removal from the home is necessary.

e. Do not suggest answers or try to push for answers that the child seems to be unwilling to give at the time; he/she may respond later.

5. The parents need to be told why the interview is taking place, and that it is the physician's legal obligation to report suspected abuse. The interview should be in private, remain objective, nonjudgmental, and unemotional.

D. Reporting.

1. Along with assessment and emergency intervention, a case of suspected maltreatment must be reported to the child protective services. Most hospitals have a multidisciplinary team or have affiliation with local teams that provide diagnostic and consultative help.

2. In all 50 states, physicians, nurses, and mental health professionals are mandated by law to report suspected incidents of child maltreatment and are given legal immunity in case the suspicion is proved to be false. In 44 of the 50 states, there are civil or criminal penalties for failure to report, and in most states, the patient-physician confidentiality is abrogated. Depending on local law, the child may be held in custody of the physician or hospital for the protection of the child, and photographs may be taken for evidence. However, the local Department of Social Services should be consulted.

E. Psychiatric treatment.
After the legal requirements have been met and care has been given, a program of continued psychiatric care and follow-up for the child and parents should be arranged.

1. New knowledge about the psychodynamics of abusers indicate that they, too, are in need of help, but there is no evidence that any particular form of therapy is more effective. Each intervention plan should be individualized to the level of the parent's severity of dysfunction and psychopathologic condition, the extent to which the parent is motivated and willing to participate in rehabilitation, and the resources available. Combinations of individual and group psychotherapy, parent teaching and training, and groups, such as Parents Anonymous, have been successful in some cases.

2. Various treatments also exist for the abused or neglected child, depending of the locality, which include therapeutic nurseries, crisis nurseries, day-care centers, support groups for sexually abused children, as well as individual and group psychotherapy. Psychologically untreated children who have been abused or neglected may have emotional disturbances as adolescents and adults, including abusive behaviors.

3. Prevention of new cases of abuse should attempt to identify the vulnerable families and children and to reduce the isolation, frustration, and poor-parenting techniques that may lead to potentially abusive situations.

IV. **Rape.**

A. **Introduction.** Rape is an act of violence and aggression. The legal definition of rape states that it is penile penetration of the victim's outer vulva against the victim's will and consent.

Seventy percent of rapists have previous criminal histories. Victims are usually threatened with violence by fists, guns, or knives and are often harmed physically in addition to being raped. Rape is highly underreported, with estimates of its incidence ranging from 50,000 to 200,000 cases per year. Females aged 10 to 29 years are most often rape victims, but cases have been reported in females aged from 15 months to 82 years. Rape usually occurs inside the victim's home or in her neighborhood. Fifty percent of rapists are strangers to their victims, and 7% of reported rapes are committed by close relatives of the victims.

B. **Syndromes.**

1. During the first few months following a rape, the victim may experience eating and sleeping disturbances, somatic symptoms, and a vast range of emotional symptoms.

2. One year after a rape, one third of all victims still report rape-related adjustment problems, such as worsened sexual relations and disturbed sleep and appetite.

3. One third of rape victims recover in a few months, but three fourths will take from 1 to 6 years to recover.

4. The acute reaction to rape has been called the "rape trauma syndrome."

5. A rape assaults the victim on many deep levels: survival, basic trust, psychic and bodily autonomy, and sexual identity. The victim thus usually experiences powerlessness and helplessness to an overwhelming degree.

6. Male rape does occur, usually in prisons and maximum-security hospitals, and the dynamic issues raised in the victim can be similar to those in female rape victims.

C. **Treatment.**

1. Supportive and short-term psychotherapy is a must for the rape victim; many victims will need more long-term psychotherapy.

2. Treatment should be provided by individuals who are experienced with treating rape victims who are sensitive to the issues created by rape. Women are often better suited to treat these women victims.

3. The help of friends and relatives should also be enlisted.

D. **Reporting.**

1. The victim will need to be examined by an M.D. for evidence of rape, to provide information to police, and to participate in legal proceedings. (These activities will often lead to restimulation of victimization feelings by focusing on the event and possibly by their prying for irrelevant information intended to incriminate the victim, such as the victim's sexual history.)

2. Many hospitals or towns have rape crisis teams who can accompany victims through the emergency room and court proceedings, in addition to being able to provide therapy and information.

V. **Spouse abuse.**

A. **Introduction.** Spouse abuse is estimated to occur in 3 to 6 million families in this country, with the vast majority of this abuse occurring against women. Husband abuse is extremely rare, and when it occurs, it usually represents a counterassault, abuse of a nonphysical nature, or elder abuse by a younger wife (see Section VI on elder abuse). Wife beating occurs in families of all racial, religious, and socioeconomic backgrounds, but it is found most frequently in families in which there is drug and/or alcohol abuse. Abusive men and abused wives tend to come from violent homes, especially those where spouse abuse had occurred.

B. **Recognition.**

1. The problem of wife battering is common enough that emergency room physicians should inquire when evaluating a woman with physical trauma, especially if she is also depressed and talks about having problems with her children.

2. Areas of the body most commonly assaulted are the head and face, the breasts, and, when pregnant, the abdomen.

3. The most common injuries are contusions and

soft-tissue injuries, with the most common weapon being a fist.

4. A diagnosis is made difficult by the wife's fear of the consequences of reporting the battering. Inquire directly in a supportive manner, while providing information about available resources, protective agencies, and therapeutic possibilities.

5. The diagnosis requires a history of only one episode of assault and is not related to possible provocative behavior.

C. **Syndromes/patterns that perpetuate continued family violence.**

1. The husband may become more threatening and/or violent when the abused wife tries to leave. The battered spouse may become more depressed and passive, unable to leave for fear of worsening her options.

2. The battered wife who desires to leave will need food, clothing, shelter, and money and may have few tools for self-sufficiency. Women have been unable to leave for fear of worsening their situation.

3. Some men feel remorse after a battering incident and then become particularly loving which gives the wife "hope" until the next episode of violence.

4. Wife battering is most destructive when the wife is most dependent, e.g., with small children or pregnant.

D. **Treatment options.** The goal is to resolve the violence in the family. The husband must participate in treatment, or the treatment must then focus on enabling the battered woman to leave the marriage. Collaboration among protective agencies, shelters, and medical and psychiatric health providers is necessary.

1. Individaul or group therapy (for each spouse separately), in conjunction with encouragement of physical separation, if necessary, are common approaches.

2. The battered woman can leave and make it known that a condition of return is her husband must receive

psychiatric/rehabilitative treatment. She might also choose supportive therapy for herself.

3. Family therapy may be an option; if so, violence must be a treatment issue, and a strictly enforced "no violence" contract must be a precondition for such therapy.

4. If the violence is a first-time occurrence after a lengthy nonviolent relationship, the batterer should be evaluated for evidence of organic brain syndrome, head trauma, systemic illness, or intoxication and treated accordingly.

E. **Reporting.**

1. Legal assistance is difficult to obtain and secure. No reporting is mandatory, and available support services are scarce.

2. The responsibility of the physician is to treat the physical and emotional wounds, to inform the victims about treatment options and available resources, e.g., shelters, therapists, and lawyers, and to prevent further violence against the victim.

3. The children of violent marriages should be assessed victims of abuse or emotional trauma.

VI. **Elder abuse.**

A. **Epidemiology.**

1. Five percent or 1 million elderly Americans are abused yearly. The growing percentage of older Americans, from 3% in 1900 to 11% in 1990, will impact on the structure of families, health care delivery, and economics.

2. The abused elder victim is most likely to be a white female, aged 70 years or older, with moderate to severe mental or physical disabilities causing her to be dependent on the family or other care givers. The patient is likely to live at home alone or with a family member.

3. The abuser tends to be the victim's son, daughter, or an unrelated care giver. There is evidence that the abuser was abused by the now-abused parent.

B. **Syndromes.**

1. **Physical abuse.** The following physical indicators should raise the suspicion of abuse.

   a. Bruises, welts, lacerations, and broken bones.

   b. Burns from cigarettes, ropes, or chemicals.

   c. Unusual marks on the body that may have been caused by blows with an instrument.

   d. Signs of sexual abuse.

2. **Psychologic abuse.** This may take the form of the following types of abuse.

   a. Verbal assaults.

   b. Infantilization.

   c. Isolation, such as by placing locks on doors and phones to prevent outside contact.

   d. The victim may often seem to be fearful in the presence of the care giver/abuser.

   e. Psychologic abuse seems to be much more prevalent than physical abuse.

3. **Financial abuse.** Care givers often handle the finances and material possessions of the elderly. Resources may be taken away from the victim and/or used without consent. The elderly patient may be forced to sign over property in return for care. With enough evidence of coercion, legal counsel may be needed.

4. **Medical neglect.** Neglect encompasses the failure to give medication at the prescribed dose and dosage schedule, to provide adequate nutrition, and to help with activities of daily living. The victim's hearing aids and glasses may be removed on purpose.

C. **Diagnosis and detection.**

1. Dependent on their caretakers, the abused elderly may be reluctant to report for fear of retaliation, removal from their home, or abandonment. The victims may not be able to report the abuse because of the mental or physical disabilities that made them dependent on a care giver or as a result of the abuse itself. Like children who are abused, elderly victims rely on their abusers.

2. If abuse is suspected, interview the patient alone, ask him/her to describe the typical day at home in detail, and ask for a history of violence in the family.

3. Home visits are extremely helpful in determining the living conditions and any evidence of abuse.

4. Intervention must be done with knowledge that the elderly competent patient may refuse intervention strategies.

D. **Treatment.** Treatment includes complete medical and psychiatric care of any physical and psychologic trauma, consideration of legal counsel for any issues of competency, finances, and durable powers of attorney, and the enlistment of the social services department. Alternatives to placement can be sought, such as increased visits by Home Health Services. The patient might choose to stay in an abusive situation if nursing homes are the only alternative.

E. **Reporting** Elder abuse is reportable in most states, but legislation varies from state to state as to which persons are mandated to report and as to the penalty for failure to report. Agencies that will receive the reports include the Department of Social Services, welfare departments, and police departments.

REFERENCES

1. Soloff P, Jewell S, Roth L: Civil commitment and the rights of the unborn. *Am J Psychiatry* 1979; 136:114–115.
2. Mackenzie T, Collins N, Popkin M: A case of fetal abuse? *Am J Orthopsychiatry* 1982; 52:699–703.
3. Kempe CH, Silverman FN, Steele BF, et al: The battered-child syndrome. *JAMA* 1962; 181:17–24.
4. Council on Scientific Affairs: AMA Diagnostic and Treatment Guidelines Concerning Child Abuse and Neglect. *JAMA* 1985; 254:796–800.
5. Fontana VJ: Child maltreatment and battered child syndromes, in Kaplan HI, Sadock BJ (eds): *Comprehensive Textbook of Psychiatry/IV*. Baltimore, Williams & Wilkins, 1985, pp 1816–1824.
6. Sanders CG: Evaluating child abuse cases: Guidelines for the physician-in-training, resident and staff physician. 1986; 32:21–33.
7. Sadock V: Special areas of interest, in Kaplan H, Sadock B (eds): *Comprehensive Textbook of Psychiatry/IV*. Baltimore, Williams & Wilkins, 1985, pp 1090–1096.
8. Carmen (Hilberman) E, Rieker P, Mills T: Victims of violence and psychiatric illness. *Am J Psychiatry* 1984; 141:378–383.
9. Rathbone-McCuan E, Goodstein RK: Elder abuse: Clinical considerations. *Psychiatr Ann* 1985; 15:331–339.
10. Rathbone-McCuan E, Voyles B: Case detection of abused elderly parents. *Psychiatry* 1982; 139:189–192.

43 | Transcultural Psychiatry

I. **Approaches to culture and psychiatry.** Psychiatry traditionally has emphasized intrapsychic factors that shape a person, and the study of culture has been the domain of anthropology and sociology. Because of increased migration and travel throughout the world, however, there has been a need for the study of psychiatry in relation to culture and ethnicity.

Ethnicity is crucial in determining identity, and despite the notion that America is a "melting pot," many ethnic groups have not "melted" and continue to maintain their ethnic values, traditions, and outlook. Rather than a melting pot, a "rainbow" or a "tossed salad" has been proposed as a more fitting description.

The aim of transcultural psychiatry is to study mental disorders in the context of an individual's culture; it aims to sort out which behaviors are considered normal and abnormal in a particular culture, as well as behaviors that are universal.

A. **Theories.**

1. **Anthropology.** Many transcultural psychiatrists have borrowed methods from anthropology to study other cultures.

a. **Emic perspectives.** These refer to socially

unique, intracultural concepts and culture-bound syndromes; the idea of cultural relativism are emic outlooks.

b. **Etic perspectives.** These are universal, cross-cultural concepts (e.g., endocrine responses or facial expressions) that are similar across cultures.

c. **Illness vs. disease.** Disease is defined as any malfunctioning of body organs and systems. Physicians treat disease. Illness may be a secondary psychosocial response to disease. Indigenous healers tend to treat illness, not disease.

2. **Sociology.**

a. Systems theory examines the relationship between groups and organizations, and the way a person acts within them.

b. Social epidemiology refers to the interaction of sociodemographic variables, such as socioeconomic status, rural vs. urban status, sex, race, marital status, religion, and mental illness.

c. The social experience of being a mental patient.

d. The interplay of life events and mental distress.

B. **Dangers of stereotyping.** Transcultural psychiatry aims to sensitize therapists and make them aware of cultural issues, differences, and nuances in the evaluation and treatment of the ethnically different client. Although cultural descriptions may sometimes be misconstrued as stereotyping, it is often helpful to have some knowledge of the ethnic group to serve as guidelines. Each person, regardless of the culture or ethnic group, needs to be evaluated and treated as an individual.

C. **Dangers of maximizing/minimizing illness because of culture.** Each medical and psychiatric symptom needs to be considered carefully, and not "written off" or assumed to be due to the patient's ethnic background. For example, many immigrants do somatize their psychiatric symptoms, but physical causes should first be ruled out.

II. The initial evaluation.

A. **Use of interpreters.** Interpreters are often needed in the initial evaluation to obtain even a cursory history from an ethnically different patient. To maximize the efficiency of the interaction and to minimize the biasing of information, it is recommended to use trained translators, if available, and to avoid family members. Even with trained personnel, psychiatric and cultural nuances may not be apparent from the translation. Experienced or not, interpreters should be educated and reminded to do the following.

1. Translate everything that is said and not to summarize what the patient or the evaluator is saying.

2. Not to impart their own values or comment.

3. Voice any problems or discomfort with the issues being discussed.

4. Ask the evaluator for clarifications.

By the same token, interpreters are valuable sources of cultural information, and they may be able to offer insight as to the process, normal behavior, and patient expectations in that culture.

B. **History.** Migration itself is a stress, and these stresses often continue to be seen for several generations of a family. In obtaining the history, the following important factors should be considered.

1. **Country of origin.**

2. **Time and circumstances of migration.** The reasons for migrating include political and/or religious persecution in the native country, and better educational or economic opportunities in the adopted country. Did the patient migrate alone, with a family or with several other families? Those persons leaving alone often give up native customs and rituals faster, but they may feel a greater loss.

3. **Race or ethnic group.** Immigrants are often grouped together by skin color and facial features, but

certain ethnic groups may be historical enemies. Consider, e.g., Japanese/Chinese or Pakistani/Indian animosities in assigning therapists or group members.

4. **Languages spoken.** English-language skills often measure acculturation, independence, and mobility. A lack of skills can lead to isolation. Note the loss or preservation of the native language. The children of migrants may speak the new language better and might be given legal or financial responsibilities that are too burdensome for their ages. This situation may lead to role reversal and disrupt the family structure.

5. **Social class and economic situation, currently and before migration.** In the process of migrating, many clients and their families lose the status that they may have had in the native country. The more educated and the more upwardly mobile the person is, the less ethnic distinction there is. But conflicts may arise between moving up socioeconomically and the loyalty to the ethnic group.

6. **Generations since migration.** These impact on the degree of acculturation and intergenerational conflicts.

7. **Rural vs. urban area.** The East and West Coasts are the usual points of entry, with secondary migration to urban areas, which tend to have ethnic neighborhoods. Rural areas may force assimilation more rapidly and cause greater stress and difficulties.

8. **Level of education.** This is often linked to social class.

9. **Family structure and dynamics.** Families migrating with young children are more often unified, but role reversal can occur, as the children are more easily acculturated. Families with adolescents have more difficulty because of less time together before the children move out on their own.

10. **Political and religious affiliations.** These may serve to unify an ethnic group, as well as to cause divisions.

11. **Intermarriage.** Many cultural and religious groups have had prohibitions against intermarriage, because of perceived threats to the survival and loss of the "purity" of the group. Intermarriage increases with duration of stay, higher socioeconomic status, and education. Successful intermarriage is more difficult the more culturally different the spouses are.

C. **Mental Status Examination.**

1. **Individual and ethnic belief systems (emic/etic perspectives).** One needs to be aware of one's own cultural limitations and of the patient's feelings of the clinician's culture. Observation is vital, but there is danger in overinterpreting nonverbal behavior. One should know the norms of culture in grooming, dress, speech, behavior, cognition, and affect, or one might, for example, view a cultural belief as a delusion. Paranoid symptoms that range from simple mistrust to psychosis occur more commonly among patients who are outside their own social milieu. Somatic complaints are increased for unclear reasons.

2. **Language.** Acquired language can relate facts, but affect is much harder to express.

3. **Proverbs.** The use of proverbs may be limited because of language and education.

D. **Physical examination.** When the history and Mental Status Examination are less than satisfactory, the physical examination becomes much more important. Assess for clinical symptoms common in the country of origin that can present as psychiatric illness, like cerebral malaria and other infections, nutritional deficiencies, and genetic dementias.

E. **Laboratory tests.** Consider drug screenings, blood counts, endocrine and metabolic tests, urinalysis, and vitamin levels.

F. **Psychologic testing.** This testing of minority and ethnically different groups has been controversial in the scientific and legal communities, because of the question of cross-cultural validity and because of past abuse of these tests. (See Chapter 3 on psychologic testing.)

1. **Minnesota Multiphasic Personality Inventory.** This has been translated into more than 100 languages. Although norms have been established for several groups and nations, the validity is debated.

2. **Zung depression scale.** This has been standardized in several languages.

3. **Cognitive-intellectual tests (IQ).** These tests are most hotly debated because of reliance on verbal skills and the inability to separate one's learning from one's culture.

4. **Hopkins 90-item checklist.** This is a general scale of psychopathology that has been translated into many languages but has not been validated.

III. **Diagnosis.**

A. **Culture-bound syndromes.**

1. **Definition.** Viewed from an emic perspective, the culture-bound syndromes are certain behavioral disturbances that occur with unusual frequency in certain societies. Prominent in the symptoms of these folk illnesses are alterations of behavior and of experience. Considered eccentric disorders in the cultures in which they are endemic, they are often dramatic and episodic.

2. **Cross-cultural aspects.** The culture-bound syndromes may not be unique to any one culture, and descriptions of similar symptoms may be found in dissimilar and geographically distinct cultures. The syndromes also have many common manifestations (etic phenomena), including anxiety, fear, amnesia, somatic complaints, social withdrawal, sleep disturbance, depression, depersonalization, thought disorder, and behavioral abnormalities.

3. **The more common syndromes.**

a. **Koro (genital retraction syndrome).** This occurs in Chinese males, who fear that the penis will be drawn into the abdomen, causing death. This syndrome may be an extension of old Chinese medical writings in which abdominal distention and penile retraction, probably due to peritonitis, would cause certain death, and the prohibitions against sexual excesses.

b. **Latah (startle matching syndrome).** This usually occurs in middle-aged women from Malaysia and Indonesia; they respond to minimal stimuli with exaggerated gestures, often throwing a held object or uttering obscenities. Similar syndromes are seen in the Ainu of Japan, in Siberia, and in French-Canada.

c. **Amok (sudden mass assault).** This classically occurs among Southeast Asian males who exhibit outbursts of violent and aggressive behavior directed toward people or objects, often involving homicide and death of the perpetrator. "Running amok" has occurred in Western societies, e.g., the Calgary (Canada) mall sniper.

d. **Bulimia/anorexia nervosa.** This occurs mostly in young North American and European females and consists of food binging, followed by purging, as in the former, or self-starvation, as in the latter, and is usually associated with depression, personality disorders, anxiety, and substance abuse (see Chapter 10 on eating disorders).

e. **Evil eye (mal de ojo).** This syndrome has been described in Mediterranean and Latin-American populations, and it consists of fitful sleep, crying, vomiting, and fever in an infant, child, or female adult. It is thought to occur when an adult stares at and admires a child too much, thereby placing a curse. The evil eye can also be caused by patting the child on the head, a behavior that is to be avoided in this population.

f. **Susto (fright).** This is often not considered a culture-bound syndrome, because it lacks an altered perception of reality. It is seen in Latin-American and Caribbean populations and consists of anxiety, anorexia, phobias, trembling, diaphoresis, tachycardia, diarrhea, vomiting, and depression; this syndrome is attributed to fright to self or to someone else.

g. Other syndromes include anthropophobia, fallen fontanelles, frigophobia, grisi siknis, and falling out. (Please refer to *The Culture Bound Syndromes*, edited by Simons and Hughes.)

4. The inclusion of anorexia and bulimia as a culture-bound syndrome may help to illustrate that these syndromes need to be seen in the context of that culture: a disorder that American psychiatrists see often might be very rare in other cultures, and vice versa.

B. *DSM III* and *DSM III-R.*

1. **International implications.** In the summary of *International Perspectives on DSM III*, *DSM III's* innovative advantage is its descriptive approach. Although etiology is important, *DSM III* does not discuss theories, which makes it useful for clinicians from various orientations, as well from different countries. The international criticisms and praise have been as follows.

a. **Multiaxial system.** Axes IV and V assume that stressors and adaptation relate to the "average" person, rather than considering the context of the situation. The addition of a cultural axis is also suggested.

b. Diagnostic criteria, in general, are seen as a major advance and appear to be valid cross-culturally for developed countries. Reliability studies from Japan, Australia, and New Zealand show similar degrees of reliability as in trials from the United States, indicating that despite language and cultural differences, *DSM III* may be valid and useful. The Structured Clinical Interview for *DSM III* has been translated into several languages.

c. For developing countries, *DSM III* seems to be less valid and practical on two points: (i) since *DSM III* relies on the American experience, it excludes several clinical syndromes seen in other countries (see Section III./A. on culture-bound syndromes); (ii) in developing countries where much of the mental health care is delivered by non-mental-health professionals or indigenous healers, the diagnostic criteria may be too cumbersome and complicated to be useful.

2. **Ongoing efforts to validate psychiatric diagnosis across cultures.** The Epidemiologic Catchment Area Study was commissioned in 1977 to study the mental health problems, diagnosed and undiagnosed, in the general population. Five cities across the United States, with specific aims to assess two major ethnic groups, blacks and Hispanics, were chosen, and results are now being released.

IV. **Therapy.**

A. **Psychotherapy.**

1. In ongoing therapy with clients of different ethnic backgrounds, be aware and open-minded about cultural and language issues. It has been recommended to address cultural differences early in the course of treatment. It has also been recommended to seek supervision from someone of the patient's background.

2. In therapy with non-English-speaking clients, a translator may be necessary for the initial interview, but not in ongoing psychotherapy. They become third parties in the treatment, with their own psychodynamic issues, e.g., religion, political, and class. Even with a patient who is fluent in the therapist's language, or if the therapist is fluent in the patient's native language, nuances can be missed. Furthermore, language can be used to resist the therapeutic process. Patients may be willing to discuss an emotional topic in a different language, thus distancing the affect from the feeling.

3. Also consider the factors reviewed under Section II./B. regarding history .

B. **Ethnopsychopharmacology.**

1. **Neuroleptics.** Compared with whites, Asians and Asian-Americans appear to require lower doses of

neuroleptics to achieve a remission. The incidence of side effects in Asians may be greater than in blacks and whites. However, not all types of neuroleptics have been studied.

2. **Antidepressants.** Studies using tricyclic antidepressants have been inconsistent in demonstrating dosage differences pharmacokinetically between different ethnic groups. Asians and blacks, compared with whites, appear to have an increased clinical response rate at equivalent doses, while data on Hispanics are equivocal. Differences in toxicity have not been well studied. Blacks may have a higher incidence of delirium developing after tricyclic antidepressant use, independent of age and plasma level, compared with whites. So far, studies using other heterocyclic agents have not been published.

3. **Anxiolytics.** Diazepam is more slowly metabolized in Asians than in whites, although no difference in sedation was found. After long-term dosing, however, a difference in sedation may occur. No other drugs in this class have been studied. Differences in side effects also have not been studied.

4. **Lithium.** Asian patients with bipolar disorder respond clinically at lower lithium blood levels as compared with white patients with bipolar disorder. (Lithium therapeutic levels of 0.4 to 0.8 mEq/L compared with 0.8 to 1.2 mEq/L.) It appears that Asian patients develop toxic symptoms at lower blood levels.

C. **Use of healers.**

1. Traditional healers, when available, may be used as an adjunct or consultant during the course of evaluation and treatment. According to Kleinman, the health care system includes not only institutions and practitioners, but also beliefs about illness, choices of treatment alternatives, and the sick role, with three subsystems: popular and family; individual and social; and professional and folk or traditional systems. The folk-healing system provides psychosocial and cultural

treatment for illness by naming and ordering the experience of illness, providing meaning for the experience, and treating the personal, family, and social problems that constitute the illness. Thus, it heals even if it is unable effectively to treat the disease. Indigenous healers tend to treat the following three types of disorders.

a. Acute, self-limiting diseases.

b. Non-life-threatening chronic diseases where the management of illness is a larger component than the biomedical treatment of disease.

c. Somatization of minor psychiatric disorders and interpersonal problems.

2. *Curanderos (an Example of Traditional Healers)*. Curanderismo is a Latin-American folk-healing system of much regional diversity with the following eight major philosophical premises.

a. Mind and body are inseparable.

b. Emotional, physical, and social balance/harmony are important.

c. The patient is an innocent victim of malevolent forces.

d. Body and soul are separable. Therefore, one can lose one's soul, which can lead to feelings of depersonalization and derealization. The curandero may treat the soul, not just the body.

e. Cure requires family participation. Interdependence is valued.

f. The natural world is not clearly distinguished from the supernatural. God, the saints, and other people may cause illnesses.

g. A sick person needs to be resocialized, especially in cases where acculturative stresses are great.

h. Healers are expected to be warm, friendly, and personable, and have a connection with the sacred.

Acculturation seems to lead to less use and belief in curanderismo, except for chronic illnesses, pediatric disorders, pain, and those maladies still classified according to traditional beliefs, like mal de ojo.

REFERENCES

1. McGoldrick M: Ethnicity and family therapy: An overview, in McGoldrick, Pearce, Giordano (eds): *Ethnicity and Family Therapy*. New York, Guilford Press, 1982.
2. Kleinman A: *Patients and Healers in the Context of Culture: An Exploration of the Borderland Between Anthropology, Medicine, and Psychiatry*. Berkeley, Calif, University of California Press, 1980.
3. Westermeyer J: Psychiatric diagnosis across cultural boundaries. *Am J Psychiatry* 1985; 142:798–805.
4. Marcos LR, Alpert M: Strategies and risks in psychotherapy with bilingual patients: The phenomenon of language independence. *Am J Psychiatry* 1976; 133:1275–1278.
5. Williams CL: Issues surrounding psychological testing of minority patients. *Hosp Community Psychiatry* 1987; 38:184–189.
6. Simons RC, Hughes CC (eds): *The Culture Bound Syndromes*. Dordrecht, the Netherlands, D. Reidel Publishing Co, 1983.
7. Spitzer RL, Williams JBW, Skodol AE (eds): *International Perspectives on DSM-III*. Washington, DC, American Psychiatric Press, Inc, 1983.
8. Lin KM: Ethnicity and psychopharmacology. *Cult Med Psychiatry* 1986; 10:151–165.
9. Kleinman A, Sung L: Why do indigenous practitioners successfully heal? *Science Medicine* 1979; 138:7–26.
10. Maduro R: Curanderismo and Latino views of disease and curing in cross-cultural medicine. *West J Med* 1983; 139:868–874.

11. Scheper-Hughes N, Stewart D: Curanderismo in Taos County, NM: A possible case of anthropological romanticism in cross-cultural medicine. *West J Med* 1979; 139:875–884.
12. Cockerham W: Sociology and psychiatry, in Kaplan H, Sadock B (eds): *Textbook of Comprehensive Psychiatry/IV*. Baltimore, Williams & Wilkins, 1985, pp 265–273.
13. Kleinman A, Good B (eds): *Culture and Depression: Studies in the Anthropology and Cross-cultural Psychiatry of Affect and Disorder*. Berkeley, Calif, University of California Press, 1985.

Index

A

Abstraction, 6
Abuse, 653–666
  of aged, 663–665
    detection, 665
    diagnosis, 665
    epidemiology, 663–664
    financial abuse, 664
    medical neglect, 664
    physical abuse, 664
    psychologic abuse, 664
    reporting, 665
    syndromes, 664
    treatment, 665
  alcohol (see Alcohol abuse)
  child, 655–659
    diagnosis, 657–658
    epidemiology, 655–656
    psychiatric treatment, 658–659
    reporting, 658
    syndromes, 656–657
  drug (see Drug abuse)
  fetal, 653–654
    drug abuse and, 654
    psychosis and, 653–654
    syndromes, 653–654
    treatment, 654
  spouse, 661–663
    recognition, 661–662
    reporting, 663
    treatment options, 662–663
Academic skills disorder, 277
Acetazolamide: interaction with lithium, 470
Acetylcholine: in affective disorders, 97
Acquired immunodeficiency syndrome (see AIDS)
Acuity, 11
Addison disease (see Hypoadrenocorticism)
ADHD
  amphetamine in, 434
  antidepressants in, 437
    dosage, 437
  antipsychotics in, 439–440
    dosage, 440
  assessment, 238
  associated features, 237
  in children and adolescents, 236–239
  clinical presentation, 236–237
  definition, 236–237
  dextroamphetamine in, 434
  diagnosis, differential, 237
  epidemiology, 237
  etiology, 237–238
  haloperidol in, 440
  imipramine in, 437
  methylphenidate in, 434
  stimulants in, 433–434
    dosage and monitoring, 434
  treatment, 238–239
Adolescence
  anxiety disorders during (see Anxiety disorders in children and adolescents)

Index

Adolescence *(cont.)*
  axis I disorders during (*see* Axis I disorders in children and adolescents)
  axis II disorders during, 272–280
  gender identity disorder during, 252
 juvenile law, 645
  mood disorders during (*see* Mood disorders in children and adolescents)
  personality disorder during, 296–297
    diagnosis, 279–280
  psychotherapy during (*see* Psychotherapy with children and adolescents)
Adrenal disease, 24–26
Affect, 7–8
Affective disorders, 93–104
  acetylcholine in, 97
  in aged, treatment, 442–446
  atypical, 94–95
  behavior, 96
  biologic factors in, 96–99
  catecholamines in, 97
  chronobiology, 99
  cognitive factors in, 96
  cortisol in, 98
  endocrine factors, 98
  etiologies, 95–99
  genetics of, 96
  growth hormone in, 98
  major, 93–94
  mixed, treatment, 102
  neurotransmitters in, 97–98
  psychiatric rating scales for, 56
  psychodynamics, 95–96
  psychologic factors in, 95
  psychosocial factors, 96
  relationship
    to eating disorders, 186–187
    to personality disorder, 291–293
  schedule for, 56
  serotonin in, 97–98
  symptoms, 96
  thyroid hormone in, 98–99
  treatment, 99–104
Affective symptoms: in schizophrenia, ECT therapy, 455
Age
  in conversion disorder, 206
  in hypochondriasis, 208–209
  mental, 37
  neuroleptic metabolic rate and, 345
  in psychogenic pain, 210
  in somatization disorder, 205
Aged, 441–453
  abuse of (*see* Abuse, of aged)
  affective disorders, treatment, 442–446
  agitation of, 446–460
    benzodiazepines for, 446
    beta-blocker for, 446–447
    neuroleptics for, 446
  anticholinergics for, doses and side effects, 448
  antidepressants for, 444
  anxiety of, 447–450
    antidepressants in, tricyclic, 447
    benzodiazepines for, 447
    buspirone in, 447–450
    MAOIs for, 447
    neuroleptics in, 447
  benztropine mesylate/trihexylphenidyl for,

doses and side effects, 448
constipation of, 453
dementia of, 451
  hydergine for, 451
depression of, with heart disease, 451–452
depression of, refractory, 443–445
  electroconvulsive therapy for, 445
  methylphenidate for, 443–445
desipramine for, 444
doxepin for, 444
dyskinesia, tardive, 452–453
fluphenazine for, doses and side effects, 448
glaucoma of, 452
haloperidol for, doses and side effects, 448
hypotension, 452
impotence, 452
insomnia in, 450
  antidepressants in, tricyclic, 450
  antihistamines for, 450
  barbiturates in, 450
  benzodiazepines for, 450
  chloral hydrate for, 450
  neuroleptics in, 450
  lithium and, 383, 443
L-triiodothyronine for, 443
mania of, 445–446
  benzodiazepines for, 446
  carbamazepine for, 445–446
  electroconvulsive therapy for, 446
  lithium for, 445
  neuroleptics for, 445
MAOIs for, 443
neuroleptics for
  dosages, 342, 448
  side effects, 448
nortriptyline for, 444
perphenazine for, doses and side effects, 448
phenelzine for, 444
prostatic hypertrophy, 452
psychopharmacology for, 441–453
psychosis of, 446–450
  benzodiazepines for, 446
  beta-blocker for, 446–447
  neuroleptics in, 446
psychotherapy with, 627–632
  modifications, 631
  resistance to cognitive work, 628–629
  resistance to empathic work, 629–630
  therapeutic relationship, 628–631
thioridazine for, doses and side effects, 448
thiothixene for, doses and side effects, 448
tranylcypromine for, 444
trazodone for, 444
Aggression: neuroleptics for, 332
Agitation
  in aged (see Aged, agitation)
  psychotic, neuroleptics in, 345
  severe, neuroleptics for, 332
Agranulocytosis: after neuroleptics, 362
AIDS: dementia complex in, 146–147
AIMS
  examination procedure, 418–419
  screen/baseline, 419–420
Akathisia, 347

Akathisia *(cont.)*
  discussion of, 415–416
  tabular data on, 348
  treatment, 421
Akinesia: tabular data on, 349
Akinetic mutism: tabular data on, 349
Akineton: for neuroleptic side effects, 350
Al-Anon, 133
Alcohol
  abuse, 115–138
    (*See also* Alcoholism)
    definition, 115–116
    history, 3–4
    psychiatric aspects, 115–138
    suicidality and, 575
  acute intoxication, 124–126
  amblyopia, 122
  amnestic disorder, 121
  dependence, definition, 116
  ethanol levels, relationship to clinical manifestations, 125
  fetal alcohol syndrome, 123–124
    congenital abnormalities in, 123–124
    ethanol in, 123
    newborn behavior in, 124
  hallucinosis, 127
    benztropine in, 127, 132
    haloperidol in, 127, 132
  interaction
    with benzodiazepines, 472
    with MAOIs, 469
    with tricyclic antidepressants, 468
  tolerance, definition, 116
  withdrawal
    delirium, 128–133
    delirium, benzodiazepines in, 130
    delirium, chlordiazepoxide in, 130
    delirium, EEG in, 84
    delirium, lorazepam in, 131
    delirium, neuroleptics in, 131
    delirium, oxazepam in, 131
    delirium, phenobarbital in, 130
    seizures, 128–133
    seizures, diazepam in, 128
    syndromes, 126–133
    syndromes, benzodiazepines in, 403
    tremulousness in, 126–127
Alcoholics Anonymous, 133
  twelve-step program of recovery, 135
Alcoholism, 25–26
  (*See also* Alcohol abuse)
  carcinoma in, 123
  cardiovascular complications, 122
  chronic
    medical complications, 122–123
    neurologic syndromes associated with, 120–122
  disulfiram in, 134–138
    monitoring schedule, 137
  gastrointestinal complications, 122
  hematologic complications, 122–123
    laboratory abnormalities, 120
  lipids in, plasma, 123
  Michigan Alcoholism Screening Test, 118, 119
  muscle in, skeletal, 123

occupational impairment in, 117–118
physical signs, 118–120
psychiatric rating scales in, 59
recognition of, 116–123
social impairment in, 117–118
symptoms, presenting, 116–117
treatment, 133–138
programs, 133–134
ALI test, 643–644
Allergy: and neuroleptics, 362
Alprazolam, 397
dosage, 402, 449
half-life, 449
Altruism: in groups, 557
Aluminum: dementia due to, 143
Amantadine
discussion of, 352
for neuroleptic side effects, 351
Amblyopia: alcohol, 122
Amiloride: interaction with lithium, 470
Aminophylline: interaction with lithium, 470
Amnesia: psychogenic, 219–220
Amnestic: organic amnestic syndrome, 167–169
Amok, 673
Amphetamine
in ADHD, 434
interactions
with MAOIs, 469
with neuroleptics, 467
Anesthesia: general, brief, for electroconvulsive therapy, 455
Anesthetic(s)
dissolved in epinephrine, interaction with tricyclic antidepressants, 468

interactions with neuroleptics, 467
for pain, 324–325
Anomalies: congenital, and lithium, 428
Anorexia
antidepressants in, 193–194
assessment, 189–191
behavioral treatment program in, 192
biopsychosocial model for, 190
cyproheptadine in, 194
diagnostic criteria, 171
epidemiology, 172
family therapy in, 193
group therapy in, 192–193
hospitalization in, criteria for, 189
monoamine disturbances in, 178–184
opiate antagonists in, 194
phenothiazine in, 194
psychotherapy in, 192–193
refeeding in, 191
complications and their treatment, 191–192
stabilization, medical, 189–191
transcultural psychiatry and, 673
treatment, inpatient, 189–194
Antabuse (*see* Disulfiram)
Anthropology: and transcultural psychiatry, 667–668
Anticholinergic(s)
action of neuroleptics, 331
for aged, doses and side effects, 448
central anticholinergic syndrome after neuroleptics, 358
CNS toxicity of neuroleptics, 331

Anticholinergic(s) *(cont.)*
  delirium, 352
    EEG in, 84
  interactions
    with neuroleptics, 466
    with tricyclic antidepressants, 468
  for neuroleptic side effects, 350
Anticoagulants: interactions with tricyclic antidepressants, 468
Anticonvulsants: in bulimia, 198
Antidepressants, 369–378
  action mechanism, 370
  in ADHD, 437
    dosage, 437
  for aged, 444
  in anorexia, 193–194
  in bulimia, 195–198
  for children, 435–437
  classification, structural, 369
  cyclic *(see* tricyclic *below)*
  dosing, 373–375
    continuing, 374
    low-unit, 374
    maximum, 374
    method, 373
  heterocyclics, 369–375
  levels, 373–374
  metabolism, 373
  in postpartum period, 429
  during pregnancy, 429
  ranking of drug effects, 371
  selection of, 372–373
  in separation anxiety disorder, 437
    dosage and duration, 437
  side effects, 370–372
  teratogenicity, 429
  in transcultural psychiatry, 676
  tricyclic
    in anxiety in aged, 447
    in depression, major, 100–101
    in insomnia in aged, 450
    interactions of, 468
    interactions with benzodiazepines, 472
    interactions with lithium, 471
    interactions with MAOIs, 469
    interactions with neuroleptics, 466–467
    overdose, 375
Antiemetics: discussion of, 344
Antihistamines
  for insomnia in aged, 450
  interactions with benzodiazepines, 472
Antimanic agents, 379–395
Antipsychotics
  in ADHD, 439–440
    dosage, 440
  in children, 437–440
  neuroleptics *(see* Neuroleptics)
  in PDD, in children, 439
    dosage, 439
  in postpartum period, 430–431
  during pregnancy, 430–431
    precaution, 431
  in schizophrenia, 438
    dosage and monitoring in children, 438
  teratogenicity, 430
  in Tourette syndrome, in children, 438–439
    dosage, 439
Anxiety
  in aged *(see* Aged, anxiety in)
  benzodiazepines in, 403
  disorders of children and adolescents, 243–249
    avoidant disorder *(see* Avoidant disorder of

children and adolescents)
overanxious disorder (*see* Overanxious disorder in children and adolescents)
separation (*see* Separation anxiety disorder)
disorders, psychiatric rating scale for, 56
dream anxiety disorder, 314–315
hierarchy, test anxiety in systematic desensitization, 518
neurosis, 288
somatized, 213–214
  diagnosis, differential, 213
  diagnostic criteria, 213
  features, clinical, 213
  features, theoretical, 213
  treatment, 214
state-trait scale, 56
in stuttering, 263
Anxiolytics
half-lives and doses, 449
in transcultural psychiatry, 676
Aphasia: in delirium, 155–156
Artane: for neuroleptic side effects, 351
Articulation disorder: developmental, 278
Assertion training, 526–527
clinical application, 526–527
Assessment: and psychotherapy, 475
A-State, 56
"A" test, 5
Ativan (*see* Lorazepam)
A-Trait, 56
Attention, 5
deficit disorder with hyperactivity disorder, stimulants in, 405–406

deficit hyperactivity disorder (*see* ADHD)
Auditory hallucinations, 10
Autism
abnormal response to sensory input in, 274
activity peculiarities, 275
clinical presentation, 274
communication disturbance, 275
course, 275
diagnosis, 275
epidemiology, 275
etiology, 276
infantile
  fenfluramine in, 435
  stimulants in, 434–435
  stimulants in, dosage, 435
social indifference in, 274
treatment, 276
uneven developmental progress in, 275
Autistic disorder (*see* Autism)
Autonomic
disturbance in delirium, 152
nervous system after neuroleptics, 360–361
Aversive therapy, 522–523
clinical application, 522
Avoidant disorder of children and adolescents, 245–246
assessment, 245–246
associated features, 245
clinical presentation, 245
definition, 245
diagnosis, differential, 245
epidemiology, 245
etiology, 245
treatment, 246
Axis I disorders in children and adolescents, 231–271
ADHD (*see* ADHD)

Axis I disorders in children and adolescents (*cont.*)
  assessment, 231–232
  conduct disorder (*see* Conduct disorder in children and adolescents)
  diagnostic categories, 236
  disorders usually first evident in infancy, childhood or adolescence, 236–269
  mood disorders (*see* Mood disorders in children and adolescents)
  oppositional defiant disorder (*see* Oppositional defiant disorder in children and adolescents)
  treatment, individualized, 235–236
Axis II disorders in children and adolescents, 272–280

B

Bacterial dementia, 147
Barbiturates
  for insomnia in aged, 450
  interactions with neuroleptics, 467
Beck Depression Inventory, 56
Beck's cognitive therapy (*see* Cognitive therapy of Beck)
Behavior
  in affective disorders, 96
  disorders, disruptive, in children and adolescents, 236–243
  imitative, in groups, 557
  interictal behavior syndrome, 161
  of newborn, in fetal alcohol syndrome, 124
  in psychiatric assessment, initial, 4–5
Behavioral
  cognitive therapy, 589
  interventions in enuresis, functional, 260
  medicine, 526
  programs for pain, 325–326
    examples of, 326–328
  -social exchange family therapy, 549
Behavioral therapy, 514–527
  definitions, 515–517
  program in anorexia, 192
Benadryl: for neuroleptic side effects, 350
Bender visual motor gestalt test, 54
Benzodiazepines, 396–404
  absorption, 397–399
  in agitation in aged, 446
  in alcohol withdrawal delirium, 130
  in alcohol withdrawal syndromes, 403
  in anxiety, 403
    in aged, 447
  cardiovascular system and, 397
  CNS and, 396
  in delirium, 157
  in depression, 404
  dosage, 401–403
  excretion, 397–399
  fate, 397–399
  hypnotic action, 404
  in insomnia in aged, 450
  interactions of, 472
    with neuroleptics, 466
  for mania in aged, 446
  in perinatal period, 431
  physical dependence, 399–400
  during pregnancy, 431
  preparations, 401–403
  in psychosis in aged, 446
  respiratory system and, 397

side effects, 401
skeletal muscle and, 397
teratogenicity, 431
therapeutic uses, 403–404
tolerance, 399–400
toxic reactions, 401
Benztropine
in alcoholic hallucinosis, 127, 132
mesylate/trihexylphenidyl, for aged, doses and side effects, 448
for neuroleptic side effects, 350
Bereavement, 577–582
Beta blocker
in agitation in aged, 446–447
in psychosis in aged, 446–447
Bethanidine: interactions with tricyclic antidepressants, 468
Bicarbonate: interaction with lithium, 470
Binge eating: etiologies, 177
Biofeedback, 564–566
applications, 565–566
definition, 564
methods, 564–565
theory, 564–565
types, 564
Biopsychosocial models: in anorexia and bulimia, 190
Biperiden: for neuroleptic side effects, 350
Bipolar disorder, 93–94
(*See also* Manic depressive disorder)
atypical, 94
depressed, 93
manic, 93
treatment, 99–100
mixed, 93
II, 94
Blockade: of dopamine by neuroleptics, 331

Blocker (*see* Beta blocker)
Blocking, 8, 505
Blood
gases, 26
pressure in hypothyroidism, 23
Body
awareness, 14–16
part identification, 14
Brain
injury, traumatic, 163
organic brain syndrome (*see* Organic brain syndrome)
tumors, 27
Breast-feeding: lithium during, 382, 427–428
Brief Psychiatric Rating Scale, 55
example of, 64–65
Brief psychotherapy (*see* Individual psychotherapy, short-term)
Bulimia
anticonvulsants in, 198
antidepressants in, 195–198
biopsychosocial model for, 190
diagnostic criteria, 171–172
epidemiology, 172–173
group therapy in, 195
hospitalization in, criteria for, 189
monoamine disturbances in, 178–184
opiate antagonists in, 198
psychotherapy in, 194–195
transcultural psychiatry and, 673
treatment, inpatient, 194–198
Buspirone
for anxiety in aged, 447–450
doses and half-life, 449

Butyrophenones
  dosages, 337
  formulations, available, 341
  potency, 337
  side effect profile, 339

C

C.A.G.E., 59
Calculations, 6
Capacities: representative tests of, 640–641
Carbamazepine, 391–393
  discontinuing, guidelines for, 393
  interactions of, 394, 473
    with lithium, 470–471
  for mania in aged, 445–446
Carcinoma
  in alcoholism, 123
  pancreas, 35–36
Cardiovascular system: and benzodiazepines, 397
Care
  emergency, 584
  of family of dying or newly deceased patient, 578–580
Catapres: for neuroleptic side effects, 351
Catastrophizing, 529
Catatonia: "lethal," 358
Catatonic symptoms: in schizophrenia, electroconvulsive therapy in, 455
Catecholamines: in affective disorders, 97
Catharsis: in groups, 558
Central nervous system
  benzodiazepines and, 396
  after electroconvulsive therapy, 462–463
  infections, 164
    chronic, 28–30

side effects of neuroleptics, non-extrapyramidal, 357
  tabular data on, 358–359
toxicity, anticholinergic, of neuroleptics, 331
Centrax: dosage, 403
Cerebral tumor, 163–164
Cerebrovascular disease, 163
Character, 282
Charcoal: activated, interaction with tricyclic antidepressants, 468
Chemical exposure: industrial, and dementia, 148
Child abuse (see Abuse, child)
Children
  antidepressants for, 435–437
  antipsychotics for, 437–440
  anxiety disorders (see Anxiety disorders of children)
  assessment, 16–17
  axis I disorders (see Axis I disorders)
  axis II disorders, 272–280
  custody of, 644–645
  depression (see Depression, in children)
  drugs for, 432–440
  gender identity disorder (see Gender identity disorders)
  juvenile law, 645
  mood disorders (see Mood disorders in children)
  personality disorder, 296–297
    diagnosis, 279–280
  play therapy for, 622–623
  reactive attachment disorder (see Reactive attachment disorder in

infancy and early childhood)
stimulants for, 432–435
Chloral hydrate: for insomnia in aged, 450
Chlordiazepoxide, 398
in alcohol withdrawal delirium, 130
dosage, 402
Chlorpheniramine: interaction with MAOIs, 469
Chlorpromazine
dosages, 336
formulations, available, 340
potency, 336
side effect profile, 338
Chlorprothixene
dosages, 337
formulations, available, 341
potency, 337
side effect profile, 339
Chronobiology: of affective disorders, 99
Cimetidine interactions
with antidepressants, tricyclic, 468
with benzodiazepines, 472
with carbamazepine, 473
Class: social, and transcultural psychiatry, 670
Clonazepam, 393
Clonidine: for neuroleptic side effects, 351
Clorazepate, 398, 402
Clozapine, 330
Cocaine, 31
withdrawal, 31
Cogentin (see Benztropine)
Cognitive
development according to Piaget, 614–617
distortions, 528
therapy (see below)
triad, 528
work, resistance of aged, 628–629

Cognitive therapy, 514, 527–535, 588–589
of Beck, 528–532
abstraction in, selective, 529
arbitrary inference, 529
assumptions and, underlying, 529–530
clinical application, 532
clinical example, 530
disqualifying the positive, 529
dysfunctional beliefs, daily log of, 530–531
jumping to conclusions, 529
labeling/mislabeling, 529
"should" statements, 529
behavioral, 589
duration, 589
feedback loop, 588
goals, 589
individual psychotherapy and, short-term, 586
interpersonal therapy and, 586–587
selection criteria, 588
theory, 588
Collagen vascular disease, 30–31
Commitment
to institution, understanding of, as capacity test, 641
involuntary, 634–637
civil, 634–635
criteria for, 635–637
Communication: in autism, 275
Competence assessment, 639
McGarry scale, 639–642
special issues in, 642
Comprehension, 15
Conditioning: operant, 516
Conduct disorder in children and adolescents, 239–243

Conduct disorder in children and adolescents (*cont.*)
assessment, 240–241
associated features, 240
clinical presentation, 239–240
definition, 239–240
diagnosis, differential, 240
epidemiology, 240
etiology, 240
treatment, 241
Confidentiality, 638
legal principles, 638–639
Confusional state, acute (*see* Delirium)
Consent: informed, 637–638
Constipation: in aged, 453
Constructions, 6
Contract: making of, as capacity test, 640
Conversion disorder, 206–208
age in, 206
with delirium, 155
diagnosis, differential, 207
diagnostic criteria, 206
EEG in, 85–91
features
 clinical, 206–207
 theoretical, 207
gender in, 206
incidence, 206
prevalence, 206
treatment, 208
Coordination abnormalities, 13
Cortisol: in affective disorders, 98
Coumarin: interactions with tricyclic antidepressants, 468
Counterconditioning, 517
negative, 517
positive, 517
Countertransference, 505
Cranial nerves: assessment, 11–12

Criminal act: responsibility for, and capacity test, 640
Crisis
acute, 571–583
intervention, 584
Culture
-bound syndromes, 672
psychiatry and, 667
Cushing's syndrome, 24
Custody: and divorce, 644–645
Cyclothymic disorder, 94
treatment, 102–103
Cylert (*see* Pemoline)
Cyproheptadine: in anorexia, 194

D

Dalmane, 398
dosage, 402
D.A.N.G.E.R.O.U.S., 58
Dangerousness standards, 634–635
Davanloo brief psychotherapy, 591
duration, 592
Death
normal response to, 577
sudden, after neuroleptics, 364
Debrisoquin: interactions with tricyclic antidepressants, 468
Decamethonium: interaction with lithium, 470
Defense(s)
insanity, 643–644
mechanisms, 505
 in neurosis and personality disorders, 291
spectrum of, 292
Defiant disorder (*see* Oppositional defiant disorder in children and adolescents)

Dehydration, 26
Delinquency: juvenile, 645
Delirium, 152–157
  alcohol withdrawal (see Alcohol withdrawal delirium)
  anticholinergic, 352
    EEG in, 84
  aphasia in, 155–156
  autonomic disturbances in, 152
  benzodiazepine in, 157
  clinical variability in, 153
  in conversion disorder, 155
  definition, 152–153
  diagnosis, differential, 155
  in dissociative disorder, 155
  drug withdrawal and, 154
  EEG in, 84–84, 153
  endocrinologic disturbances in, 153
  etiology, 153–154
  evaluation, 156
  features, major clinical, 152–153
  infection in, 153
  intellectual impairment in, 152
  intoxication and, 154
  intracranial processes in, 154
  lorazepam in, 157
  mood alterations in, 153
  motor abnormalities in, 152
  neuroleptics in, 157
  nutritional deficiencies and, 154
  perception in, disturbed, 152
  psychiatric problems in, 154
  with psychosis, manic, 155
  in schizophrenia, 155
  sleep-wake cycle abnormalities in, 153
  systemic disturbances in, 153
  temporal variability, 153
  thought content disturbance in, 153
  treatment, 156–157
  tremens (see Alcohol withdrawal delirium)
  vs. dementia, 154
  workup, 156
Delivery: and lithium, 382
Delusions, 9
Demanders: entitled, psychotherapy of, 599–601
Dementia, 139–152
  AD in, 142
  in aged, 451
  AIDS and, 146–147
  aluminum causing, 143
  bacterial, 147
  characteristics, 143–144
  chemical exposure and, industrial, 148
  cortical, 141–142
  definition, 139
  diagnostic workup, 150–151
  dialysis, 147
  drugs in, 148
  early-stage, and personality disorder, 296
  EEG in, 84
    findings, 86–87
  electrolyte disturbances and, 147
  encephalopathy and chronic uremic, 148
    liver, 148
  endocrinologic abnormalities and, 147
  etiology, 142–150
  extrapyramidal syndromes, 144–150
  Fahr disease and, 146

Dementia *(cont.)*
  features
    major clinical, 139–141
    mixed, 142
  genetic factors in, 143
  histopathologic findings, 142–143
  Huntington disease and, 145
  hydrocephalic, 149
  hypoxia and, 147
  Jakob-Creutzfeldt disease and, 146
  metals in, 148
  multi-infarct, 143
  myelin disease and, 150
  nutritional deficiencies and, 147
  Parkinson disease and, 144–145
  pathogenesis, 144
  porphyria and, 148
  spinocerebellar degeneration and, 146
  stage
    early, 140
    final, 140–141
    middle, 140
  subcortical, 141–142
  supranuclear palsy and, progressive, 145
  traumatic, 150
  treatment, 151–152
  with tumor, 150
  uremia and, 147
  vs. delirium, 154
  Wilson disease and, 145
Denial, 505
  self-destructive deniers, psychotherapy of, 601–602
Depersonalization
  disorder, 220–221
  neurosis, 288
Depression
  in aged (*see* Aged, depression of)
  atypical, 94–95
    treatment, 102
  Beck Inventory for, 56
  benzodiazepine in, 404
  in children, 436
    antidepressant dosage, 436
    antidepressant duration, 436
    antidepressant monitoring, 436
    desipramine in, 436
    imipramine in, 436
  electroconvulsive therapy in, 455
  Hamilton Scale for, 56
    example of, 73–79
  with heart disease in aged, 451–452
  in Huntington disease, 164
  in hydrocephalus, 164
  in interictal psychiatric disorder, 159
  inventory, example of, 70–72
  major, 94
    MAOIs in, 101
    TCAs in, 100–101
    treatment, 100–102
  in Parkinson disease, 164
  somatized, 213–214
    diagnosis, differential, 213
    diagnostic criteria, 213
    features, clinical, 213
    features, theoretical, 213
    treatment, 214
  in supranuclear palsy, progressive, 164
  Zung scale, and transcultural psychiatry and, 672
Depressive neurosis, 288
Dermatosis: and neuroleptics, 362
Desensitization, systematic, 517–518

clinical application, 520
desensitization proper, 519
hierarchy construction, 518
hierarchy, test anxiety, 518
Desipramine
for aged, doses and side effects, 444
in depression in children, 436
Development
abnormality
in habit disorder, 269
in stereotypy, 269
changes, major, 607
cognitive, according to Piaget, 614–617
disorders of, 272–279
pervasive, 274–276
specific, 276–279
specific, assessment, 276–277
specific, diagnosis, 277–278
specific, diagnosis, differential, 277
specific, evaluation, 277
specific, treatment, 278–279
history, 4
intellectual, according to Piaget, 614–617
lines of Anna Freud, 610–613
phases of groups, 556
psychosocial stages, according to Erikson, 615
three aspects of, 610–617
Dexedrine (*see* Dextroamphetamine)
Dextroamphetamine
in ADHD, 434
discussion of, 412
dosage, 411

Dextromethorphan: interaction with MAOIs, 469
Diagnosis, 1–91
psychotherapy and, 475
Dialysis dementia, 147
Diazepam, 398
in alcohol withdrawal seizures, 128
dosage, 402
Dibenzoxazepines
dosages, 337
formulations, available, 341
potency, 337
side effect profile, 339
Diet: during monoamine oxidase inhibitors, 376–377
Difficult patients (*see* Psychotherapy with difficult patients)
Digit span, 5
Dihydroindolones
dosages, 337
formulations, available, 341
potency, 337
side effect profile, 339
Diphenhydramine: for neuroleptic side effects, 350
Diphenylbutylpiperidines
dosages, 337
formulations, available, 342
potency, 337
side effect profile, 339
Directive psychotherapy (*see* Psychotherapy, directive)
Disability: grave, and involuntary commitment, 635–636
Disaster victims, 580
Disipal: for neuroleptic side effects, 350
Displacement, 505

696 Index

Disruptive behavior disorders: in children and adolescents, 236–243
Dissociation, 505
Dissociative disorders, 216–230
  with delirium, 155
Dissociative states: EEG in, 85–91
Disulfiram
  in alcoholism, 134–138
  monitoring schedule, 137
Diuretics: thiazide, interaction with lithium, 470
Divorce
  custody and, 644–645
  understanding of, as capacity test, 641
Dopamine
  blockade by neuroleptics, 331
  interaction with MAOIs, 469
Double simultaneous stimulation, 12
Doxepin: for aged, doses and side effects, 444
Drawing tests: projective, 50–51
Dream anxiety disorder, 314–315
Droperidol
  discussion of, 344
  dosages, 337
  formulations, available, 341
  potency, 337
  side effect profile, 339
Drug(s)
  abuse
    fetal abuse and, 654
    history, 3–4
    suicidality and, 575
  for children, 432–440
  dementia and, 148
  in enuresis, 435
    dosage, 435
  interactions, 465–473
    with carbamazepine, 394
    with lithium, 387–388
    with neuroleptics, 364, 366–367
  in medical illness presenting as psychiatric illness, 21
  psychosis due to, 112–113
  psychotropic (see Psychotropic drugs)
  withdrawal (see Withdrawal)
DTs (see Alcohol withdrawal delirium)
Dusky vs. US, 639
Dying patient: psychotherapy of, 597–599
Dyskinesia
  tardive, 352–356
    in aged, 452–453
    definition, 352–353
    description, 352–353
    detection, early, 356
    diagnosis, differential, 353, 354–355
    discussion of, 417–420
    informed consent for neuroleptics, 353
    neuroleptic dose reduction in, 356
    neuroleptic withdrawal in, 356–357
    oral-facial movements in, 352–353
    prevention, 353–356
    restricting neuroleptics, 353
    stimulants and, 413
    treatment, 356–357, 421–422
  withdrawal, 353
Dyssomnias, 308–314
Dysthymia
  family therapy in, 104
  treatment, 103–104

Dysthymic disorder, 94
Dystonia, acute, 347, 415
  as neuroleptic extrapyramidal side effect, 347
  after neuroleptics, 348
  treatment, 420–421

E

Eating
  binge, etiologies, 177
  disorders, 171–202
    associated features, 174–175
    classification, 171–172
    complications, medical, 178, 179–180
    development, psychodynamic factors, 187–189
    endogenous opiate peptides in, 184–185
    epidemiology, 172–173
    evaluation, 173–175
    evaluation, clinical, 175–178
    family theories, 188–189
    history in, 175–176
    history in, family, 176
    laboratory tests in, 176
    mental status examination in, 176
    monoamines in, 178–184
    neuroendocrine changes in, 178, 182–183
    neurotransmitter systems in, 178–185
    outcome, 199–200
    physical examination in, 176
    premorbid personality and, 187
    presentation, clinical, 173–175
    presentation, modes, 173
    prognosis, 198–199
    psychodynamic theory, 187–188
    psychological tests in, 177–178
    relationship to affective disorders, 186–187
    treatment, 524–525
"Ecstasy," 31
ECT (see Electroconvulsive therapy)
Education: and transcultural psychiatry, 670
EEG (see Electroencephalography)
Elderly (see Aged)
Electroconvulsive therapy, 454–463
  adverse effects, 462–463
    systemic, 462
  anesthesia, brief general, 455
  central nervous system after, 462–463
  contraindications, 455–466
  in depression, 455
    in aged, 445
  electrode placement, 460
  evaluation, pretreatment, 457–460
  indications, 455
  informed consent for, 456–457
  intracranial pressure and, 456
  involuntary, 457
  maintenance, 463–464
  in mania, 455
  in mania, acute, 393
    in aged, 446
  myocardial infarction and, 455–456
  number of treatments, 461–462
  precautions, 455–456
  preparation for, 456–457
  in schizophrenia, 455

Electroconvulsive therapy *(cont.)*
  seizure and the electrical stimulus, 461
  spacing of treatments, 461–462
Electroencephalography, 81–91
  in conversion disorders, 85–91
  in delirium, 83–84, 153
  in dementia, 84
    findings, 86–87
  in dissociative states, 85–91
  in endocrinologic states, 88–90
  in neuroleptic malignant syndromes, 84
  normal patterns, 82–83
  in nutritional states, 88–90
  in organic mental disorders, 83–85
  in pseudoseizures, 85–91
  in seizures, 85–91
    hysterical, 85–91
  in sleep disorders, 91
  of sleep stages, 306
  in toxic/metabolic disorders, 84–85
    findings, 88–90
Electrolyte(s), 26
  alteration and lithium, 382
  disturbances and dementia, 147
Elimination disorder, 257–260
Emergency care, 584
Emic perspectives: and transcultural psychiatry, 667–668
Emory model: classes of psychogenic pain disorder, 321
Empathic work: resistance of aged, 629–631
Encephalopathy
  liver, 25
  uremic, chronic, 148
  Wernicke, 120–121
Encopresis, functional, 257–258
  assessment, 258
  associated features, 257
  clinical presentation, 257
  definition, 257
  epidemiology, 257
  etiology, 257
  treatment, 258
    primary, 258
    secondary, 258
Endocrinologic
  abnormalities and dementia, 147
  disturbances in delirium, 153
  states, EEG in, 88–90
Endogenous opiate peptides: in eating disorders, 184–185
Enflurane: interactions with neuroleptics, 467
Entitled demanders: psychotherapy of, 599–601
Enuresis
  drugs in, 435
    dosage, 435
  functional, 258–260
    assessment, 259–260
    associated features, 259
    behavioral interventions, 260
    clinical presentation, 258–259
    definition, 258–259
    diagnosis, differential, 259
    epidemiology, 259
    etiology, 259
    pharmacotherapy, 260
    psychotherapy, 260
    treatment, 260
  imipramine in, 435
  sleep-related, 316
Ephedrine: interaction with MAOIs, 469

Epilepsy, temporal lobe, 157–158
  personality disorder and, 296
Epinephrine interactions
  with antidepressants, tricyclic, 468
  with neuroleptics, 467
EPS (*see* Extrapyramidal symptoms)
Erikson, Erik
  eight ages of man, 613–614
  psychosocial stages of development, 615
Erythromycin: interaction with carbamazepine, 473
Ethanol
  in fetal alcohol syndrome, 123
  level, relationship to clinical manifestations, 125
Ethnicity: and transcultural psychiatry, 669–670
Ethnopsychopharmacology, 675–678
Ethopropazine: for neuroleptic side effects, 350
Etic perspectives: and transcultural psychiatry, 668
Evaluation, 1–91
Evil eye, 673
Experiential psychotherapy (*see* Psychotherapy, experiential)
Expert witness: psychiatrist as, 646
Exploratory psychotherapy (*see* Psychotherapy, exploratory)
Extinction, 516
  in sexual dysfunction treatment, 521–522
Extraocular movements, 11

Extrapyramidal
  effects of neuroleptics, 348–349
    acute, 347–352
    acute, agents used to treat, 350–351
    prophylactic treatment, 347–352
  symptoms, 414–423
    definition, 414–415
    pathogenesis, 414–415
    treatment, 420–424
    treatment, guidelines to, general, 422–423
    types of, 415–420
  syndrome and dementia, 144–150
Extremities (*see* Limb)
Eye: evil, 673

F

Face: movement abnormality in tardive dyskinesia, 352–353
Factitious disorder, 210–212
  diagnosis, differential, 211–212
  diagnostic criteria, 210–211
  features
    clinical, 211
    theoretical, 211
  treatment, 212
Fahr disease: and dementia, 146
Family
  assessment, 17
  of dying or newly deceased patient, care of, 578–580
  functioning, six main dimensions of, 545
  history (*see* History, family)
  issues in stuttering, 263
  law/child custody, 644–645

Family (cont.)
  primary, corrective recapitulation of, in groups, 557
Family therapy, 490–491, 538–551
  in anorexia, 193
  behavioral-social exchange, 549
  circumplex model, 544
  contraindications, relative, 491
  diagnostic formulation, 542–546
  diagnostic formulation, development of, 540
  in dysthymia, 104
  enabling factors, 490–491
  experiential, 551
  family assessment, 538–546
    current functioning of family, 539–540
    practical considerations in, 538–540
  family feedback, 540
  family history, review of, 540
  family life cycle, 541–542
  family systems, 550
  Fischer's schema (see Fischer's schema)
  genogram in
    construction of, 540
    example of, 540–541
  goals, 547–551
  greet the family, 539
  identification of stated problem, 539
  integrated, 543–544
  join the family, 539
  models, 547–551
  practice, 542–543
  preinterview task, 538–539
  preparation for, 538–539
  psychodynamic, 549–550
  recommendations for, 540
  strategic, 548
  structural, 547
Family: and transcultural psychiatry, 670
Feedback
  family, 540
  loop in cognitive therapy, 588
Feelings: rating scales, example of, 63
Fenfluramine: in autism, infantile, 435
Fetus
  abuse (*see* Abuse, fetal)
  alcohol syndrome (*see* Alcohol, fetal alcohol syndrome)
  exposure to lithium, 427
Finger-to-nose, 13
Fischer's schema, 546
  controls, 546
  cultural aspects, 546
  developmental aspects, 546
  emotions, 546
  needs, 546
  sanctions, 546
  structural descriptors, 546
Flooding and implosive therapy, 523–524
  clinical application, 524
  modeling, 524
Fluid alteration: and lithium, 382
Fluphenazine
  for aged, doses and side effects, 448
  decanoate, discussion of, 343–344
  dosages, 336
  ethanoate, discussion of, 343
  formulations, available, 340
  potency, 336
  side effect profile, 338
Flurazepam, 398
  dosage, 402

Folate, 27
Folstein Mini-Mental State Examination, 55
Forensic psychiatry, 634–646
Free association, 507
Freud, Anna
  developmental lines, 610–613
  diagnostic profile, 610–613
Fright syndrome, 673–674
Frontal lobe syndrome
  convexity syndrome, 293
  orbital-medial syndrome, 293–296
  personality disorder and, 293–296
"Frontal systems" tasks, 14
Fundi, 11
Furosemide: interaction with lithium, 471

G

Gait/station, 13
Gases, 26
  blood, 26
Gender
  in conversion disorder, 206
  distribution of somatization disorder, 205
  in hypochondriasis, 208–209
Gender identity disorders, 247–252
  of adolescence and adulthood, nontranssexual type, 252
  in children, 249–251
    assessment, 250
    treatment, 250–251
  epidemiology, 248
  etiology, 248–249
Gender: in psychogenic pain, 210
Genetic
  descriptive relationships in neurosis and personality disorders, 291
  factors in dementia, 143
  theory in schizophrenia, 108
Genetics: of affective disorders, 96
Genital retraction syndrome, 672–673
Genogram (*see* Family therapy, genogram)
Geriatrics (*see* Aged)
Glaucoma: in aged, 452
Global Assessment Scale, 55
  example of, 60–62
Grandiose, 9
Grasp: abnormal, 13
Grief
  acute, 577–582
    care of family of dying or newly deceased patient, 578–580
    reaction in emergency room setting, 578
  pathologic, 577
Group(s)
  for Advancement of Psychiatry, 544–546
  cohesiveness, 557–558
  corrective recapitulation of primary family in, 557
  developmental phases, 556
  dynamics, intrapsychic, 555
  existential factors in, 558
  imparting information, 557
  interactions, dyadic, 555
  interpersonal experiences and, 557
  level phenomena, 555
  membership, 554
  organizational parameter differences, 554–555
  processes, 555–556
  structure, 554–555

Group(s) *(cont.)*
  therapeutic impact of, 556–558
  therapist, beginning, guidelines for, 560
Group therapy, 491–493, 552–560
  in anorexia, 192–193
  in bulimia, 195
  conceptualizing, 555–556
  contraindications, 559
    relative, 492–493
  as educational, 553
  enabling factors, 492
  focus, 553
  forms of, 552–555
  goals, 553
  group-centered approach, 553–554
  indications, 558–559
    relative, 491–492
  leadership style, 552–553
  precaution for, 558
  supportive, 553
  teaching skills, 553
  theoretical orientation, 555
Growth hormone: in affective disorders, 98
Guanethidine: interactions with tricyclic antidepressants, 468

H

Habit disorder, 268–269
  abnormal development in, 269
  assessment, 269
  associated features, 268
  biochemical abnormality in, 269
  clinical presentation, 268
  definition, 268
  diagnosis, differential, 268
  epidemiology, 268–269
  neurologic abnormalities in, 269
  psychiatric disorder feature of, 269
  psychosocial abnormality in, 269
  treatment, 269
Halazepam, 398
  dosage, 402
Halcion: dosage, 403
Haldol *(see* Haloperidol*)*
Hallucinations
  auditory, 10
  olfactory, 10
  visual, 10
Hallucinogens, 31
Hallucinosis
  alcoholic *(see* Alcohol hallucinosis*)*
  organic, 169–170
Haloperidol
  in ADHD, 440
  for aged, doses and side effects, 448
  in alcoholic hallucinosis, 127, 132
  decanoate, discussion of, 344
  dosages, 337
  formulations, available, 341
  potency, 337
  side effect profile, 339
  in Tourette syndrome in children, 439
Halstead-Reitan neuropsychological battery, 52
Hamilton Depression Scale, 56, 73–79
Hand sequences, 14
Healers: in transcultural psychiatry, 676–678
Heart disease: with depression in aged, 451–452
Heel-to-shin, 13
Hepatolenticular degeneration, 27–28
Hepatotoxicity: of neuroleptics, 363

History
- alcohol abuse, 3–4
- developmental, 4
- drug abuse, 3–4
- in eating disorders, 175–176
- family
  - in anorexia, 186
  - bulimia, 186
  - in eating disorders, 176
  - in medical illness presenting as psychiatric illness, 21
- medical
  - family, 3
  - past, 3
- in medical illness presenting as psychiatric illness, 20–21
- occupational, 4
- of present illness, 3
- psychiatric, 2
  - family, 3
  - past, 3
- social, 4
- suicidality and, 574

HIV, 29–30
Homicidal ideation, 9
Homicide scale, 58
Hope: instillation of, 557
Hopkins 90-item checklist: and transcultural psychiatry, 672
Hormone(s)
- growth, in affective disorders, 98
- thyroid, in affective disorders, 98–99

Human immunodeficiency virus, 29–30
Huntington disease
- dementia and, 145
- depression in, 164

Hydergine: for dementia in aged, 451
Hydrocephalus
- with dementia, 149
- depression in, 164

Hyperactivity (see ADHD)
Hyperadrenocorticism, 24
- laboratory findings, 24
Hypercarbia, 27
Hypersomnia, 311–313
- primary, 313
- related
  - to another mental disorder, 311–312
  - to known organic factor, 312–313
Hyperthyroidism, 23
Hypertrophy: of prostate in aged, 452
Hypervitaminosis, 27
Hypnosis, 566–569
- applications, 567–569
- definition, 566
- history, 566–567
- methods, 567
- theory, 567
Hypnotic action: of benzodiazepines, 404
Hypnotics
- nonbarbiturate, interactions with neuroleptics, 467
- sedative, interaction with benzodiazepines, 472
Hypoadrenocorticism, 24
- diagnosis, 25
- exam, 24
- history, 24
- laboratory findings, 24–25
Hypochondriasis, 208–209
- age in, 208–209
- diagnosis, differential, 209
- diagnostic criteria, 208
- features
  - clinical, 209
  - theoretical, 209
- gender in, 208–209
- incidence, 208–209
- prevalence, 208–209
- treatment, 209
Hypotension

Hypotension *(cont.)*
  in aged, 452
  orthostatic, after neuroleptics, 357
Hypothyroidism, 23
  blood pressure in, 23
  examination, 23
  history, 23
  pulse in, 23
  thyroid size and texture in, 23–24
Hypovitaminosis, 27
Hypoxia: and dementia, 147
Hysterical
  neurosis *(see* Neurosis, hysterical)
    dissociative type *(see* Dissociative disorders)
  "seizures:" EEG in, 85–91

I

Iatrogenic intoxication, 31
Ibuprofen: interaction with lithium, 470
Ideas: flight of, 8
Ideation
  homicidal, 9
  suicidal *(see* Suicidal ideation)
Identification
  in groups, 557
  projective, 506
Identity
  disorder, 265–266
    assessment, 266
    associated features, 265
    clinical presentation, 265
    definition, 265
    diagnosis, differential, 265
    etiology, 265–266
    treatment, 266
  gender *(see* Gender identity)
Imipramine
  in ADHD, 437
  in depression in children, 436
  in enuresis, 435
  in separation anxiety disorder, 437
Implosive *(see* Flooding and implosive therapy)
Impotence: in aged, 452
Inapsine *(see* Droperidol)
Inderal: for neuroleptic side effects, 351
Individual psychotherapy, 489–490
  brief *(see* short-term *below)*
  contraindications, relative, 490
  enabling factors, 489–490
  indications, relative, 489
  short-term, 584–593
    approaches, general, 585
    cognitive therapy in, 586
    directive, 586–589
    directive, overview, 586–587
    directive vs. exploratory, 585–586
    exploratory *(see below)*
    goals, 585
    major divisions, 585
    not for acutely unstable patients, 584
    symptom reduction in, 586
    time restriction, discussion of, 584–585
  short-term, exploratory, 589–592
    duration, 592
    duration, Davanloo, 592
    duration, Malan, 592
    duration, Mann, 592
    duration, Sifneos, 592
    exploratory vs. directive, 585–586
    goals, 591
    major schools, four, discussion of, 589–590

selection criteria, 590
techniques, 591
techniques, Davanloo, 591
techniques, Malan, 591
techniques, Mann, 591
techniques, Sifneos, 591
theory, 590–591
Indomethacin interactions
  with lithium, 470
  with neuroleptics, 467
Industrial chemical exposure: and dementia, 148
Infant
  autism (*see* Autism, infantile)
  reactive attachment disorder (*see* Reactive attachment disorder in infancy)
  rumination disorder (*see* Rumination disorder of infancy)
Infarction
  multi-infarct dementia, 143
  myocardial, lithium after, 382
Informed consent, 637–638
  for electroconvulsive therapy, 456–457
  for neuroleptics, 353
Insanity defense, 643–644
Insight, 7, 507–508
Insomnia, 308–311
  in aged (*see* Aged, insomnia in)
  primary, 311
  related
    to another mental disorder, 309
    to known organic factor, 309–311
  transient, treatment, 310
Institutionalization, 636
Intellect, 6–7

test, 7
Intellectual
  development according to Piaget, 614–617
  impairment in delirium, 152
Intellectualization, 506
Intelligence
  classification, 39
  quotient, 37
    classification, 39
  scale, Wechsler (*see* Wechsler adult intelligence scale)
  tests, 37–41
  transcultural psychiatry and, 672
Interictal behavior syndrome, 161
Interictal psychiatric disorder, 159–161
  depression in, 159
  evaluation, 161–162
  with psychosis, schizophreniform, 159–161
  treatment, 162–163
  workup, 161–162
Intermarriage: and transcultural psychiatry, 671
Interpersonal therapy
  cognitive therapy and, 586–587
  discussion, 587–588
  duration, 588
  goals, 587
  selection criteria, 587
  techniques, 587–588
  theory, 587
Interpretation, 508
Interpreters: in transcultural psychiatry, 669
Intervention(s)
  crisis, 584
  after crisis, acute, 571–583
  decisions concerning, 481
Interview: Structured Clinical, 56

Intoxication, 31–33
  delirium and, 154
  iatrogenic, 31
  lithium, approach to, 390
  water, 26
Intracranial
  pressure and electroconvulsive therapy, 456
  processes in delirium, 154
Involuntary
  commitment (*see* Commitment, involuntary)
  treatment, 634–637
Iproniazid: interactions with neuroleptics, 467
IQ, 37
  classification, 39
Isoflurane: interactions with neuroleptics, 467
Isolation, 506
Isoniazid: interaction with carbamazepine, 473

J

Jakob-Creutzfeldt disease: and dementia, 146
Jaw jerk, 12–13
Judgment: as test of intellect, 7
Juvenile
  delinquency, 645
  law, 645

K

Kaolin: interaction with tricyclic antidepressants, 468
Kemadrin: for neuroleptic side effects, 351
Ketamine: interaction with lithium, 471
Kidney insufficiency: and lithium, 383
Knowledge: general fund of, 6
Koro, 672–673

Korsakoff psychosis, 121

L

Labeling, 529
Labor: and lithium, 382
Language
  disorders, 278–279
    developmental expressive, 278
    developmental receptive, 278
  testing of, 15
  transcultural psychiatry and, 670, 671
Latah, 673
Law
  family, 644–645
  juvenile, 645
Leukodystrophy: metachromatic, 30
Leukoencephalopathy: progressive multifocal, 30
Leukopenia: after neuroleptics, 362
Levarterenol: interaction with MAOIs, 469
Levodopa, interaction
  with benzodiazepines, 472
  with MAOIs, 469
  with neuroleptics, 467
Librium (*see* Chlordiazepoxide)
Life cycle: family, 541–542
Limb
  command, 14
  drift, 12
  imitation, 14
  object, 14
Lipids: plasma, in alcoholism, 123
Lithium, 379–395
  adverse effects, 385–387
  for aged, 443
  alternative agents, 389–395
  anomalies and, congenital, 428

breast-feeding and, 427–428
description, 379
dosage regimen, initial, 384
drug interactions with, 387–388
effects on laboratory values, possible, 386
fetal exposure to, 427
indications, 379–380
interactions of, 470–471
  with antidepressants, tricyclic, 468
  with carbamazepine, 473
  with neuroleptics, 466
intoxication, approach to, 390
levels for various conditions, 385
in mania in aged, 445
pharmacokinetics, 380–381
precautions, 381
during pregnancy, 427–429
  guidelines for use, 428–429
risk with, significant, 382–383
side effects, management, 386–387
in transcultural psychiatry, 676
treatment guidelines, 381–385
Liver encephalopathy, 25
  dementia and, 148
Lorazepam, 398
  in alcohol withdrawal delirium, 131
  in delirium, 157
  dosage, 402, 449
  half-life, 449
Loxapine
  dosages, 337
  formulations, available, 341
  potency, 337
  side effect profile, 339
Loxitane (see Loxapine)
Luria-Nebraska test battery, 52–53

M

Magnification, 529
Malan brief psychotherapy, 591
  duration, 592
Mal de ojo, 673
Malingering, 212–213
  diagnosis, differential, 212–213
  diagnostic criteria, 212
  features
    clinical, 212
    theoretical, 212
  treatment, 213
Malnutrition, 36
Malpractice: in psychiatry, 645–646
Mania
  acute ECT in, 393
  in aged (see Aged, mania)
  electroconvulsive therapy in, 455
  in Wilson disease, 164
Manic
  depressive disorder (see Bipolar disorder)
  episode, treatment, 99–100
  psychosis with delirium, 155
Mann bried psychotherapy, 591
  duration, 592
Mannitol: interaction with lithium, 470
MAOI (see Monoamine oxidase inhibitors)
Marchiafava-Bignami syndrome, 25–26

Marital therapy, 490–491
  contraindications, relative, 491
  enabling factors, 490–491
Marriage
  intermarriage and transcultural psychiatry, 671
  spouse abuse (see Abuse, spouse)
  understanding of, as capacity test, 640
MAST, 118, 119
McGarry scale: in competence assessment, 639–642
McNaghten case, 643
MDMA, 31
Medical history (see History, medical)
Medical illness
  presenting as psychiatric illness, 20–36
    general appearance, 22
    history, 20–21
    onset, 21
Medication (see Drugs)
"Medication patient:" and psychotherapy, 489
Medicine: behavioral, 526
Melancholia: with depression, electroconvulsive therapy in, 455
Mellaril (see Thioridazine)
Memory, 6
  recent, 6
  remote, 6
Mental age, 37
Mental illness (see Psychiatric illness)
Mental retardation, 272–274
  assessment, 274
  associated features, 273
  definition, 272
  diagnosis, 272–273
  epidemiology, 273
  etiology, 273–274
  treatment, 274
Mental status
  examination, 4–16
    in eating disorders, 176
    of OBS vs. psychiatric illness 35
    in transcultural psychiatry, 671–672
  interictal, 28
Meperidine: interaction with MAOIs, 469
Mephentermine: interaction with MAOIs, 469
Mesoridazine
  dosages, 336
  formulations, available, 340
  potency, 336
  side effect profile, 338
Metals: and dementia, 148
Metaraminol: interaction with MAOIs, 469
Methylphenidate
  in ADHD, 434
  in depression in aged, 443–445
  discussion of, 412
  dosage, 411
  interaction with MAOIs, 469
Michigan Alcoholism Screening Test, 118, 119
Migration: and transcultural psychiatry, 669–670
Mini-Mental State: example of, 66–69
Minimization, 529
Minnesota Multiphasic Personality Inventory, 41–46
  advantages, 45–46
  interpretation, 42–45
  in personality disorders, 57
  problems, 45–46
  scales, 43–45

transcultural psychiatry and, 672
MMPI (see Minnesota Multiphasic Personality Inventory)
Mnemonic(s)
  clinically useful, 57–59
  for somatization disorder screening symptoms, 204
Moban (see Molindone)
Model(s)
  biopsychosocial, in anorexia and bulimia, 190
  circumplex, in family therapy, 544
  of family therapy, 547–551
Modeling
  in flooding and implosive therapy, 524
  in groups, 557
Molindone
  dosages, 337
  formulations, available, 341
  potency, 337
  side effect profile, 339
Monitoring
  in ADHD of stimulants, 434
  in depression in children, with antidepressants, 436
  of disulfiram, 137
  in schizophrenia in children, antipsychotics used, 438
Monoamine oxidase inhibitors, 375–378
  in affective disorders in aged, 443
  for anxiety in aged, 447
  in depression, major, 101
  diet during, 376–377
  dosing, 378
    schedule for, 378
  indications, 378

interactions of, 469
medication restrictions during, 376–377
during pregnancy, 429
Monoamines: in eating disorders, 178–184
Mood, 7
  alterations in delirium, 153
  disorders (see below)
  organic mood syndrome, 163
Mood disorders
  in children and adolescents, 232–234
    assessment, 233–234
    associated features, 233
    clinical presentation, 232–233
    diagnosis, differential, 233
    epidemiology, 233
    etiology, 233
    treatment, 234
Mortality (see Death)
Motor
  abnormalities in delirium, 152
  activity, 4–5
    abnormal, 4–5
  Bender visual motor gestalt test, 54
  skills disorder, 278
  system
    assessment, 12
    limb drift, 12
    strength, 12
    tone, 12
  tic disorder (see Tic disorder, motor, chronic)
Mouth: dry, after neuroleptics, 357
Movement(s)
  abnormalities, 12
  neuroleptics in, 332
  rapid alteration, 13
  rapid alternation, 13
  whole-body, 14

MPD, 221–227
  associated features, 223
  clinical presentation, 221–223
  diagnosis, differential, 227
  diagnostic assessment, 223–224
  epidemiology, 224–225
  etiologic theories, 225–226
  treatment, 226–227
Multiple personality disorder (*see* MPD)
Multiple sclerosis, 34–35
  mood disturbance in, 164
Muscle, skeletal
  in alcoholism, 123
  benzodiazepines and, 397
Mutism
  akinetic, tabular data on, 349
  elective, 263–275
    assessment, 264
    associated features, 264
    clinical presentation, 263–264
    definition, 263–264
    diagnosis, differential, 264
    epidemiology, 264
    etiology, 264
    treatment, 264–265
Myelin disease: with dementia, 150
Myocardial infarction
  electroconvulsive therapy and, 455–456
  lithium after, 382

N

Naming, 15
Naproxen: interaction with lithium, 470
Narcolepsy: stimulants in, 406
Narcotics, interactions of
  with benzodiazepines, 472
  with neuroleptics, 466
Navane (*see* Thiothixene)
Neoplasia (*see* Tumors)
Nerve: cranial, assessment, 11–12
Nervous system
  autonomic, after neuroleptics, 360–361
  central (*see* Central nervous system)
Neurobiology: of starvation, 185–186
Neuroendocrine changes: in eating disorders, 178, 182–183
Neuroleptics, 330–368
  action
    anticholinergic, 331
    mechanism, 331
  age affecting metabolic rate, 345
  for aged, doses and side effects, 342, 448
  for aggression, 332
  in agitation
    in aged, 446
    severe, 332
  in alcohol withdrawal delirium, 131
  in anxiety in aged, 447
  classification, 332–345
  CNS side effects, non-extrapyramidal, 357
  in delirium, 157
  depot, 343–344
  description, 332–345
  documenting need for, 353
  dopamine blockade by, 331
  dosages, 336–337, 342
    for elderly, 342, 448
    equivalent, 342–343
    minimal effective dose for shortest time, 353
    reduction in tardive dyskinesia, 356

extrapyramidal effects (see Extrapyramidal effects of neuroleptics)
formulary, 340–342
half-lives, 345
hepatotoxicity, 363
history, 330
informed consent for, 353
in insomnia in aged, 450
interactions of, 466–467
  with benzodiazepines, 472
  with other drugs, 364, 366–367
  with lithium, 470
maintenance, 346–347
malignant syndrome, 358, 412–423
  clinical features, 424
  definition, 424
  EEG in, 84
  treatment, 424–425
in mania in aged, 445
in movement disorder, 332
nonpsychiatric uses, 332
overdose, 365
parkinsonism as side effect, 348–349
pharmacokinetics, 345
for physical interventions, 346
potency, 336–337
prescription of, methods of, 345–347
psychopharmacologic interventions with, 345–346
in psychosis
  in aged, 446
  agitation of, 345
  functional, 331
in schizophrenia in children, 438
for sedation, 346
side effects, 332, 347–365
  in aged, 448
  non-extrapyramidal CNS, tabular data on, 358–359
  peripheral, 357–364
  peripheral, tabular data on, 360–363
  profiles, 338–339
  summary of, 364–365
sudden death after, 364
target symptoms, 331–332, 333
terminology, 330
therapeutic levels, rapid attainment of, 345–346
in thought disorder, 332
toxicity, 352
  CNS, anticholinergic, 331
in transcultural psychiatry, 675–676
treatment uses, 331–345
withdrawal, 365
  in tardive dyskinesia, 356–357
Neurologic assessment, 10–16
Neurologic syndromes: associated with chronic alcoholism, 120–122
Neuropsychological tests, 51–52
  comprehensive test batteries, 52–54
  specialized approach, 53–54
Neurosis, 287
  anxiety, 288
  depersonalization, 288
  depressive, 288
  hysterical
    conversion type, 289
    dissociative type (see Dissociative disorders)
  obsessive-compulsive, 289
  personality disorder and, 289–291

Neurosis *(cont.)*
   defense mechanisms and spectrum of illness, 291
   differences, 290–291
   genetic descriptive relationships in, 291
   overview of spectrum of illness, 291
   similarities, 289–290
   phobic, 289
Neurosyphilis, 29
Neurotic disorder, 287
   DSM III-R and, 288
   relationship to personality disorder, 286–297
   relationships of, 294–295
Neurotic process, 287–288
Neurotransmitter(s)
   in affective disorders, 97–98
   hypothesis in schizophrenia, 108–109
Newborn: behavior in fetal alcohol syndrome, 124
Niacin, 27
Nightmare disorder, 314–315
Noncompliant patient: psychotherapy of, 599–602
Norlex: for neuroleptic side effects, 350
Nortriptyline: for aged, doses and side effects, 444
Nose: stuffiness after neuroleptics, 357
Novacaine: interaction with MAOIs, 469
Nutrition
   deficiency
     in delirium, 154
     dementia and, 147
   states, EEG in, 88–90

O

Obsessional thoughts, 9
Obsessive-compulsive neurosis, 289
Occupational
   history, 4
   impairment in alcoholism, 117–118
O'Connor vs. Donaldson, 634–635
Olfactory
   examination, 11
   hallucinations, 10
OMD: signs of, 21–23
Operant conditioning, 516
   for pain, 327–328
Ophthalmologic manifestations: of neuroleptics, 361
Opiate
   antagonists
     in anorexia, 194
     in bulimia, 198
   peptides, endogenous, in eating disorders, 184–185
Oppositional defiant disorder in children and adolescents, 241–243
   assessment, 242
   associated features, 242
   clinical presentation, 242
   definition, 242
   diagnosis, differential, 242
   epidemiology, 242
   etiology, 242
   treatment, 242–243
Oral
   /lingual orientation, 14
   movement abnormality in tardive dyskinesia, 352–353
Orap *(see* Pimozide*)*
Orbital-medial syndrome, 293–296
Organic amnestic syndrome, 167–169
Organic brain syndrome, 139–170

lithium and, 383
psychiatric rating scales for, 56
Organic disorder
mental, EEG in, 83–85
psychiatric, neuroleptics in, 331
relationship to personality disorder, 293–296
signs and symptoms, to both organic and psychiatric illness, 34
Organic hallucinosis, 169–170
Organic mood syndrome, 163
Organic patient: psychotherapy of, 595–597
Organic personality syndrome, 165–167
Orphenadrine: for neuroleptic side effects, 350
Orthostatic hypotension: after neuroleptics, 357
Overanxious disorder in children and adolescents, 246–247
assessment, 247
associated features, 246
clinical presentation, 246
definition, 246
diagnosis, differential, 246–247
epidemiology, 247
etiology, 247
treatment, 247
Overdose
antidepressants, tricyclic, 375
neuroleptics, 365
Overgeneralization, 529
Oxazepam, 398
in alcohol withdrawal delirium, 131
dosage, 403, 449
half-life, 449

P

Pain, 12, 317–328
anesthetics for, 324–325
assessment, 318–320
behavior programs in, 325–326
examples of, 326–327
chronic pain-associated features, 321–322
common pain syndromes, 322–323
operant conditioning for, 327–328
pharmacologic therapy, 326
physical medicine for, 325
psychogenic, 209–210
age in, 210
diagnosis, differential, 210
diagnostic criteria, 209–210
disorder, 320–321
disorder, Emory model of classes, 321
features, clinical, 210
features, theoretical, 210
gender in, 210
treatment, 210
psychotherapy for, supportive, 326–327
treatment, 323–328
admission criteria, 323
initial steps, 324
modalities, 324–326
Palmomental abnormalities, 13
Palsy
pseudobulbar, mood disturbance in, 164
supranuclear, progressive dementia in, 145
depression in, 164
Pancreas: carcinoma, 35–36
Pancuronium: interaction with lithium, 470

Paranoid, 9
Parasomnia, 314–318
  NOS, 316
Parkinsonism, 347
  dementia in, 144–145
  depression in, 164
  discussion of, 416–417
  as side effect of neuroleptics, 348–349
    agents used to treat, 350–351
    tabular data on, 348
  treatment, 421
Parsidol: for neuroleptic side effects, 350
Patients
  difficult (see Psychotherapy with difficult patients)
  dying, psychotherapy of, 597–599
  "medication patient" and psychotherapy, 489
  noncompliant, psychotherapy of, 599–602
  organic, psychotherapy of, 595–597
  rights of, 642–643
  violent, psychotherapy of, 602–603
Pavor nocturnus, 315
Paxipam: dosage, 402
PCP, 31
PDD
  antipsychotics in, in children, 439
  dosage, 439
  thioridazine in, in children, 439
Pellegra, 25
Pemoline
  discussion of, 412
  dosage, 411
Perception, 10–16
  deficits, 26
  in delirium, 152
Permitil (see Fluphenazine)

Perphenazine
  for aged, doses and side effects, 448
  dosages, 336, 448
  formulations, available, 341
  potency, 336
  side effect profile, 338
Perseveration, 8
  tests for, 15
Personality
  abnormal, 282–283
    criterion list, multidimensional, 284
  alteration, 161
  characteristics of, 281–282
  as consistent, 282
  definition, 281
  disorder(s), 281–303
    during adolescence, 296–297
    in children, 296–297
    classification, 283–286
    definition, 281
    diagnosis, 297
    diagnosis during adolescence, 279–280
    diagnosis in children, 279–280
    diagnosis, differential, 298–302
    diagnostic criteria for three clusters of disorders, 285
    DSM III-R, accepted, 283
    DSM III-R, provisional, 283–286
    features, distinguishing, 298–302
    features, major, 298–302
    MMPI in, 57
    multiple (see MPD)
    neurosis and (see Neurosis, personality disorder and)
    relationship(s) of, 294–295

relationship to affective disorder, 291–293
relationship to neurotic disorders, 286–297
relationship to organic disorders, 293–296
relationship to psychosis, 286–287
relationship to psychotic disorders, 286–297
sadistic, 286
self-defeating, 286
treatment, 297
normal, 282–283
criterion list, multidimensional, 284
organic personality syndrome, 165–167
origin of, 282
as pervasive, 282
premorbid, and eating disorders, 187
stable, 282
test, objective, 41–51
traits, definition, 281
types, definition, 281
Personalization, 529
Pharmacotherapy, 329–473
in enuresis, functional, 260
Phenelzine: for aged, doses and side effects, 444
Phenobarbital: in alcohol withdrawal delirium, 130
Phenothiazines
aliphatic, 336
formulations, available, 340–341
side effect profile, 338
in anorexia, 194
dosages, 336
formulations, available, 340–341
potency, 336
in schizophrenia in children, 438
side effect profile, 338
Phenylbutazone: interaction with lithium, 470
Phenylephrine: interaction with MAOIs, 469
Phenytoin: interactions with tricyclic antidepressants, 468
Pheochromocytoma, 33–35
Phobic neurosis, 289
Photosensitivity: after neuroleptics, 357–364
Physical appearance, 4–5
Piaget: concept of intellectual development, 614–617
Pica, 200–201
clinical features, 201
complications, medical, 201
epidemiology, 201
etiologic theories, 201
evaluation, 201
treatment, 201
Pigmentary retinopathy: after mellaril, 357
Pimozide
discussion of, 344
dosages, 337
formulations, available, 342
potency, 337
side effect profile, 339
Piperazine
dosages, 336
formulations, available, 340
potency, 336
side effect profile, 338
Piperidine
dosages, 336
formulations, available, 340
potency, 336
side effect profile, 338
Piroxicam: interaction with lithium, 470

Plantar responses, 13
Play therapy: with children, 622–623
Political affiliation: and transcultural psychiatry, 670
Polyneuropathy: in alcoholism, 121
Porphyria, 33
  dementia and, 148
Postpartum psychosis, 113
Praxis, 14
Prazepam, 398
  dosage, 403
Pregnancy
  antidepressants during, 429
  antipsychotics during, 430–431
    precaution, 431
  benzodiazepines during, 431
  lithium during, 382, 427–429
    guidelines for use, 428–429
  MAOI during, 429
  psychotropic drugs during, 426–431
Premack, 517
Premorbid personality: and eating disorders, 187
Procaine hydrochloride: interaction with MAOIs, 469
Procainamide: interactions with tricyclic antidepressants, 468
Procyclidine: for neuroleptic side effects, 351
Projection, 506
Projective identification, 506
Prolixin (see Fluphenazine)
Propoxyphene: interaction with carbamazepine, 473
Propranolol
  discussion of, 352
  for neuroleptic side effects, 351
Prostate: hypertrophy in aged, 452
Proverbs, 6–7
Pseudobulbar palsy: mood disturbance in, 164
Pseudodementia, 148–149
Pseudoephedrine: interaction with MAOIs, 469
Pseudoepilepsy, 159
Pseudoseizure, 159
  differentiation from seizure, 160
  EEG in, 85–91
Psychiatric aspects: of seizures, 157–163
Psychiatric assessment, 2–19
  chief complaint, 2–3
  history (see History)
  initial, 2–19
    appearance, general, 4–5
    attitude toward interviewer, 5
    behavior, general, 4–5
Psychiatric disorder (see Psychiatric illness)
Psychiatric history (see History, psychiatric)
Psychiatric illness, 92–328
  interictal (see Interictal psychiatric disorder)
  involuntary commitment and, 635
  medical illness presenting as (see Medical illness presenting as psychiatric illness)
  mental status exam of OBS vs. psychiatric illness, 35
  organic
    EEG in, 83–85
    neuroleptics in, 331

signs and symptoms, to both organic and psychiatric illness, 34
Psychiatric problems: in delirium, 154
Psychiatric rating scales, 55–90
  affective disorder, 56
  alcoholism, 59
  anxiety disorders, 56
  brief, 55
    example of, 64–65
  organic brain syndromes, 56
  in psychosis, 55–56
Psychiatric ward: admittance to, and suicidality, 576–577
Psychiatrist: as expert witness, 646
Psychiatry
  culture and, 667
  forensic, 634–646
  malpractice and, 645–646
  transcultural (see Transcultural psychiatry)
Psychoanalytic psychotherapy, 508
Psychodynamic psychotherapy, 504–513
  criteria that favor the use of, 512
  definitions, 505–509
  family, 549–550
  practice, contributors to field of, 512–513
  preparing patient for therapy, helpful hints, 511–512
  theory of, contributors to field of, 512–513
  therapy process, 509–512
    beginning, 510
    goals, 509–510
    middle, 510
    termination, 510–511
Psychogenic amnesia, 219–220

Psychogenic fugue, 218
Psychogenic pain (see Pain, psychogenic)
Psychological tests, 37–54
  in eating disorders, 177–178
  projective, 46–51
  transcultural psychiatry and, 671–672
Psychomotor
  agitation, 4
  retardation, 4
  seizure, 157–158
Psychoneurosis (see Neurosis)
Psychosis, 286
  in aged (see Aged, psychosis)
  agitation in, neuroleptics for, 345
  atypical, 112–114
  brief reactive, 112
  with depression, electroconvulsive therapy in, 455
  drug-induced, 112–113
  fetal abuse and, 653–654
  functional, neuroleptics in, 331
  as iatrogenic intoxication, 32
  Korsakoff, 121
  manic, with delirium, 155
  nonaffective, 105–114
  postpartum, 113
  psychiatric rating scales in, 55–56
  refractory, in schizophrenia, 111
  relationship to personality disorder, 286–287
  schizophreniform, with interictal psychiatric disorder, 159–161
Psychosocial abnormality: in stereotypy and habit disorder, 269

718 *Index*

Psychosocial stages: of development according to Erikson, 615
Psychotherapy, 474–632
  with aged (*see* Aged, psychotherapy with)
  in anorexia, 192–193
  brief (*see* Individual psychotherapy, short-term)
  in bulimia, 194–195
  characteristics, 481–502
  with children and adolescents, 607–626
    assessment, 617–620
    background, 607–617
    characteristics, 608–610
    communication for, alternative forms, 608
    contrasted with psychotherapy of adults, 607–608
    developmental lines of Anna Freud, 610–613
    diagnosis, 619–620
    diagnostic profile of, Anna Freud, 610–613
    early adolescence, 623–624
    Erikson, Erik, eight ages of man, 613–614
    Erikson, Erik, psychosocial stages of development, 615
    gathering information, 617–618
    goals, 608–610
    indications for psychotherapy, 620–621
    initiating therapy, 622
    late adolescence, 625
    midadolescence, 624
    Piaget's concept of intellectual (cognitive) development, 614–617
    play therapy, 622–623
    summarizing data, 618–619
    treatment recommendations, 620
  choosing the appropriate, 475–503
  cognitive (*see* Cognitive therapy)
  conceptual hypotheses checklist, 480
  conceptualizing the "issues," 479–480
  concomitant use of other therapeutic modalities, 488–502
  contraindications, relative, 498
  diagnosis, communication of, 477–478
  with difficult patients, 594–606
    dying patient, 597–599
    entitled demanders, 599–601
    noncompliant patient, 599–602
    organic patient, 595–597
    self-destructive deniers, 601–602
    somaticizers, 594–595
    suicidal patient, chronically, 603–605
    violent patients, 602–603
  directive, 494–495, 497–498
    clinical data, 497
    contraindications, relative, 495
    enabling factors, 495
    indications, relative, 494
    purpose/goal, 497
    techniques, 497–498
  in enuresis, functional, 260
  experiential, 495
    clinical data, 500
    enabling factors, 495
    family, 551

indications, relative, 495
purpose/goal, 500
role of therapist, 500
techniques, 501
exploratory, 493–494, 496–497
clinical data, 496
contraindications, relative, 494
enabling factors, 493–494
indications, relative, 493
purpose/goal, 496
role of therapist, 496
"schools" and their proponents, 496–497
techniques, 496
family (see Family therapy)
first stage of assessment and diagnosis, 475
format, 486
selection criteria for, 489–502
goals, 481–486
group (see Group therapy)
individual (see Individual psychotherapy)
interpersonal (see Interpersonal therapy)
major psychotherapies, overview of, 498–502
marital (see Marital therapy)
"medication patient" and, 489
no treatment as a disposition, 488–489
patient characteristics and, 481
therapeutic implications of, 484–485
presenting problem and, 480
conceptualization of, and initial therapeutic implications, 482–483
psychiatric evaluation for, 475–476

psychoanalytic, 508
psychodynamic (see Psychodynamic psychotherapy)
is psychotherapy for everyone? 488–489
"schools" and their proponents, 500
second stage, 475
setting, 486
supportive, 498, 501–502
clinical data, 501
enabling factors, 498
group, 553
indications, relative, 498
for pain, 326–327
purpose/goal, 501
role of therapist, 501
"schools" and their proponents, 502
techniques, 502
techniques, 487–488
selection criteria, 493–495
timing, 487
transcultural, 675
treatment recommendations, communicating, 477–478
Psychotic disorder, 286
relationship(s) of, 294–295
to personality disorder, 286–297
Psychotropic drugs
interactions, 465–473
during pregnancy, 426–431
Pupils, 11

Q

Quinidine: interactions with tricyclic antidepressants, 468

R

"Rabbit" syndrome: tabular data on, 349

Race: and transcultural psychiatry, 669–670
Rape, 659–661
  reporting, 661
  syndromes, 660
  treatment, 660
  victims, 581–582
Rational emotive therapy, 532–535
  ABCs of, 534
  clinical application, 534–535
  philosophy of, 533–534
  techniques, 534–535
Reaction formation, 506
Reactive attachment disorder in infancy and early childhood, 266–268
  assessment, 267
  associated features, 267
  clinical presentation, 266–267
  definition, 266–267
  diagnosis, differential, 267
  etiology, 267
  treatment, 268
Reading disorder: developmental, 277
Recovery: spontaneous, 516–517
Refeeding, 36
  in anorexia (*see* Anorexia, refeeding in)
Reflexes, 12–13
  abnormal, 13
Regression, 506
Reinforcement
  partial, 516
  positive, in sexual dysfunction treatment, 521–522
Reinforcers, 516
Relaxation training, 519, 561–564
  applications, 563–564
  definition, 561
  methods, 561–563
  theory, 561–563
  types, 561
Religion: and transcultural psychiatry, 670
Religious, 9
Repetition, 15
Repression, 506
Resistance, 508–509
Respiratory system: and benzodiazepines, 397
Restoril: dosage, 403
Restraint (*see* Seclusion and restraint)
RET (*see* Rational emotive therapy)
Retardation (*see* Mental retardation)
Retinopathy: pigmentary, after mellaril, 357
Rhythm
  speech, 5
  tapping, 14
Right(s)
  /left orientation, 14
  of patient, 642–643
  to treatment, 636–637
    refusal of, 637
Rinne test, 11
Ritalin (*see* Methylphenidate)
Root: abnormal, 13
Rorschach test, 46–49
  content areas, 48
  determinants, 48
  examples, 49
  location, 47–48
  popular responses, 48–49
  scoring, 47
Rumination disorder of infancy, 201–202
  clinical features, 202
  complications, 202
  diagnosis, differential, 202
  epidemiology, 202
  etiologic theories, 202
  management, 202

Ruminative thoughts, 9

S

Sadistic personality disorder, 286
S.A.D. P.E.R.S.O.N.S., 57–58
SADS, 56
Schedule: for affective disorders and schizophrenia, 56
Schizoaffective illness: treatment, 102
Schizophrenia, 105–114
    antipsychotics in, 438
        dosage and monitoring in children, 438
    biologic and genetic theory, 108
    catatonic type, diagnosis, 107
    in children, phenothiazines in, 438
    with delirium, 155
    diagnosis, 105–108
    disorganized type, diagnosis, 107
    electroconvulsive therapy in, 455
    epidemiology, 108
    EPS in, 111
    etiologies, postulated, 108–109
    "negative" symptoms, and neuroleptics, 332
    neuroleptics in, in children, 438
    neurotransmitter hypothesis, 108–109
    outcomes, statistical, 111
    paranoid type, diagnosis, 107
    "positive" symptoms, and neuroleptics, 331–332
    psychosocial precipitants, 109
    residual type, diagnosis, 108
    schedule for, 56
    TD in, 112
    thioridazine in, in children, 438
    treatment, 109–114
        acute occurrence, 109–110
        first break, 109
        nonacute, 110–111
    undifferentiated type, diagnosis, 107
Schizophreniform psychosis, 159–161
SCIDS-II: psychiatric rating scales in, 57
Sclerosis, multiple, 34–35
    mood disturbance in, 164
Seclusion and restraint, 647–652
    contraindications, 649–650
    definitions, 648
    history, 647–648
    incidence, 649
    indications, 649–650
    prevalence, 649
    techniques, 650–651
Sedative(s)
    hypnotics, interaction with benzodiazepines, 472
    neuroleptics as, 346
Seizure(s), 28
    alcohol withdrawal, 128–133
    control, 162
    differentiation from pseudoseizure, 160
    EEG in, 85–91
    hysterical, EEG in, 85–91
    partial, complex, 157–159
        clinical characteristics, 157–159
        definition, 157
        treatment, 162
    psychiatric aspects of, 157–163

Seizure(s) *(cont.)*
  psychomotor, 157–158
  threshold decrease after neuroleptics, 359
Self-defeating personality disorder, 286
Self-destructive deniers: psychotherapy of, 601–602
Sensorium, 5–6
  orientation, 5
Sensory system: assessment, 12
Sentence completion test, 51
Separation anxiety disorder, 243–245
  assessment, 244
  associated features, 243–244
  antidepressants in, 437
    dosage and duration, 437
  definition, 243
  diagnosis, differential, 244
  epidemiology, 244
  etiology, 244
  imipramine in, 437
  treatment, 244–245
Serax *(see* Oxazepam)
Serentil *(see* Mesoridazine)
Serial 7's, 6
Serotonin: in affective disorders, 97–98
Sexual dysfunction treatment, 520–521
  clinical application, 521
  token economies, 521–522
Sick sinus syndrome: lithium during, 382
Sifneos brief psychotherapy, 591
  duration, 592
Similarities: as test of intellect, 7
Singing, 15
Sinus: sick sinus syndrome, lithium during, 382

Skeletal *(see* Muscle, skeletal)
Sleep, 304–316
  definition, 304
  deprivation, 307–308
  disorder, 304–316
    DSM III-R classification, 308–316
    EEG in, 91
  normal cycle, 304–307
    EEG in, 306
    major theories, 304
    physiology, 304–305
    stages, 305–307
  -related enuresis, 316
  terror disorder, 315
  variations in cycle, 307–308
  -wake cycle abnormalities in delirium, 153
  -wake schedule disorder, 313–314
Sleepwalking disorder, 315–316
Snout: abnormal, 13
Social-behavioral exchange family therapy, 549
Social history, 4
Social impairment: in alcoholism, 117–118
Social skills: development in groups, 557
Sociology: and transcultural psychiatry, 668
Sodium
  bicarbonate interaction with lithium, 470
  chloride interaction with lithium, 470
Somatic, 9
Somaticizers: psychotherapy of, 594–595
Somatization, 507
  in anxiety *(see* Anxiety, somatized)
  in depression *(see* Depression, somatized)
  disorder, 203–206

age in, 205
diagnosis, differential, 206
diagnostic criteria, 203–205
features, clinical, 205
features, theoretical, 205–206
gender distribution, 205
incidence, 205
prevalence, 205
screening symptoms, mnemonic for, 204
treatment, 206
Somnambulism, 315–316
Spectinomycin: interaction with lithium, 470
Speech, 5
automatic, 15
disorders, 261–263, 278–279
cluttering (see below)
stuttering (see Stuttering)
disorders, cluttering, 261
assessment, 261
associated features, 261
clinical presentation, 261
definition, 261
diagnosis, differential, 261
treatment, 261
fluent, 5
halting, 5
rate, 5
rhythm, 5
spontaneous, 15
Spinocerebellar degeneration: and dementia, 146
Spironolactone: interaction with lithium, 470
Splitting: definition, 507
Spontaneous recovery, 516–517
Spouse abuse (see Abuse, spouse)

Stanford-Binet, 37–38
problems, 38
Startle matching syndrome, 673
Starvation: neurobiology of, 185–186
State-trait anxiety scale, 56
Stelazine (see Trifluoperazine)
Stereotyping: and transcultural psychiatry, 668
Stereotypy, 268–269
abnormal development in, 269
assessment, 269
associated features, 268
biochemical abnormality in, 269
clinical presentation, 268
definition, 268
diagnosis, differential, 268
epidemiology, 268–269
neurologic abnormalities in, 269
psychiatric disorder feature of, 269
psychosocial abnormality in, 269
treatment, 269
Stimulants, 405–413
action mechanism, 409–410
in ADHD, 433–434
dosage and monitoring, 434
in attention deficit disorder with hyperactivity disorder, 405–406
in autism, infantile, 434–435
dosage, 435
for children, 432–435
controversial uses, 406–407
dosages, 411
dyskinesia and, tardive, 413

Stimulants *(cont.)*
  guidelines for, clinical, 410–413
  in narcolepsy, 406
  questionable uses, 406–407
  side effects, 407–409
Structured Clinical Interview, 56
Stuttering, 261–263
  anxiety in, 263
  assessment, 262–263
  associated features, 262
  clinical presentation, 261–262
  definition, 261–262
  diagnosis, differential, 262
  emotional sequelae in, 263
  epidemiology, 262
  etiology, 262
  family issues in, 263
  treatment, 263
Sublimation, 507
Succinylcholine: interaction with lithium, 470
Sudden death: after neuroleptics, 364
Suicidal gesture, 575–576
Suicidal ideation, 9
  active, 10
  passive, 10
Suicidal patient: chronically, psychotherapy of, 603–605
Suicidality, 571–577
  admittance
    to general hospital ward, 576
    to psychiatric ward, closed, 576–577
    to psychiatric ward, open, 576
  alcohol abuse and, 575
  chief complaint, 574
  drug abuse and, 575
  history of present illness, complete, 574

Suicide
  risk factors for, 572–573
  scale, 57–58
Sulindac: interaction with lithium, 470
Supportive psychotherapy *(see* Psychotherapy, supportive)
Supranuclear *(see* Palsy, supranuclear)
Susto, 673–674
Symmetrel: for neuroleptic side effects, 351

T

Tapping
  reciprocal, 14
  rhythm, 14
Taractan *(see* Chlorprothixene)
Tarasoff vs. UC Reagents, 638
TAT *(see* Thematic apperception test)
TCA *(see* Antidepressants, tricyclic)
T-cell lymphotropic virus III, 29–30
Temazepam, 399
  dosage, 403
Temperament, 282
Temperature, 12
  dysregulation after neuroleptics, 359
Temporal lobe
  epilepsy, 157–158
    personality disorder and, 296
  syndromes, 27
Teratogenicity
  antidepressants, 429
  antipsychotics, 430
  benzodiazepines, 431
Tetracycline: interaction with lithium, 470
Thematic apperception test, 49–50
  instructions, 49

interpretation, 49–50
Theophylline: interaction with lithium, 470
Therapeutic alliance
  do's and dont's for, 478
  establishing, 475–478
Therapeutic inquiry, 476–477
Therapeutic interventions (*see* Interventions)
Therapeutic relationship: and psychiatric evaluation, 475–476
Therapeutic techniques: choice of, 476
Thiamine, 27
Thiazide diuretics: interaction with lithium, 470
Thinking
  all-or-nothing, 528–529
  "masturbatory," 529
Thioridazine
  for aged, doses and side effects, 448
  dosages, 336
  formulations, available, 340
  in PDD in children, 439
  potency, 336
  in schizophrenia in children, 438
  side effect profile, 338
Thiothixene
  for aged, doses and side effects, 448
  dosages, 337
  formulations, available, 341
  potency, 337
  side effect profile, 339
Thioxanthenes
  dosages, 337
  potency, 337
  side effect profile, 338–339
Thorazine (*see* Chlorpromazine)
Thought(s), 8–10
  circumstantiality, 8
  content, 9–10
    disturbance in delirium, 153
    poverty of, 9
  disorder
    examples of, 334–335
    formal, neuroleptics in, 332
  disorganization and neuroleptics, 332
  form, 8
  ideas of reference, 9
  loosened associations, 8
  obsessional, 9
  ruminative, 9
  tangentiality, 8
Thyroid
  disease, 23–24
  hormone in affective disorders, 98–99
Tic disorders, 252–257
  motor, chronic, 254–255
    clinical presentation, 254–255
    definition, 254–255
    etiology, 255
    treatment, 255
  transient, 254
    assessment, 254
    diagnosis, differential, 254
    epidemiology, 254
    treatment, 254
  vocal, 254–255
    clinical presentation, 254–255
    definition, 254–255
    etiology, 255
    treatment, 255
Tourette disorder, 255–257
  antipsychotics in, in children, 438–439
    dosage, 439
  assessment, 256
  associated features, 255–256
  clinical presentation, 255

Tourette disorder *(cont.)*
  definition, 255
  diagnosis, differential, 256
  epidemiology, 256
  etiology, 256
  haloperidol in, in children, 439
  treatment, 256–257
    pharmacotherapy, 256–257
    psychosocial, 256
Toxic/metabolic disorders: EEG ink, 84–85, 88–90
Toxicity
  of benzodiazepines, 401
  CNS, anticholinergic, of neuroleptics, 331
  hepatotoxicity of neuroleptics, 363
  neuroleptic, 352
    anticholinergic CNS, 331
Transcultural issues, 17–18
Transcultural psychiatry, 667–679
  antidepressants, 676
  anxiolytics in, 676
  diagnosis, 672–675
  evaluation, initial, 669–672
  healers in, 676–678
  history, 669–671
  interpreters in, 669
  laboratory tests, 671
  lithium in, 676
  mental status exam in, 671–672
  migration, 669–670
  neuroleptics, 675–676
  physical exam, 671
  psychologic testing, 671–672
  psychotherapy, 675
  sociology and, 668
  stereotyping in, 668
  theories, 667–668
Transference, 509
Transsexualism, 251–252
  assessment, 251–252
  treatment, 252
Tranxene, 402
Tranylcypromine: for aged, doses and side effects, 444
Traumatic
  brain injury, 163
  dementia, 150
Trazodone: for aged, doses and side effects, 444
Trial: standing of, as capacity test, 640
Triamterene: interaction with lithium, 470
Triazolam, 399
  dosage, 403
Tricyclic (*see* Antidepressants, tricyclic)
Trifluoperazine
  dosages, 336
  formulations, available, 341
  potency, 336
  side effect profile, 338
Trihexphenidyl: for neuroleptic side effects, 351
Triiodothyronine: with tricyclic antidepressants, 468
L-Triiodothyronine: for aged, 443
Trilafon (*see* Perphenazine)
Trioxanthenes: formulations, available, 341
Tumors
  brain, 27
  cerebral, 163–164
  with dementia, 150
Two-point discrimination, 12

U

Unconscious, 509
Universality, 557
Urea: interaction with lithium, 470
Uremia

dementia and, 147
with encephalopathy, chronic, 148

V

Valium (see Diazepam)
Valproic acid, 393
Verapamil, 395
Vessels
  cerebral, disease, 163
  collagen vascular disease, 30–31
Vibration, 12
Violence scale, 58
Violent patients: psychotherapy of, 602–603
Virus(es)
  human immunodeficiency, 29–30
  T-cell lymphotropic, III, 29–30
Visual
  Analog Scale, 56
  hallucinations, 10
Vitamin B_{12}, 27
Vocal activity: abnormal, 4–5
Vocal tic disorder (see Tic disorder, vocal)

W

Water, 26
  intoxication, 26
Weber test, 11
Wechsler adult intelligence scale, 38–41
  assessment, general, 40–41
  diagnostic uses, 40
  interpretative approach, 38–39
  scoring, 38
Wechsler memory scale, 54
Weight loss: differential diagnosis, 177
Wernicke encephalopathy, 120–121
Wernicke-Korsakoff syndrome, 25
Will: making of, as capacity test, 640
Wilson disease, 27–28
  dementia in, 145
  mania in, 164
Withdrawal
  alcohol (see Alcohol withdrawal)
  cocaine, 31
  drug, and delirium, 154
  dyskinesia, 353
  neuroleptics, 365
    in tardive dyskinesia, 356–357
Witness
  expert, psychiatrist as, 646
  understanding responsibility of, as capacity test, 641
Word list, 15
Writing disorder: developmental expressive, 277

Z

Zomepirac: interaction with lithium, 470
Zung depression scale: and transcultural psychiatry, 672